Professional Learning in Nursing

Professional Learning in Nursing

Jenny Spouse

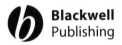

© 2003 by Blackwell Science Ltd,
a Blackwell Publishing Company
Editorial Offices:
Osney Mead, Oxford OX2 0EL, UK
    Tel: +44 (0)1865 206206
Blackwell Science, Inc., 350 Main Street,
Malden, MA 02148-5018, USA
    Tel: +1 781 388 8250
Iowa State Press, a Blackwell Publishing
Company, 2121 State Avenue, Ames, Iowa
50014-8300, USA
    Tel: +1 515 292 0140
Blackwell Publishing Asia Pty Ltd, 550 Swanston
Street, Carlton South, Victoria 3053, Australia
    Tel: +61 (0)3 9347 0300
Blackwell Wissenschafts Verlag,
Kurfürstendamm 57, 10707 Berlin, Germany
    Tel: +49 (0)30 32 79 060

First published 2003 by Blackwell Science Ltd

Library of Congress
Cataloging-in-Publication Data
Spouse, Jenny.
    Professional learning in nursing / Jenny Spouse.
      p. ; cm.
    Includes bibliographical references and index.
    ISBN 0-632-05991-5 (alk. paper)
    1. Nursing–Study and teaching (Continuing
education) 2. Career development. I. Title.
    [DNLM: 1. Education, Nursing, Continuing.
    2. Professional Role. WY 18.5 S765p 2002]
    RT76 .S68 2002
    610.73′071′5—dc21
                                    2002074439

ISBN 0-632-05991-5

A catalogue record for this title is available
from the British Library

Set in 10.5/12.5 pt Sabon
by SNP Best-set Typesetter Ltd., Hong Kong
Printed and bound in Great Britain by
MPG Books Ltd, Bodwin, Cornwall

For further information on
Blackwell Science, visit our website:
www.blackwell-science.com

Dedication

To Helen, Grace, Jack, Marie, Nicola and Ruth whose contribution made this book possible, and also to Petra and Natalie who were there at the beginning of the story.

Table of Contents

Preface   *ix*
Acknowledgements   *xiii*

1   Introducing Professional Learning in Nursing   **1**
1.1 Nurse education 1971–1989   1
1.2 Reforming nurse education   5
1.3 Organisation of the book   9
     References   10

2   Researching Nurses' Professional Learning   **13**
2.1 The context of the research   14
2.2 The curriculum   15
2.3 The research design   18
2.4 The research participants   19
2.5 Data collection   22
2.6 Analysing the data   26
2.7 Quality assurance activities   30
     References   31

3   Case Studies of Professional Development   **34**
3.1 Helen   34
3.2 Marie   49
3.3 Nicola   63
3.4 Jack   75
3.5 Grace   91
3.6 Ruth   107
     References   123

4   Being a Nurse   **124**
4.1 Images of being a nurse   124
4.2 Caring and intimacy   133
     References   136

5   Feeling Like a Nurse   **137**
5.1 The nature of socialisation   138

5.2 Disconfirmation   143
5.3 Confusion   146
5.4 Impression management   149
5.5 Equilibrium   153
5.6 Feeling and acting like a nurse   155
     References   157

6   **Learning to be a Professional**   **158**
6.1 Learning to relate to patients and their carers   159
6.2 Developing technical knowledge   164
6.3 Learning to bundle nursing activities together   169
6.4 Developing professional craft knowledge   171
6.5 Learning to manage feelings and emotions   173
6.6 Learning to cope with ethical dilemmas   176
6.7 Developing the essence of nursing and therapeutic action   178
6.8 Developing interprofessional relationships   180
6.9 Developing professional knowledge   183
     References   184

7   **Supporting Professional Development**   **185**
7.1 Breaking through   185
7.2 Mentorship   190
7.3 Explaining good mentorship   199
7.4 Learning by flying solo   203
7.5 Learning through story-telling   206
7.6 Learning through assessment of theory and practice   209
7.7 Students' professional development   210
     References   211

8   **Enhancing Nurses' Professional Learning**   **213**
8.1 Conceptualising nurse education   214
8.2 Researching nurses' professional learning   217
8.3 Curriculum issues   220
8.4 Conceptualising mentorship in nurse education   222
8.5 Research and the future professional development of nurses   226
     References   228

Index   230

Preface

With increasingly stringent professional regulation throughout all the healthcare professions, practitioners are being subjected to greater scrutiny than ever before. Nurses constitute the majority of professional practitioners, working in hospitals, clinics, homes, prisons, schools, occupational health departments and so on. Many practitioners continue their education after their initial qualification of registered nurse to prepare them for working in such specialist settings. Their foundation for such learning is gained in their pre-registration programme, which since 1989 has taken place in higher education settings. This move has provoked much controversy, with traditionalists urging a return to the old days where nursing students constituted the majority of the workforce in hospital settings. The poor standards of care that such arrangements engendered and the high levels of stress that caused more than 30% of students to leave before qualifying and another 30% within a year are forgotten.

With demographic changes to our population and more career opportunities for girls especially, governments throughout the world are concerned about recruiting sufficient nursing staff to meet staffing needs of their healthcare services. Poaching staff from neighbouring countries is not the solution but merely a stopgap and often leads to other problems caused by cultural and language differences. An effective health service needs practitioners who are capable of providing effective care in response to the technological advances in medical science and the higher needs and expectations of the public. Without highly skilled nursing practitioners able to care for patients effectively, much expensive technology will be wasted. The cost of inadequate practice arising from ignorance is reflected in human misery and escalating litigation costs caused by iatrogenic disorders that are mostly avoidable with good nursing care and resources.

One strategy to address this issue has been to transfer nurse education into higher education and Project 2000 was the first step towards this. It was revolutionary in its conceptualisation, requiring a completely different approach to nurse education both in the clinical setting and the classroom. One of the reasons why it was not as successful as hoped was that insufficient money was available to invest in the clinical setting and as a result students were not given the kind of support that was needed. Nearly fifteen years later further radical changes to nurse education are being implemented, largely to increase recruitment by widening the entry gate to people wishing to become nurses and making arrangements for studying more flexible and family friendly. New partnership courses are designed to involve patients and clinicians at all levels of policy making throughout the educational processes. The courses also provide more time for nursing entrants to make the social and intellectual adjustments of learning to become professional nurses by removing them entirely from the labour force numbers. For many nursing students, learning how to care for strangers suffering physical and emotional disorders is challenging and distressing. For other entrants it is adapting to the social expectations of becoming professional nurses and learning how to individualise care for patients rather than treating them like work objects, which is what happens when there are too few staff with too much work.

Supernumerary status allows nursing students to learn everyday professional craft knowledge from their clinical mentors by working in partnership with them and their patients. It provides time for students to follow patients through their healthcare pathway and so develop a profound understanding of professional healthcare without the exhausting and stressful demands of dealing with unrealistic workloads. It also permits nursing students to increase their capability in a measured and supervised manner that maintains their enthusiasm and ensures effective supervision and support. As a result they are able to integrate formal classroom knowledge with practical experiences and become effective practitioners who are more likely to remain in the profession. Such an approach reduces strains on clinical staff and providing the skill mix and staffing levels meet quality assurance standards for the clinical setting, they will be less exhausted and have more time for their own professional development.

Whilst all nurse educators and clinical practitioners have undergone professional preparation to become registered practitioners, it is often difficult to remember the needs of students as individuals when working under pressure. Despite calls for evidence-based practice there is little research about the experiences of nursing students to inform policy makers and educators (both clinical and university staff). As a result most courses are based on custom and practice and placements are designed to respond to requirements laid down by the European Union and professional statutory organisations. These in turn are often based on earlier workforce requirements rather than as a result of research-based evidence as to what constitutes educationally and professionally sound clinical experiences. In many countries throughout the European Union, North America and Australasia, nurse education is at degree level. Indeed England will soon be one of the few countries in the western world where pre-registration nurse preparation is not at degree level. Preparation at degree level has been available to nurses in England for over forty years, but only to a small number of entrants. In contrast to many diplomas in nursing courses, degree courses are always over subscribed.

This focus of this book is on the experiences of eight nursing students who entered a nursing degree programme in the United Kingdom. The material is derived from a longitudinal research project undertaken for a doctoral award and is concerned with the students' experiences of learning in clinical settings.

They represent a sample of the population of people who enter nursing every year. Three started their programme after leaving school, one had a gap year working overseas, another had intermitted for a year, come back for a year, and then intermitted again. The other three students were mature entrants. One was a single mother who had completed an access course and had extensive experience of working as a healthcare assistant, another was a registered mental-health nurse fulfilling his ambition to become an adult trained nurse. The third left a successful career in the business world to become a nurse. All of them faced considerable adjustments whilst learning to become nurses. Not all of them completed the programme and this book contains case studies of the five who did in Chapter 3. The subsequent Chapters draw on material from all eight entrants. In Chapters 4 to 7, I examine what led these people to want to become nurses, how they learned the necessary professional knowledge and the factors that supported their progress and development. In Chapter 8, I discuss my conclusions arising from these findings and make some recommendations for the future.

Research-based evidence is a key aspect of any scholarly endeavour and Chapter 2 provides an overview of the research process in sufficient detail to allow readers to judge whether the study was conducted in such a way to provide robust evidence to support these findings and my assertions. The names given to the students in the text are pseudonyms and as far as possible were chosen by the students themselves.

I hope this book will be of interest to many readers. Students from around the world have read the case studies and found them enormously helpful. For many they provided a catalyst to express pent up feelings about their own experiences, and gave them reassurance that they were after all normal people and not 'going mad' as one American student phrased it. This implies that learning to become a nurse is very much the same whatever continent or country you are in. It also indicates the nature of the process of learning to be a nurse.

Hopefully people contemplating nursing as a career will read the book to give them firmer ground on which to make their decisions and if they decide that nursing is their chosen path, that it will help to support them through their studies.

I hope mentors and clinical practitioners will find time to dip into the book, especially Chapters 4 to 7 as they provide some insights into how nursing students can be supported during their clinical placements. No less importantly I hope my colleagues in educational institutions will also find the book helpful and that they will be able to use parts of it when planning their programmes, teaching their students and generally mulling over ways of supporting their students.

Perhaps most importantly I do hope people who are instrumental in creating policies and deciding funding for nurse education read this book. Lay people in particular have great difficulty in understanding what it is that nurses do. Practitioners do not have a language for describing their experiences, so I hope this

book is able to make a small contribution to increasing understanding and promoting a better environment for student nurses and practitioners of the future.
Indeed our future healthcare depends on it.

I very much hope this book provides a basis for much discussion as it is the best
way to advance our understanding and I look forward to receiving your comments and being able to engage in dialogue with you.

Jenny Spouse

Acknowledgements

Figure 3.6a 'Split demands', that also appears in Figure 5.1e, Ruth: 'Split demands', was first published in *Nursing Times Research* 5(4) 253–61 (2000). My thanks goes to the publishers for allowing me to reproduce it here.

Chapter 1
Introducing Professional Learning in Nursing

Most nurses remember their student experiences. Inevitably some aspects remain more vivid than others. Many people remember wondering whether they should quit before they got dismissed especially during their first six months of training when they struggled to come to terms with such unfamiliar people, the language, the role and dealing with other people's dispositions. Memories of spending hours discussing various clinical incidents which friends encounter are important and meaningful. Key landmarks include first attempts at performing various intimate tasks for a patient of the opposite gender, watching how some staff relate to patients, or the shame of making a mistake in front of a senior nurse. Many ward sisters and staff nurses have struggled with balancing inappropriate staffing levels and the particular skill mix of staff with the needs of seriously ill or post-operative patients, and being too busy to think about the special needs of students. However, with increasing knowledge and education many qualified nurses have a better understanding of their educational role as well as of their clinical role.

We have very little knowledge about how nurses learn, and without such knowledge, it is difficult to teach students in clinical practice. Through research activities we are beginning to develop models of conditions which facilitate learning in clinical practice. But most knowledge currently in use has been derived from theories and practices designed for classrooms and schoolteachers, or from recreational educational activities which have in turn been divined from laboratories or schoolrooms. This book is concerned with trying to answer questions about how nurses learn in practice and the contributing factors to their professional development.

1.1 Nurse education 1971–1989

Whilst considering the current professional development of nurses it is unwise to ignore factors which have brought the profession through several momentous changes. In designing future curricula it is inevitable that contextual and historical influences will continue to dominate their design and implementation. Their successful outcome depends largely upon the quality of mentor support and the educational guidance provided to large numbers of students on an individual basis by clinical practitioners. Other models of educational support to students in their clinical placements have been found to be both unrealistic and ineffective in the past. This is due to the inevitable difficulties faced by external individuals (such as academics, clinical teachers or even lecturer–practitioners) making incidental clinical visits to their students. As a result the success of implementing new educational policies rests largely on staff working in clinical settings.

Researching nurse education

The role and function of the registered nurse first began to be systematically examined with a series of research projects commissioned by the Department of Health and Social Security (DHSS) and published as monographs by the Royal College of Nursing (RCN) in 1971. It was the first time that a systematic examination of nursing practice had been undertaken and it was designed to develop quality assurance tools concerned with significant general nursing practices. These published studies had considerable influence on discussions about the practice of nursing and the role of nurses, leading to more detailed studies of the role of the ward sister and the nature of nursing. Within the second series of commissioned research was an investigation into the role of the nurse by Anderson (Anderson 1973). Her findings led to recommendations that care should be individualised and students be given more formal teaching by ward sisters on how to meet the emotional needs of patients (Anderson 1973). Anderson's concerns were later amplified by Smith (Smith 1992) whose research demonstrated the emotional difficulties nursing students experience when supporting patients.

Alongside the dissemination of results from these early research projects, a review of the role and educational preparation of nurses and midwives was published. The report of this Committee on Nursing recommended radical reforms to nurse education that were not allowed to languish and be forgotten as so many earlier reports had been. It made recommendations for sweeping changes to the structure of nursing and midwifery education and practice (DHSS 1972). One recommendation was a common initial preparation programme for all health-care professionals with opportunities for transfer between different career choices and for stepping in and out without loss of academic credit. Of greatest concern was the recruitment and retention of nursing and midwifery staff, in order to justify the heavy cost of training and mitigate the attrition of these professionals from the National Health Service (NHS). These recommended developments in nurse preparation were strongly supported by a small but influential body of university trained nurses, not least the Registrar of the General Nursing Council (GNC), and a number of principals of nursing schools. The recommendations were slowly implemented piecemeal into the legislature with creation of the United Kingdom Central Council (UKCC) and the four National Boards of Nursing, Midwifery and Health Visiting. Their establishment led to an unprecedented funding of research into practice and education by the UKCC, the National Boards and the Royal College of Nursing. The RCN commissioned a study into the future of nurse education that reported in 1985. It identified concerns that reflected findings from so many earlier reports, namely:

* the dependence of service delivery upon nursing students for labour, and the consequent small number of qualified nurses available to supervise
* the integration of theory and practice
* the unrealistically heavy demands upon nurse–teachers
* the high attrition rates from nurse education programmes either before or immediately following registration
* demographic changes and competing demands for traditional entrants to nursing.

From this report came recommendations that nurse education should be transferred into higher education and that students be supernumerary (RCN 1985). Numerous other reports urged government to remove the staffing commitment of nursing students by making them supernumerary, but hospital matrons and governments concerned about the implications of high staffing costs ignored their advice (reviewed in Rafferty, Allcock et al. 1996).

Debates raged between educationalists and influential practitioners about the nature of practice and the supervision of students in clinical practice. Central to their concern was a belief that students were ill-prepared for their role as registered nurses (Alexander 1982; Bendall 1971, 1975, 1976; Gott 1984).These research studies indicated that the quality of practice was inadequate and that students were ill-prepared to link educational theory with professional practice. Several proposals were made to reconcile the problem and these were mainly concerned with three aspects of nurse education: changing the resources (at different times) by making entry requirements higher, lower or broader; reorganising the structure of programmes and the curriculum into a modular system; and redefining the role of nurse–teachers. The professional statutory body of the time (the General Nursing Council for England and Wales) made several recommendations aimed at reducing dependence on student labour including ensuring that there should be sufficient staff on duty to provide adequate supervision of students. But without extra funding from the government such recommendations were almost impossible to implement.

In response to the growing diversity of medical practice and beliefs that nursing students should experience care in a variety of settings, the curriculum content was broadened and their placements made more frequent, with subsequent effects on hospital staffing. Student nurses began to become less attractive as a workforce; a new role of clinical teacher was instituted to provide teaching in the clinical setting. Lack of funding for nurse education resulted in high student–teacher ratios, and the itinerant nature of students, affected the degree to which these new clinical teachers could be used. Shortage of teaching staff meant clinical teachers were used to supplement classroom teachers, or to cover large groups of students as they worked their way around the hospital, resulting in few opportunities for effective clinical teaching. The few clinical teachers who worked in the specialities used for nurse training, such as paediatrics and geriatrics, were able to become respected members of the clinical team, knowledgeable about the patients and credible in the classroom (House & Sims 1976; Kirkwood 1979).

Current thinking about nurse education relied on beliefs that students would transfer and consolidate classroom learning when working in the wards. Subsequent clinical education was provided by the ward sister or a visiting tutor with formal tutorials or occasionally a demonstration of technical skills (Reid 1985a). All nurse–teachers had previously held positions of responsibility (normally at Charge Nurse/Ward Sister level) as a precondition to acceptance on a mandatory teacher preparation programme along with possessing suitable academic qualifications in their subject area. Thus teachers represented experienced and senior members of the profession. Their preparation was frequently through generic teacher preparation programmes and so the pedagogical knowledge they brought to nurse education reflected current educational practices and favoured the status of students as learners rather than workers.

Learning in clinical settings

Most students saw learning as taking place on the wards and this was endorsed by the preface in the syllabus of training published by the General Nursing Council (GNC 1969). In this official document, nursing was identified as essentially a practical art which would predominantly be learned in the wards. Teaching was expected to be provided by didactic methods, discussions and project work. There was little reference to teaching of theoretical material in this syllabus until the English and Welsh National Boards (ENB) published their first syllabus dated 1977, and recommended that knowledge, skills and attitudes be synthesised to support a code of professional practice (ENB 1977). The checklist of skills had been removed and an outline of competency was provided. With the introduction of Project 2000 and transfer into higher education, this democratic approach to professional education continued and responsibility for curriculum development was devolved to individual departments providing nursing and midwifery programmes.

Studies investigating nurse education in the early 1980s prior to introduction of Project 2000, confirmed the extent to which students' undertook a clinical workload where care was often delegated on a task-allocation basis. These found that more than 66% of students' time was spent either working alone or with another unqualified staff member such as an auxiliary or a junior student. Only 11% of their time was spent alongside a registered nurse (Burkey 1984; Reid 1985a; Jacka & Lewin 1987). Jacka and Lewin identified the importance of good supervision and grounding in the students' first year otherwise they were unlikely to develop good practices later. Students resorted to procedure books to help them undertake practical tasks, but Reid identified that this only occurred in 'good' wards (Reid 1985). As in earlier studies, students' educational contact with trained staff was often in relation to unfamiliar technical procedures, which were more highly valued (Fretwell 1982; Reid 1985; Smith 1992). Interestingly little reference is made to how nursing students developed the sort of organisational skills they needed whilst undertaking their student work and, more critically, those they needed when they became qualified nurses. Hughes' (Hughes 1951) ethnographic study of contemporary American nursing practices in task allocation, recognised that nursing was more than just a bundle of tasks and needed management skills.

1.2 Reforming nurse education

Introduction of project 2000

Under the traditional system of nurse training the United Kingdom healthcare system functioned on a student 'replacement system'. With 30,000 entrants to nurse training each year they provided 20% of the total healthcare (although a much higher percentage in hospital wards). Whilst on average 90% of these entrants completed their course, only 65% actually registered (UKCC 1986). With such unsatisfactory statistics of the state of nurse training and escalating demographic and healthcare changes, it was essential to transform existing nurse training into an academic programme. Students and staff had to move from the often stifling monotechnic culture of schools of nursing attached to hospitals and be able to engage in broader fields of education. It was essential for students to develop the necessary intellectual and research-based clinical skills to care for people in the twenty-first century whilst gaining academic recognition for their achievements. Recommendations for radical reform were only accepted and implemented after much careful consideration by the whole profession, led by the UKCC and supported with research initiated by the UKCC and other professional organisations including the RCN.

An important impetus to change in nurse education was provided by the Report of the Commission on Nursing Education, known as the Judge Report (RCN 1985). This took advice from specially commissioned researchers and argued that nurse education should take account of demographic and social changes in the structure of the population and competing career opportunities for women. The government and the profession had to find more attractive ways of preparing nurses if the nation's future healthcare needs were to be met. Transferring nursing and midwifery education into higher education and turning initial preparation into an undergraduate programme would, they argued, substantially contribute to this and expose nurse educators and students to a more liberal and academic environment.

It was a bold and unprecedented strategy that fortunately was given government support and thus money to finance some of the changes. In approving the new programme the DoH estimated that at 1987 prices, it would cost an additional £580 million over 14 years to implement. The majority of this extra cost was to recruit new staff to replace nursing students (Brown 1992). In attempting to ensure that the new programme would be approved, the UKCC agreed a compromise which reduced 100% fulltime student status to 80%. This ensured that service-dependency on student labour continued, albeit just for the final year of their programme. Experimental programmes of nurse education had been conducted in a small number of university departments throughout the United Kingdom and had demonstrated how degree and diploma course students were more likely to continue in nursing for longer than those prepared in the old traditional system.

Many of the difficulties anticipated by the UKCC and the Commission on Nursing Education in over-reliance on student labour by service providers, high attrition rates and limited recruitment were realised (White, Riley et al. 1993; Wilson Barnett, Butterworth et al. 1995). But implementation of Project 2000 courses also took place during times of radical changes to the NHS resulting in a reduction in student places, short-term contracts or the unemployment of newly qualified nurses. Recruitment fluctuated according to local and government policies and in 1994/5 annual intakes of students commencing pre-registration nursing or midwifery programmes had fallen to 12,000 new students (ENB 1994), but by 2000 had reached over 21,000 in the NHS (DoH 2001). Project 2000 transformed nurse education for many reasons. By 1994 all pre-registration courses had transferred into higher education settings and were offered at either diploma or degree level. Nursing students from different parts of the professional register shared a common foundation programme and the curriculum was less disease orientated and was also more concerned with the social and emotional aspects of health and healthcare in homes as well as hospitals.

Problems concerned with recruitment in a highly competitive labour market and public as well as management expectations of newly qualified nurses led to further research and reforms of their preparation. The ambitions of Project 2000 had been undermined by service requirements and continuing change in health and educational provision (UKCC 1999). Government policies moved closer towards the earlier recommendations of nursing review bodies and midwifery education (RCN 1985; UKCC 1986) calling for common elements in preparatory programmes for all healthcare professionals with greater flexibility of access and egress (NHSE 1998; DoH 1999). To attract more people from a wider range of educational and cultural backgrounds entry had to be more flexible and programmes had to meet the needs of people who could not afford to study full-time. They also had to give credit to prior relevant experience and include pathways to qualification that acknowledged such earlier experiences. Standards to be achieved were identified at two points in the nursing programme: the end of the common foundation programme; and prior to admission to the professional register. These provided a means for students to exit their programme at a point prior to registration without loss of academic or professional credit; they could then use this credit towards completing their professional award at a later date. The UKCC undertook an investigation into nursing and midwifery education to see what needed to be done.

Fitness for practice and purpose

Professional practice and professional education was becoming increasingly a topic for public domain debate. Public concerns about the professional conduct of several groups of healthcare practitioners were highlighted by various scandals associated with abuse of their privileged position, misinformation and failure to address at an early stage interprofessional practice issues and difficulties. At the same time and nearly eleven years after the first Project 2000 intakes the UKCC Commission on Nursing and Midwifery Education (UKCC 1999) delivered its evaluation of Project 2000. It made recommendations for the future of nursing and midwifery education 'that enabled fitness for practice based on healthcare need'. In addition to recommending development of better data collection and statistical information for workforce planning the report covered three particular areas: increasing flexibility; achieving fitness for practice; and working in partnership.

Increasing flexibility

Recommendations to increase the flexibility of educational provision were designed to compensate for the shortfall in traditional (18 year-old female) recruits to nursing; and to make nursing and midwifery education more attractive and sustainable to people from a wider range of educational and cultural backgrounds. To achieve this programmes had to provide more flexible entry points and requirements, give academic recognition for successful completion of the (shorter) first year common foundation programme and allow intermission or exit from the course. Students were to be given more time to decide which branch programme they wished to follow. The working party recommended expansion of graduate preparation for several reasons. These were partly to meet government demands for increased participation in higher education, and partly to meet the need for a more flexible workforce with appropriate intellectual and clinical skills. In an increasingly competitive labour market, young people had higher career expectations that undergraduate preparation was seen to meet.

Achieving fitness for practice

Recommendations were concerned with quality assurance activities associated with clinical and educational issues. These included: subject benchmarking of core, specialist and transferable outcomes to meet Quality Assurance agency standards for academic awards. Support for learners in clinical settings to be developed through effective structures, including partnership arrangements and agreements between service and education providers and between mentors and students. Clinical settings were to develop transparent and explicit outcomes for students' clinical education that enabled effective monitoring of student achievements and fitness for practice. Course structures and processes were to be designed to foster integration of knowledge, skills and attitudes, where appropriate, using a range of pedagogical and technological strategies. Placements were to be used on the basis of their prespecified educational value and reflect the total healthcare needs of service users. Ensuring that students were exposed to high standards of practice and appropriate educational support was the responsibility of the Commission for Health Improvement (CHI), the agency directly responsible to the Department of Health. Importantly the Commission recommended that students were to have a period of practice towards the end of their programme designed to prepare them for their future role and that they should be supervised by specifically prepared practitioners. On employment newly-qualified nurses and midwives were to have a period of induction and preparation for their new role.

Working in partnership

The commission identified several groups with whom partnership activities needed to be developed and enhanced. At a strategic level these partnerships needed to include the private and independent sectors in order to identify overall workforce requirements and funding of education. Relevant government departments of the four countries were to develop common policies and standards for the preparation of healthcare assistants that reflected current and future health and social care needs. The Commission recognised the need for close working relationships between healthcare providers and education providers in programme provision. This was to be reflected at all stages including recruitment of students, curriculum planning and staff development for their educational role, either as mentors, preceptors or lecturers. Teaching was to be undertaken by collaborative teams of experts drawn from service and education. Clinical settings were to be selected and developed for their educational value, which was to be made explicit and evaluated. Funding was to take account of these additional costs including the costs of preparing mentors and preceptors, development of clinical staff roles and funding exchanges of service and education staff.

The Commission made two further recommendations that were reviewed and reported on by the Post Commission Group in 2001 (UKCC 2001). These recommendations were concerned with reviewing the continuing relevance of the four-branch programmes in meeting contemporary healthcare needs and provision of opportunities for students from different healthcare professions to learn with and from each other. Since these recommendations the pace of change accelerated and the impetus for interprofessional learning became a driving force for partnership curricula (as they became known).

Regulation of healthcare practitioners

Professional regulatory bodies and government departments undertook a radical review of the regulation of healthcare practitioners leading to the demise of the four national boards and the UKCC. In their place a new interim Nursing and Midwifery Council (NMC) was established in 2002, with responsibility for monitoring the profession and protecting the public by setting standards and monitoring the quality assurance (QA) of preregistration education and other programmes leading to recordable and registerable qualifications throughout the UK. Under the new arrangements England became the only nation that decided not to have an all-graduate profession at the point of entry to the professional register. New education bodies for each of the three nations of Wales, Scotland and Northern Ireland were appointed to support the work of the Nursing and Midwifery Council to carry out its work. In England QA work is through the (new) Learning and Personal Development Division. To achieve its responsibilities for regulating and monitoring standards of education leading to recordable or registerable qualifications, the Nursing and Midwifery Council (NMC) works in partnership with other QA organisations. The Commission for Health Improvement in England and Wales has responsibility for monitoring practice and educational standards in clinical settings, whilst Scotland and Northern Ireland have their own organisations (Northern Ireland Practice and Education Council and the Clinical Standards Board for Scotland). Congruent with the NMC's mission to protect the public and ensure that lay perspectives are reflected at every level, all programmes have lay members on their curriculum development and management boards and this is monitored periodically (UKCC 2002).

1.3 Organisation of this book

In exploring how nurses develop their professional knowledge this book has three parts. Chapter 2 explores the research that informs this text and the context in which it arose. This includes a brief discussion of the choice of a naturalistic research approach influenced by phenomenological and constructivist perspectives of reality and experience, followed by a brief overview of the research design, choice of data collection methods and data analysis. Four different strategies for data collection were used: interviews, observation, document analysis and illuminative art. Narrative is becomingly increasingly recognised as a powerful means of exploring reality and so interviews conducted frequently over a long period were an obvious choice, as perhaps were documentary and observational data. Illuminative art was chosen as a result of seeing unexpected characterisations of experience through drawings and paintings in the literature (Bentley 1989; Durkin, Perach et al. 1989). There is little evidence of using projective imagery in naturalistic research and its use in this study provided a powerful source of information. Data derived from this research method are offered where relevant throughout the book. Chapter 2 contains descriptions of the research methods, data analysis and the quality assurance strategies used to safeguard both the participants and the data.

Following this is Chapter 3 containing six case studies of the participants who ultimately completed their programme, providing individual accounts of what it is like to become a nurse. One male who had been a psychiatric nurse, and four female participants wanted to be adult branch nurses. Another female wanted to be a children's nurse and the sixth planned to be a mental health nurse. Three were mature students being more than 22 years old when they started and three had come straight from school. All these participants had engaged in some form of nursing or care experience before starting the programme. Each case study has been presented in a slightly different format to acknowledge the individuality of each participant, and Nicola's case study is the most distinctive. Specific issues arising from each student's experience raise have been discussed within the individual's case study. Other more general aspects are discussed in subsequent chapters.

Chapters 4 to 7 are concerned with the major themes arising from data generated from all eight participants in the research, as well as data from interviews with some of the students' mentors. In discussing this material, I have sought to address four research questions concerned with investigating pre-registration nursing students' professional development. Chapter 4 considers the conceptions students held on entry and how these appeared to frame their professional development and approach to patient care. Chapter 5 examines the kinds of knowledge and understanding students acquired whilst learning to nurse and in particular their knowledge of how they felt about learning to become nurses. Their illuminative art was particularly revealing in uncovering this knowledge and has been used to illustrate the discussion. Acquisition of functional knowledge has preoccupied nursing for a long time and Chapter 6 explores how students acquired the seven forms of knowledge they believed they needed and developed over the programme.

Perhaps many people will not be surprised to know how much students' development was influenced by the quality of mentorship support. Mentorship from a registered nurse working in the placement was singularly the most important influence and the kinds of activities that make good mentoring are explored here. Although this was the most important factor promoting students' clinical development it was not the only factor and these other factors will be also be discussed. Of particular interest was the importance of peer support through story-telling or narratives that helped students begin to think and talk like nurses. Little attention has been paid to this area in the literature to date.

Finally Chapter 8 sets out to reexamine conceptions of nurse education and professional development and explores how curriculum development and future research could be further developed.

References

Alexander, M.F. (1982) Integrating theory with practice: an experiment evaluated. In: *Advances in Nursing Education*. (ed. M.S. Henderson) 56–80. Churchill Livingstone, London.

Anderson, E.R. (1973) *The role of the nurse*. Royal College of Nursing and National Council of Nurses of the United Kingdom, London.

Bendall, E. (1971) A Nursing Dilemma. *Nursing Times* March 18 (Occasional Paper No. 11): 41–4.

Bendall, E. (1975) *So You Passed, Nurse: An exploration of some of the assumptions on which written examinations are based.* Royal College of Nursing of the United Kingdom, London.

Bendall, E. (1976) Learning for reality. *Journal of Advanced Nursing*, **1**: 3–9.

Bentley, T. (1989) Talking Pictures. *Nursing Times* (Occasional Paper) **85** (31): 58–69.

Brown, J. (1992) *Nursing education: Implementation of Project 2000.* Report by the Comptroller General and Audit General. National Audit Office, London.

Burkey, B.P. (1984) Student nurses' perceptions of training. University of Manchester, Manchester.

DoH (1999) *Making a difference. Strengthening the nursing, midwifery and health visiting contribution to health and healthcare.* Department of Health, London.

DoH (2001) *Investment in Reform for NHS staff – Taking forward the NHS Plan.* Department of Health. HMSO, London.

DHSS (1972) *Report of the Committee on Nursing.* London, Department of Health & Social Security. Chair, Lord Briggs.

Durkin, J., Perach, D., et al. (1989) A model of art therapy supervision enhanced through art making and journal writing. In: *Advances in Art Therapy.* (eds H. Wadesdon, J. Durkin, D. Perach) 390–432. John Wiley, New York.

ENB (1977) *Syllabus of Training: Professional Register – Part 1* (Registered General Nurse) amended 1977. English and Welsh National Boards for Nursing, Midwifery and Health Visiting, London.

ENB (1994) *The Eleventh Annual Report submitted to the Secretary of State for the period 1 April 1993–31 March 1994.* English National Board for Nursing Midwifery and Health Visiting, London.

Fretwell, J. (1982) *Ward teaching and learning: Sister and the learning environment.* Royal College of Nursing of the United Kingdom, London.

GNC (1969) *Syllabus of subjects for examination and record of practical instruction and experience for the Certificate of General Nursing.* Reprinted 1973. General Council for England and Wales, London.

Gott, M. (1984) *Learning nursing: A study of the effectiveness and relevance of teaching provided during student nurse introductory course.* Royal College of Nursing of the United Kingdom, London.

House, V., Sims, A. (1976) Teachers of nursing in the United Kingdom: A description of their attitudes. *Journal of Advanced Nursing* **1**: 495–505.

Hughes, E.C. (1951) Studying nurses' work. *The American Journal of Nursing* **51** (5): 294–5.

Jacka, K., Lewin, D. (1987) *The Clinical Learning of Student Nurses.* NERU Report no. 6, Kings College University of London, London.

Kirkwood, L. (1979) The clinical teacher. *Nursing Times Occasional Papers* May 3rd **75** (12): 59–61.

NHSE (1998) *Widening access to nursing and midwifery education and training.* NHS Executive, Leeds.

Rafferty, A.-M., Allcock, N. et al. (1996) The theory–practice gap: taking issue with the issue. *Journal of Advanced Nursing* **23**: 685–91.

RCN (1985) *The education of nurses: A new dispensation.* Commission on Nursing Education. Royal College of Nursing of the United Kingdom, Chair: Dr Harry Judge, London.

Reid, N.G. (1985) The effective training of nurses: Manpower implications. *International Journal of Nursing Studies* **22** (2): 89–98.

Reid, N.G. (1985a) *Wards in Chancery: Nurse training in the clinical area.* Royal College of Nursing of the United Kingdom, London.

Smith, P. (1992) *The Emotional Labour of Nursing.* Macmillan, Basingstoke.

UKCC (1986) *Project 2000. A new preparation for practice.* United Kingdom Central Council for Nursing, Midwifery and Health Visiting. Chair: Margaret D. Green, London.

UKCC (1999) *Fitness for Practice. The UKCC Commission for Nursing and Midwifery Education*. United Kingdom Central Council for Nursing, Midwifery and Health Visiting. Chair: Sir Leonard Peach, London.

UKCC (2001) *Fitness for practice and purpose*. The Report of the UKCC's Post Commission Development Group. United Kingdom Central Council for Nursing, Midwifery and Health Visiting; Chair: Valerie Morrison: 94, London.

UKCC (2002) New arrangements for the quality assurance of professional education. Register (38): 10–11, London.

White, E., Riley, L. (1993) *A detailed study of the relationship between teaching, support, supervision and role modelling in clinical areas within the context of Project 2000 courses*. Kings College London & University of Manchester. Research commissioned by the English National Board for Nursing, Midwifery and Health Visiting, London.

Wilson Barnett, J., Butterworth, T. et al. (1995) Clinical support and the Project 2000 nursing student: factors influencing this process. *Journal of Advanced Nursing*, **21**: 1152–8.

Chapter 2

Researching Nurses' Professional Learning

In this chapter we consider some contextual information about the students' course. This includes an outline of the curriculum, the clinical placements and some information about the support they received. Later on I shall describe the research design, how the data was collected, analysed and presented and some of the issues surrounding research of this kind.

Many earlier developments in nurse education have evolved from research that has been conducted rather like a photographer taking cumulative snapshots of a scheme. Research studies have mostly been short term, intensive investigations sampling students' experiences at different points in their programmes. The kind of information they captured was often influenced by political perspectives such as difficulties in recruitment and retention of nursing and midwifery staff. Researchers pursued their work using a range of theoretical and disciplinary beliefs. As a result we have a series of snapshots of nursing education over the past forty or so years, pasted into a somewhat fragmented and incomplete album of information.

Few studies have attempted to describe and understand the professional growth of nurses from the moment they embark on their career. In taking account of these earlier studies I decided to attempt a more holistic perspective and map the entire learning experience of a few students. I also wanted to evaluate an imaginative and innovative programme leading to nurse registration. By undertaking this it was anticipated that we could develop a better understanding of initial nurse preparation and so be able to develop a theoretical framework to inform the future provision of nurse education. To understand how nursing students develop their professional knowledge several perspectives were needed, and four broad questions were used to frame the research design reported here:

- what conceptions of nursing do students hold on entry to nursing and how do these frame their professional development?
- what kinds of knowledge and understanding do students acquire whilst learning to nurse and how do they believe they learn to become nurses? How is their practice influenced?
- what are the major factors that facilitate their learning to nurse? What is the nature and extent of supervisory, peer, personal and activity factors?

- how can the professional development of nurses be better understood and what are the implications for the design, organisation and funding of nurse education?

These questions reflected some of the preoccupations of earlier researchers and some of the current trends in nursing education. They also reflect my own experiences of being a nurse and a nurse educator. The questions carry my assumption that people wishing to nurse hold some preconceptions about their future role and how they will carry it out. It also assumes that such preconceptions influence how people learn to nurse and indeed whether they complete their programme. Other assumptions embedded in the questions are that learning a practical, professional activity is more sophisticated and complex than learning a pure subject such as physics, geography or literature for example, and is multifaceted. These questions assume that learning to become a nurse requires students to draw on a variety of sources of information and support, but so far we have little evidence of this or understanding about what these resources are. To research these questions a flexible and responsive research design was needed that was underpinned by a suitable belief system or philosophy.

2.1 The context of the research

The student's programme was innovative for several reasons. In particular it was influenced by Donald Schön's (Schön 1983) work on reflective practice. Students were expected to use an action-inquiry approach to their practice experiences and write them up reflectively so as to provide evidence of meeting standards for progression through the foundation programme and their branch programme. This form of problem-based learning was student driven and directly related to their clinical experiences. The programme had the largest intake of students taking a preregistration nursing degree in Britain. It provided students from diverse social and educational backgrounds with opportunities to study at degree level. They followed a four-year modular degree programme as recommended in the report of the Commission on Nursing Education (RCN 1985).

Entry access to the programme was wide, whilst meeting standards set by the professional statutory body (the then United Kingdom Central Council for Nurses, Midwives and Health Visitors). Students could intermit and rejoin the programme within the time limit specified by this professional statutory body and the European Union. Such flexibility helped students coping with family or financial difficulties to take their programme over a longer time. Some students came directly from school, some via the local further education college after completing an access course, whilst others gave up jobs to fulfil their lifelong ambition to nurse.

Being full-time students on a four-year programme meant they could participate in university life, enjoy the same vacations as other students in the university and if they wished, work in their vacations to supplement their meagre student grants. Three-year nursing degree courses require students by contrast, to attend for a longer academic year in order to meet professional requirements and to accumulate sufficient hours of practice and theory. Consequently they have less time to integrate with other university students and less time to supplement their grants. The advantage of being full-time students is that their supernumerary status frees them to work alongside clinical practitioners, rather than be relied upon as pairs of hands and be left to struggle on their own (White 1993; Wilson Barnett, 1995).

The course curriculum was equally divided 50:50 between theory and clinical practice. Student placements were weekly and integrated with formal academic activities throughout an academic year of three, ten-week terms. For the duration of each clinical placement students were allocated to their own qualified nurse prepared to give mentor support. With guest or supernumerary role, students had the (relative) freedom to negotiate clinical days around their university programme and the availability of their mentor. By structuring clinical placements in this manner, students' educational needs became central to the placement, rather than service needs. This matched recommendations by the report of the UKCC Commission on Nursing and Midwifery Education (UKCC 1999), unlike earlier nurse education programmes including the Diploma in Higher Education (otherwise known as Project 2000). Students' placements were strictly prescribed to meet educational and professional requirements of the European Union and the professional statutory body.

Liaison between clinical and educational staff responsible for particular modules of learning was through clinically-based lecturer–practitioners (Lathlean 1995). These practitioners were appointed to clinical settings, taking a clinical and educational lead in ensuring that placements met the required standards and that placement mentors were adequately prepared for their role. They also taught students about their clinical speciality and participated in marking students' clinical assignments, known as learning contracts.

By working as supernumerary students in clinical settings they could work alongside experienced professionals or work under distant supervision according to their learning needs and capability. Brown and his colleagues (Brown *et al.* 1989) describe this approach to learning in practice as cognitive apprenticeship. Apprenticeship of this type includes sponsorship to a community of practice (the clinical team), participating in legitimate practice activities alongside their mentor and engaging in debriefing discussions about their practice experiences.

2.2 The curriculum

The students' first-year programme focused on inducting students to university life, concepts of health and the nature of nursing work as well as the underpinning sciences. In their second term, students had a community placement supported by a healthcare practitioner. They were allocated to a family within the community and given the project of exploring how people's lifestyle influenced their ability to be healthy. Subsidiary aims were to help students develop inter-personal skills and begin to learn how to conduct an interview and make an assessment of health.

Students did not see this experience as being clinical practice or nursing, which they associated with hospital wards. For many students these visits were a culture shock as they provided a first glimpse into different social environments from their own. Also in their first year they visited a hospital ward in their proposed specialist branch of nursing. Such observation experiences helped students appreciate the sort of work they would be undertaking after their foundation programme and assisted their reaching a final decision about career choice.

In their second year, students worked in a range of clinical settings sampling all the different branches of nursing and midwifery. These placements included visiting a mother and baby unit, caring for older people, working in community homes of people with learning disabilities or placements for people with mental health needs, as well as caring for children and adults. On average students spent eight to ten days in each placement, spread over four weeks, giving a total of 19–22 clinical days over a ten-week term. In one module they had three place-ments: two of eight days and one of three days; in another they had 22 days. These placements were supplemented by lectures and tutorials from clinical specialists led by lecturer–practitioners and generic theoretical modules, such as 'Understanding Families' and 'Law and Ethics'. When students reached their third and fourth years, they were allocated to clinical placements in their chosen field for a whole term and received seminars and key lectures each week. Sometimes their placements were up to 30 kilometres away and negotiating their clinical visits around their academic timetable often meant fitting their place-ments in over weekends. This did not necessarily provide the best opportunity to get to grips with busy clinical settings but it did provide a calmer atmosphere for learning.

Supervision in placement settings

Throughout the course and in each clinical placement, supervision was provided by a nominated member of the unit's healthcare team (a nurse, midwife or health visitor) known as a mentor. This practitioner continued with a normal caseload and was an experienced practitioner. Mentorship was usually provided by staff nurses, but towards the end of their programme students were often mentored by a charge nurse or ward sister. Students had to identify and negotiate with their mentor suitable times to work on the same shifts. This was often a delicate bal-ancing act between the mentor's duty times and the students' required attendance at university for concurrent modular activities. Changes in a mentor's shift times totally disrupted any opportunity for mentor and student to work together, as their mentor was the main educational and social contact within a clinical area, and students saw the relationship as pivotal to their success in achieving module learning outcomes. Because of the large number of students and the small number of placements, students did not take modules in the same sequence; consequently it was exceptional when any of the students were allocated to the same placement. As it happened, Helen and Jack shared a number of the same placements in their second and third years. Similarly, Marie and Nicola went to the same ward for their children's placements, with very different experiences. Ruth and Jack also shared the same placement for their acute surgical nursing module.

Table 2.1 *(Sequence and length of clinical placement modules over the course)* provides an overview of the pattern of students' Common Foundation Programme as well as their third and fourth year branch practice modules. Sequencing of these modules was not fixed except for a double final (practice-

Table 2.1 Sequence and length of clinical placement modules over the course.

	Practice Module & number of days in practice Term 1	Practice Module & number of days in practice Term 2	Practice Module & number of days in practice Term 3
Year 1 10 Modules in total		Individual and Family Health 5 days	Community Health Studies 10 days
Year 2 10 Modules in total	The Growing Child 8 + 10 + 2 days	Adult Health & Disorders 10 + 10 days	Elderly Adult Health & Disorders 22 days
Year 3 **Mental Health** Nursing	Adult Mental Health I	Adult Mental Health II	Therapeutic Approaches to Psychiatric Nursing
Year 4 **Mental Health** Nursing	Care of the Elderly with Psychiatric Disorders	Special Care in Psychiatric Nursing	Management of Care in Nursing
Year 3 **Children's** Nursing	Mastering Childhood	Children's Nursing Practice 1	Children's Nursing Practice 2
Year 4 **Children's** Nursing	Children's Nursing Practice 3 (double module)	Children's Nursing Practice 4 (double module)	Children's Nursing Practice 5 (double module)
Year 3 **Adult** Nursing	Acute & Crises Care	Experience of Physical Impairment, Disability & Handicap	Loss, Adjustment & Dying
Year 4 **Adult** Nursing	Accident & Emergency Nursing	Patient's experience of Illness or Specialist, Advanced Nursing Skills	Management of Care in Nursing

based) management module, taking place in the last term of their course. Modules were each deemed to require 110 hours of student effort in the first year and 120 hours of student effort in subsequent years. Over each term students took the equivalent of four modules, so a single module of 120 hours included ten days or 75 hours of practice. Modules that were practice-based were assessed using students' action-inquiry reports generated from their practice experiences and drawing on relevant literature. These statements of learning, or Learning Contracts as they were called were verified as representing the student's clinical experiences, by their mentor and lecturer–practitioner.

2.3 The research design

To understand how nursing students developed their professional knowledge a research approach was needed that elicited participants' thoughts and feelings when learning in clinical settings. The key focus was to learn about students' experiences from their perspective and not to impose any external ideas. With no evidence of any earlier work in this area it was difficult to anticipate any pitfalls, so a flexible research approach was needed that allowed different data collection methods to be used in responding to how the study developed and its findings. The focus was on students' clinical learning activities and how their experiences contributed to this, so the research took place in natural settings. Moving between data collection methods and the data itself provides more opportunities to really understand the breadth and depth of participants' experiences. The philosophical framework that seemed most appropriate for such an iterative process between researcher and researched was one described by Schwandt (Schwandt 1994) as constructivist–naturalistic. It has two strands, ethnography and phenomenology. Ethnographic research uses a variety of data sources, such as fieldwork, documents and interviews. Phenomenology seeks to capture the essence of phenomena, such as sleep, being listened to and so on. This is achieved through detailed descriptions of preconscious reflections, commonly obtained either from verbal or written descriptions. But Van Manen (Van Manen 1991) argues that other forms of data can also be used, such as poetry, art or observation. Using this approach to investigate human experiences in naturalistic settings is supported by other authorities such as Miles and Huberman (Miles & Huberman 1984). They recommend using case studies to illustrate findings so that future readers can decide whether they match their own experiences. This QA strategy of confirmabilty and transferability to other people's experiences provides credibility and dependability to the data. Choosing a longitudinal, collaborative approach with a small group of students provided more opportunity to understand the whole process of students' professional development. It also enabled flexibility and greater sensitivity to the data as the research progressed (Denzin 1989). By starting the project at the start of the students' programme I planned to capture their thoughts and feelings about nursing relatively untainted by influences from their programme. The research project was in two phases. An initial sensitising process for myself as well as the participants took place whilst students were on their first-year community placements. The second phase covered the remaining part of their course.

2.4 The research participants

Selecting research participants for a longitudinal study depends upon several factors, the most important being their enthusiasm to be part of the process and commitment to remain for the whole four years. They needed to participate in the research whilst at the beginning of their programme and this gave a short time to negotiate with potential participants. A third important consideration was the timing of their first practice placement. A small sample was going to be the most manageable for this study but it posed the threat of becoming non-viable and the data having limited trustworthiness if informants dropped out. Something that was likely to happen over a four-year period as Robinson and Marsland describe (Robinson & Marsland 1994). A sample group was chosen of between 6 and 10 students, to accommodate attrition if it occurred. This sample size constituted 15% of the whole intake of nursing students, and by selecting from a random sample it was likely to produce a cross-section of the whole group. Approximately 60% of the students in that year's intake were planning to become adult nurses, 16% midwives and the remaining 24% either children's, mental health or learning disability nurses. Ten students taking a community placement in their second term were approached by letter and invited to participate in the study and attend a meeting to discuss what it entailed. The letter gave details of the research and addressed a number of questions concerned with confidentiality, possible implications of participating in the study for their own programme, the extent and nature of the commitment being sought and how the data materials would be handled and used.

Following a preliminary meeting where we discussed these issues, six students were recruited to the study. They received a contract and consent form that had been approved by the Head of School and Reader in Nursing and which contained these details. Participants were asked to return one copy and keep the second copy for their own records. Serendipitously, these students represented a cross-section of the intake of nurses. They were all women, aged between 19 and 26 and had differing experiences of working in care-giving situations prior to starting their nursing degree course. They also intended to qualify on different parts of the professional register. Two planned to become children's nurses, a third, a mental health nurse and the other three planned to become adult nurses (see Table 2.2). One of these students left at the end of her first year and another two students were recruited. Jack, a male student who had previously qualified as a psychiatric nurse and Petra who had intermitted from the course for a year and worked as a healthcare assistant before rejoining the course. She later intermitted again along with Grace, one of the original six students at the end of their second year.

Table 2.2 Entry characteristics of students in case studies.

Pseudonym	Age on entry	Previous nursing experience	Family connection with therapeutic care	Branch of nursing
Helen	20	Care assistant in nursing homes for 4 years & 1 year working in an overseas orphanage	None	Adult nursing
Grace	27	Healthcare assistant, pupil nurse for Enrolled Nursing	None	Adult nursing
Jack	26	Left (RGN) nursing course in 2nd year; completed RMN	Grandfather good at massage	Adult nursing
Marie	18	As a patient when a child	None	Children's nursing
Nicola	18	Some occasional help in a nursing home for the elderly	Close family, doctors or nurses	Mental Health Occupational Therapy preference
Ruth	26	Volunteer assistant for a lady who was physically disabled	Both parents were nurses	Adult nursing

Student participation – ethical issues

As identified earlier, students were encouraged to think carefully about the possible implications of participating in the research study. We discussed the aims and processes of the study as well as ethical issues and confidentiality, their rights and their freedom to opt out. In their first term all the students had successfully completed a module assignment on research methods and had considered these aspects in detail. As a result they had been able to use this knowledge when drawing up their form of consent to participate in the research. It is possible that they entered the study feeling better informed than perhaps most research participants. Decisions about confidentiality were explored and agreed with the students, including the use of pseudonyms to preserve the identity of their mentors and any other people whose names were mentioned in their conversations. Students also chose their own pseudonym.

A basic premise of the study was the importance of having a collaborative partnership with the student participants. This included discussing the research design, negotiating times and venues for interviews to take place and the other forms of data collection. Heron's (Heron 1981) strong model of participation is suited to critical theory and emancipatory research, whilst his weak model engages participants in a democratic relationship, but acknowledges their role as

Table 2.3 Issues associated with the researcher–participant relationship.

Problem	Rationale	Strategy
Differential in status and thus concern to prevent power-coercion of students that could jeopardise the investigation.	Lecturer status within the same department of the university as the students' course.	Engage in no further academic relationship with the students' programme.
Congruence of students' expressed experiences with those that have been lived.	Students may construct a version influenced by their perception of my needs or their perception of our relationship.	Discuss this concern with the students, checking with them when a situation or statement occurs that seems inconsistent or dissonant with earlier accounts.
Participants may feel unable to give frank criticism of my analysis of the data.	Concern for the power relationship.	Discuss the importance of openness and honesty in the data analysis, and try to behave in a way that is congruent.

participants rather than as co-researchers. This approach reflects the real dilemmas presented by age and status differentials, some of which are expressed in Table 2.3. Cassell and Wax (Cassell & Wax 1980) discuss the researcher influence on participants and argue that essentially the relationship should be beneficial to them. Cassell (Cassell 1982) further explores the ethics of the researcher relationship by offering four dimensions, concerned with: the researcher's relative personal power, influence of setting, influence of context and influence of interaction. My own position as a senior lecturer in the school inevitably created an asymmetrical power relationship with the students. I shared these concerns with them and we discussed any possible implications and strategies that could be used to protect them. The outcome of these discussions was written into their consent form. Congruent with this desired democratic approach to the research process, students were fully informed about the nature and purpose of the research activity at every stage and their continuing consent was discussed and agreed. They were encouraged to collaborate in a democratic manner as described by Heron, by participating in decision-making processes and to collaborate by verifying transcript summaries and drafts of their case studies.

On occasions students may have believed I could influence their course in some way and they may have slanted their conversations with this intention. In reality I had no influence over the course and this was made clear to them. However, my knowledge as a nurse and a lecturer meant I was able to offer information that could help them develop a broader perspective on aspects of the course they found perplexing; much as Oakley (Oakley 1981) did with her research participants when investigating motherhood. Throughout the research process I tried to develop and maintain a humanistic and feminist approach of genuineness and warm regard for the participants as fellow equals, although it was clear that a number of different relationships would exist between us.

2.5 Data collection

A variety of data collection methods were used to provide as comprehensive a picture of students' experiences as possible. The main sources of data were interviews that took place with students individually and in focus groups. Sometimes individual interviews were preceded by an observation of a student's practice, or after they had completed a piece of illuminative artwork (Spouse 2000). Students also provided copies of their written clinical assignments. These were written reports of their action inquiries written up as critical incidents using problem based learning of their clinical practice experiences and were written reflectively and analytically. A summary of the different methods of collecting data along with their rationale can be found in Table 2.4.

Table 2.4   Planned data collection methods and their purpose.

Data collection method	Phase in the research	Purpose to gain access to:
1. *Focus groups discussions*	Phase 1 Term 2 of first year & term 3 of final year	Personal background, students' images, beliefs, understandings, pre-course and course experiences of nursing in the community
2. *Individual interviews*	Phase 1 & 2 (2–3 times a term)	Students' personal images, beliefs, understandings, experiences
3. *Observation of practice*	Phase 2 throughout students' programme	Accounts of students' learning & discussion of experiences
4. *Illuminative artwork*	Phase 2 at end of term	What it feels like to be a nursing student – students' tacit understandings of learning to nurse
5. *Learning Contract analysis*	Phase 2	A third perspective on students' learning experiences
6. *Interviews with mentor*	Phase 2	Incidentally, following observation. Used to gain a second perspective on observed clinical practice

Interviews

Semi-structured in-depth interviews were the principal approach to data collection. From the beginning of their second year students were invited to talk about their clinical experiences two or three times each term of their programme. These conversations focused on clinical practice issues they found meaningful or important and they explored how they knew what to do or what helped them learn how to perform. Their thoughts, feelings and actions were important to the whole process of learning to be a nurse and to do nursing. At the beginning of the study, in the second term of their first year, students participated in four focus group discussions. These took place at the same time as their first clinical visits. In the focus groups, students discussed why they chose nursing as a career and how they felt about the course, their first impressions of nursing and their clinical experiences. Towards the end of their programme they participated in another focus group to consider their progress and their future plans and aspirations. An important part of the focus group meetings were the picnic lunches that helped break the ice and gave students time to relax and get to know each other. These early meetings also helped us all get used to the idea of participating in research activity and using tape recorders and microphones.

Negotiating interviews

Once the study was established interviews were arranged by telephone and we negotiated the most suitable venues to meet. Mostly students chose to visit my office, which was away from the main university site, but also convenient for their clinical placements, though sometimes they found it easier to meet in their home or their clinical setting. Refreshments and comfortable surroundings that were free from interruption helped them feel at ease; giving students encouragement to take the lead during interviews helped them to say what they wanted to say about the topic without external pressure, and it also increased the authenticity of their accounts. Interviews were introduced by asking each student to describe their clinical experiences and then elaborate on particular points, to confirm understanding. The tape recorder was started at the beginning of interviews and it was positioned close to them so they could stop it whenever they wanted. When the audio-recordings were transcribed students were given copies of the data and the summary to review and correct.

Illuminative artwork

Supplementing the interviews was students' illuminative artwork (Spouse 2000). This gave them an alternative means of expressing what it felt like to become nurses. Having a different form of 'language' helped them reach experiences that perhaps were too difficult to bring to mind and talk about, but once displayed visually students could begin to find the necessary words to describe their experiences. There is a wealth of literature relating to using images and art in education (Hirst 1973; Read 1943); in nursing (Bentley 1989; Cortazzi & Roote 1973); in psychiatry (Anderson 1977; Naumberg 1966); and in psychology (Maslow 1963) which provided a solid basis for using this technique. Preparing students for using illuminative art included discussing an article about a supervisory relationship between two occupational therapists who used art to express their feelings (Durkin, Perach et al. 1989). When students agreed to try this approach I also participated in the first group session with the students.

We agreed that the purpose of using artwork was to stimulate further memories and language rather than as a source in itself of detailed critique and analysis. After this trial students agreed to use this as a supplementary form of data collection when they came to their end-of-term interview. Before each of these interviews I would check that they were happy to create a picture. Once they got used to the process and felt comfortable about using paints, coloured pens or crayons they would come to their session saying they had been thinking about what they wanted to create. These end-of-term art activities were sandwiched between two 45-minute interviews. The first interview explored their clinical experiences and the second discussed the images. This second interview often developed further their earlier reflections on their clinical experiences, and introduced new memories and feelings that might otherwise have been overlooked.

Documentary sources of data

Several phenomenological researchers used documentary sources of information when investigating a range of different phenomena such as 'Really feeling understood' (Van Kaam 1959), 'Experiences of coronary artery surgery' (Trumbull 1993), 'Sexual passion' (Jager 1978). Using documents that students needed to produce as part of their assessment of practice, provided a verified source of additional information. These documents were known as Learning Contracts. They were students' reflective and analytical explorations of critical incidents from their clinical practice that were evaluated by their mentor who knew the student during their clinical placement. Having the authenticity of students' accounts verified in this way proved data that was valid. It also meant this source of data did not impose an additional, research-generated burden on participants.

Observation of practice

Using direct observation to collect alternative information about a phenomenon provided a sense of the reality of students' experiences in clinical practice that could be explored further through subsequent discussion and is advocated by several ethnographers and phenomenologists such as Becker and Geer (Becker & Geer 1969) and Van Manen (1990). Following up an observation with an interview immediately afterwards provided better opportunities to probe students' understanding and experiences of their own practice. Students took responsibility to get the necessary permissions from their clinical manager for me to come and watch them, which gave them a control over the event that was congruent with the collaborative philosophy we were using. Most of the time this process worked very effectively, though on a couple of occasions difficulties arose (see Spouse 1997) that provided a different and valuable perspective on their placement experiences and how they learned to become nurses.

Entering the field, ethical considerations and procedures

Gaining access

As indicated earlier, negotiating to enter the field was a delicate process and required negotiation on several levels. Permission to undertake the research had been granted by the school through its various committees. Further permission was needed to enter clinical settings and observe students in practice. This was obtained through the same education committee members. When students entered their specific clinical field or branch of their programme (adult, child, mental health) permission was gained from the relevant branch committee and the appropriate service manager for the clinical area. These prescribed procedures were carried out, but didn't necessarily provide rights of access. Other researchers describe similar experiences (see, for example, Burgess 1984). Depending upon beliefs about the locus of power, whether it resides with the researcher or the researched could raise concerns about the students being manipulated by the researcher. Trying to maintain a humanistic approach, I sought to empower participants by giving them opportunities to refuse entry on whatever pretext they wished. Some of their mentors may have felt compromised by this approach, or they may have preferred me to approach them personally. However only one mentor mentioned this in the seventeen visits and this is when the student forgot to make arrangements because she was preoccupied with other things. During clinical observation visits and following the interview both mentor and student had access to my notes and to all the information the visit generated. Mentors were assured that confidentiality would be respected.

Patient consent

When patients were involved in the observation, the student and mentor explained that I was a nurse undertaking research into how students gave nursing care and checked whether the patient was willing to have me present during the procedure. If they gave their consent (and all the patients gave it freely) I would follow up this explanation by introducing myself and asking if I could be present. In none of the observations did I attempt to disguise myself by wearing a uniform, or a white coat, which could have associated me as a member of the hospital staff. Patients who were involved in these observations were articulate and alert and were considered to be in a mental state able to give their consent. When observing the children's nurse, consent was gained from the child's parent. In the mental health field, access was considered by the student's mentor to be inappropriate because of the risk of a patient misinterpreting the nature of the request. Alternative methods of recording the student's activities were considered, such as wearing a radio microphone, but after discussion with the ward manager this was rejected for the same reasons.

A second reason to refuse entry, given by one mentor was that the student had not been on the ward long enough to be observed. This was made despite repeated assurances from the student that she would welcome my coming to observe her. There were other concerns about access to researching mental health nursing that have been identified by researchers such as Strauss et al. (Strauss, Schatzman et al. 1964) who identified the strategies of role definition and boundary maintenance, practised by healthcare professionals in psychiatric institutions studied in the United States in the 1960s. My experiences echoed those described by Cassell (Cassell 1988) when researching up and the difficulties of finding access to the powerful gatekeepers.

2.6 Analysing the data

The volume and distribution of data accumulated over the project illustrated in Table 2.5 shows that it needed careful management and that I needed to be sure that it remained congruent with my chosen constructivist paradigm. Three particular aspects of the data analysis had to be considered. These were the intersubjective meaningfulness of students' actions; development of explanations that

Table 2.5 Summary of data collected from all participants.

Student	Interviews – Individual: Focus Group	Observation of practice	Learning Contracts	Illuminative Artwork
Helen	12 : 5	1	4	4
Grace	6 : 2	2	0	3
Jack	16 : 0	4	7	8
Marie	18 : 5	3	3	7
Nicola	15 : 5	1	3	6
Ruth	23 : 6	5	7	7
Natalie	2 : 4	–	–	–
Petra	3 : 0	1	1	2
TOTAL	95 + 6	17	25	37

were both contextually and temporally sensitive and thirdly to arrive at theory construction derived from meaningfulness that reflected the cultural and social norms which existed for the students (Halfpenny 1989). Students' transcripts and learning contracts were read several times not only to get a sense of the significance of what they were saying, but also to check that the initial categories assigned remained congruent. From these, short summaries were developed and shared with the relevant student and then draft case studies prepared. Over the four years several case studies of each student was refined and developed further until we both felt they fully represented the important elements of each individual's experiences. These had to be both sufficiently rich or 'thick' as to be transferable or recognisable by other nursing students and demonstrably trustworthy (Lincoln 1985; Moustakas 1994).

Presenting the findings

Developing the case studies

Drawing on interview data, written materials from their learning contracts and observation reports the students' case studies were created to reflect each student's personal experience. My first attempt at writing a case study drew on literature concerned with professional education and constructs of socialisation, technical knowledge, schema and personal knowledge – see for example Ruth's case study in Spouse (Spouse 1994). However these theoretical frameworks did not explain the complexities of Ruth's professional development. Neither did the case study meet the three criteria identified earlier. As a result these first attempts were abandoned and a more reflexive and sensitive approach to students' narratives was used to generate constructs drawn from the data. So a second round of data analysis was undertaken using these constructs to address the research questions and these provided the framework for writing each students' case study.

Each case study underwent four or five drafts whilst I tried to represent the essence of each student's experience and professional learning. Students reviewed their own drafted case study and their comments and suggestions were sought and incorporated. Differences were partly due to whether they wanted to be a children's nurse, a mental health nurse or an adult nurse. Although over their first two years they took the same programme, the timing of each module differed slightly and their clinical placements also differed, either because the settings were different or because they encountered different mentors and different patients.

Students' case studies rely on their own words either to illustrate key points or, in Nicola's case study, to tell her own story. Each case study represents a unique flavour of the student's personality and responses to their experiences as they progressed through their programme. Nicola's story is the most idiosyncratic and perhaps reflects her particular way of thinking and learning to become a mental health nurse. In mental health nursing the ability to develop relationships with clients and the quality of these relationships are important components of the therapeutic relationship. As with the other branches of nursing caring is also concerned with how nurses use themselves in a therapeutic manner. In mental health this is expressed through social interactions more often than through physical care and technical dexterity. In the early stages of students' stories they were concerned with technical aspects of care, and once these were mastered they felt more able to relax into forming professional care relationships. An explanation for this could be that students were concerned for patients' safety and they were conscious that this could be jeopardised if they made a technical mistake.

Deciding how to order the case studies was problematic because of the choices that it offered. Should all four adult nursing students be located together, or the stories of the three older and the three younger students be juxtaposed? Controversially, should the stories of heroism, conviction, confusion and self-doubt be set in contrast? Perhaps it may be argued that all the case studies reflect the different strengths of each of these students and in particular the heroism that could not have been anticipated when students first agreed to participate in the study.

Helen's story opens the sequence. It reflects the struggle she experienced throughout her journey to become a nurse, which in many ways reflects that of the others and in other respects is special to her. Subsequently several nursing students from different parts of the world have read her case study and found it matched their own experiences. Being close in age, but different in temperament, Marie's experiences of becoming a children's nurse follow. These two are followed by their contemporary, Nicola whose very different account explores what it is like to become a mental health nurse. All three enjoyed the emotional and social support of fellow students and nursing peers, which seems to have helped them make their transition to become nurses. By contrast, the three older students, Grace, Ruth and Jack relied upon different support networks. Jack and Grace both started the course having had a considerable amount of nursing experience and training and it is interesting to compare their experiences with those of the others. Grace experienced a number of setbacks and eventually at the end of her second year decided to take a break from the programme. Ruth and Jack had less distractions, nevertheless they faced a range of challenges and difficulties associated with their earlier life experiences. Jack was less concerned about developing his technical skill but more concerned with adjusting to the social mores of adult nursing. Ruth on the other hand, entered nursing from the business world and brought a refreshing outer-worldliness which led her to question and challenge not only her experiences but her whole being and to compare them with the stories of her nursing parents with whom she had grown up.

To give some indication of each students' stage in their programme, every narrative has been given a label that states the point reached in their programme. In sequence, this identifies the student by pseudonym, the number interview and the point in their programme, e.g. (Helen 8, year 3 term 3). From this label the reader can develop a view of each students' development as they progressed. An additional identifier has been added to note the number of the narrative in the case study. This number is referred to in subsequent chapters to illustrate a particular student's experience or point.

Answering the research questions

Through writing the students' case studies, I became increasingly conscious of the dominant themes that influenced their development. Some were anticipated, the role of the mentor, the value of peer support, others were initially considered to be less important owing to the number of items relating to the categories, such as learning contracts and the lecturer–practitioner. What emerged as being significant, was the nature of the activities students were given and their context. The mentor's role was seen as highly complex and instrumental in providing both a social, affective and educational value to their development. Existing studies of nursing education had indicated the importance of a clinical instructor or mentor but had not provided any theoretical basis for their importance. Nor had they illuminated what actually took place during mentor–student interactions. Nursing educational textbooks using behavioural and humanistic theories provided little guidance. These failed to explain what seemed to be taking place. It was necessary to return to the literature to find possible explanations for what was happening.

A second issue was the implicit discussion of students' learning or acquisition of professional knowledge. In addressing the research questions it became necessary to review the twelve categories that had been developed from the first round of data analysis (see Table 2.6).

A category 'learning the essence of nursing' emerged from this classification and was associated with the category of students 'flying solo'. Data was extracted and placed into category files for each student. Rolls of wallpaper lining were used to map the categories and their entry locations. Eventually these were displayed on four sheets, each two-foot square. This visual display of categories made it possible to recognise the dominating themes immediately. Using this new framework and relevant literature in an iterative fashion, the research questions were then addressed and this is how the data are discussed in the following chapters.

Table 2.6   Categories of data.

Images of nursing and nurses	Learning to relate theory and practice
Learning technical procedures	Flying solo
Learning to relate to clients	Learning from narrative
Coping with feelings, ethical dilemmas, empathy	Learning from mentors
Learning through practice	Relating to team members
Learning the role of a nurse	Learning contracts

2.7 Quality assurance activities

Member checking

A vital part of any research is to demonstrate that the data has been collected in a rigorous and exhaustive manner as befits the study. Another important quality aspect is to make sure that data represents the thoughts and feelings of the research participants. Without this confirmation then the material is potentially faulty and any findings can only be tentative. To promote these important quality measures and to ensure accuracy and fidelity throughout the study students read and commented on all their transcripts. This gave them opportunities to reconsider what they had said and whether it was what they had meant. The same principle applied to developing each student's case study. Throughout the study after each new development in their case study, they collaborated in verifying the content and the interpretations. A further check was made to establish whether case studies portrayed the branch specialities adequately and the expertise of specialist nurses' was utilised. In one situation a specialist mental health nurse identified a lack of emphasis on the personal growth in Nicola's story. A factor that had permeated the data but which I had not recognised or valued as particularly significant. This aspect was subsequently given recognition in her case study. Since then other colleagues and students from around the world have read the case studies and have found they could identify with individual experiences. Nurse educators who read them believed they could recognise students they had encountered (not these particular students) and also with Jack's experiences.

Trustworthiness

Qualitative research has long been criticised for lacking qualities that have been espoused and cherished by deterministic researchers. In some studies where issues of validity, reliability and replicability are desirable different research approaches are used and the context of the data collection is pre-determined. In conducting a research study with the intention of defining truths rather than 'truth', different procedures are needed and the researcher becomes a participant in the process rather than an experimenter or quasi-objective recorder. As in this qualitative research study the integrity of the findings and my research activities must be demonstrated, if only to respect the effort and time contributed by the participants. One of the most effective strategies, prescribed by Lincoln (Lincoln & Guba 1985) was member checking which the earlier paragraph described. A second concern identified by some authors for example Calderhead (Calderhead 1997) is the veracity of student accounts. Trustworthiness was addressed in a number of ways using the following strategies:

- students were invited to volunteer to participate and were given a written assurance that their programme would not be affected if they chose to withdraw

- confidentiality was assured and data management was discussed with them fully
- the initial focus group interviews enabled a sense of group identity and development of trust and rapport
- the length of the study required considerable commitment from the students and investment of self
- students were fully conversant with the objectives of the study and were closely involved in its design and progress
- the purpose of the study was to explore their perceptions of their experiences of becoming nurses. This acknowledged multiple realities and thus no single truth. It was accepted that at different stages in their development, students could view their experience differently, but this would not invalidate their earlier perceptions.

Anonymity

Secondly, there is the question of anonymity and confidentiality. As Johnson (Johnson 1982) identifies, keeping an institution secret is probably impossible simply by the nature of its programme. Disguising place names and those of all the participants helps to ensure that a level of responsibility has been discharged, unless the instances are exceptional.

In identifying and addressing these issues, my concern was that these students should benefit from participation rather than suffer from its consequences. It is possible that through narrating their experiences they were able to create greater meaning from them than perhaps they may have done otherwise (Hutchinson et al. 1994) Student reports indicated that they did find engagement in the process beneficial. It is hoped that their success following completion of their degree and professional registration will continue to be enhanced by their contributions.

References

Anderson, W. (1977) *Therapy and the Arts: Tools of consciousness.* Harper Colophon, New York.

Becker, H.S., Geer, B. (1969) Participant Observation and Interviewing: a comparison. *Issues in Participant Observation: A text and reader.* (eds G.J. Macall, J.L. Simmons), pp. 322–41. Addison Wesley, Reading MA.

Bentley, T. (1989) Talking Pictures. *Nursing Times*, Occasional Paper 85 (31): 58–69.

Brown, S.J., Collins, A., Duguid, P. (1989) Situated cognition and the culture of learning. *Educational Researcher* 18 (1): 32–42.

Burgess, R.G. (1984) Starting research and gaining access. In: *In the Field.* (ed. R.G. Burgess), pp. 31–52. Chapman and Hall, London.

Calderhead, J., Shorrock, S.B. (1997) *Understanding Teacher Education: Case studies in the professional development of beginning teachers.* Falmer Press, London.

Cassell, J. (1982) Harms, benefits, wrongs and rights in fieldwork. In: *The Ethics of Social Research: Fieldwork regulation and publication.* (ed. J.E. Sieber), pp. 7–31. New York, Springer-Verlag, New York.

Cassell, J. (1988) The relationship to observed when studying up. In: *Studies in Qualitative Methodology*. (ed. R.G. Burgess), pp. 89–108. JAI Press Inc., London.

Cassell, J., Wax, M.L. (1980) Editorial introduction: Towards a moral science of human beings. *Social Problems* **27** (3): 259–64.

Cortazzi, D., Roote, S. (1973) Don't talk, draw. The use of illustrations in learning from critical incidents in patient care. *Nursing Times* **69** (35): 1134–6.

Denzin, N.K. (1989) *The Research Act: A theoretical introduction to sociological methods.* Prentice Hall, Englewood Cliffs.

Durkin, J., Perach, D. et al. (1989) A model of art therapy supervision enhanced through art making and journal writing. In: *Advances in Art Therapy*. (eds H. Wadesdon, J. Durkin, D. Perach), pp. 390–432. John Wiley, New York.

Halfpenny, P. (1989) The analysis of qualitative data. *Sociological Review* **27** (4): 799–825.

Heron, J. (1981) Philosophical basis for new a paradigm. In: *Human Inquiry: A source book for new paradigm research*. (eds P. Reason, J. Rowan), pp. 19–35. John Wiley and Sons, Chichester.

Hirst, P. (1973) Literature and the fine arts as a unique form of knowledge. *Cambridge Journal of Education* **3** (Michaelmas): 118–32.

Hutchinson, A.A., Wilson, M.E., Wilson, H.S. (1994) Benefits of participating in research interviews. *Image: Journal of Nursing Scholarship* **26** (2): 161–4.

Jager, B. (1978) Towards a phenomenology of the passions. In: *Existential Phenomenological Alternatives for Psychology*. (eds R.S. Valle, M. King), pp. 341–57. Oxford University Press, New York.

Johnson, C.G. (1982) Risks in the publication of fieldwork. In: *The Ethics of Social Research: Fieldwork, regulations and publication*. (ed. J.E. Sieber). Springer-Verlag, New York.

Lathlean, J. (1995) *The Implementation and Development of Lecturer–Practitioners in Nursing*. Oxford University Press, Oxford.

Lincoln, Y.S., Guba, E.G. (1985) *Naturalistic Inquiry*. Sage Publications Inc., Newbury Park.

Maslow, A. (1963) The creative attitude. In: *Therapy and the Arts: Tools of consciousness*. (ed. W. Anderson). Harper Colophon, London.

Miles, A.M., Huberman, M.B. (1984) *Qualitative Data Analysis: A source book of new methods*. Sage Publications Inc., Newbury Park.

Moustakas, C. (1994) Phenomenological research methods. Sage Publications, Thousand Oaks.

Naumberg, M. (1966) *Dynamically Orientated Art Therapy: Principles and practices*. Grune and Stratton, London.

Oakley, A. (1981) Interviewing women: A contradiction in terms. In: *Doing Feminist Research*. (ed. H. Roberts), pp. 30–61. Routledge & Kegan Paul, London.

RCN (1985) *The Education of Nurses: A new dispensation. Commission on Nursing Education*. Royal College of Nursing of the United Kingdom, Chair: Dr Harry Judge, London.

Read, H. (1943) *Education Through Art*. Faber and Faber, London.

Robinson, S., Marsland, L. (1994) Approaches to the problem of respondent attrition in a longitudinal panel study of nurses' careers. *Journal of Advanced Nursing* **20**: 729–41.

Schön, D. (1983) *The Reflective Practitioner: How professionals think in action*. Arena Ashgate Publishing Ltd, Aldershot, Hants.

Schwandt, T.A. (1994) Constructivist, interpretivist approaches to human inquiry. Chapter 7. In: *Handbook of Qualitative Research*. (eds N.K. Denzin, Y.S. Lincoln), pp. 118–37. Sage Publications Inc., Thousand Oaks.

Spouse, J. (1994) Development of professional knowledge in nursing students. In: *Improving Student Learning: Theory and practice*. (ed. G. Gibbs), pp. 419–39. Oxford Centre for Staff Development, Oxford.

Spouse, J. (2000) Talking pictures: Investigating personal knowledge through illuminative art-work. *Nursing Times Research* **5** (4): 253–61.

Strauss, A., Schatzman, L. et al. (1964) *Psychiatric ideologies and institutions.* Transaction Books, New Brunswick.

Trumbull, M. (1993) *The experience of undergoing coronary artery by-pass surgery: A phenomenological investigation.* (Doctoral dissertation). Dissertation Abstracts International, The Union Institute.

UKCC (1999) *Fitness for Practice.* The UKCC Commission for Nursing and Midwifery Education. United Kingdom Central Council for Nursing, Midwifery and Health Visiting. Chair: Sir Leonard Peach, London.

Van Kaam, A.L. (1959) Phenomenal analysis exemplified by a study of the experiences of 'Really feeling understood'. *Journal of Individual Psychology* **May**: 66–72.

Van Manen, M. (1991) *Researching the lived experience: A human science for action sensitive pedagogy.* The Althouse Press, London, Ontario.

White, E., Riley, L. et al. (1993) *A detailed study of the relationship between teaching, support, supervision and role modelling in clinical areas within the context of Project 2000 courses.* Kings College London & University of Manchester. Research commissioned by the English National Board for Nursing, Midwifery and Health Visiting, Manchester.

Wilson Barnett, J., Butterworth, T. et al. (1995) Clinical support and the Project 2000 nursing student: factors influencing this process. *Journal of Advanced Nursing* **21**: 1152–8.

Chapter 3
Case Studies of Professional Development

3.1 Helen

Helen started the (adult) nursing degree course at the age of 20 having spent a year working in a South American orphanage. She had already decided that she wanted to become a nurse and had spent much of her spare time working in a nursing home for the elderly. Her decision had been influenced by a childhood hospital experience. Like many people who choose nursing as a career, Helen found it difficult to articulate her reasons, other than the desire to care for people.

> When I had my tonsils out at about seven I thought the nurse was really nice. It's just something I'd wanted to do. I wanted to do something positive for people rather than going into sales and manipulating people for money. (I want to be) Someone who has the confidence to know what they're doing, but is also caring for the patient and has a good sense of humour.
> (Helen 9: year 3 term 3)   (Narrative 1)

With the help of her parents, Helen started voluntary work at a nearby nursing home to see if she would enjoy the work. Initially she went in to chat to the residents and later when she was older she was employed to work at weekends and school holidays.

3.1a Helen's images of what it is to be a nurse

As she became more familiar to the nursing home staff Helen was allowed to work unsupervised and to take on more and more of the personal nursing care for the residents. Becoming familiar with how her colleagues worked and with the daily routines of the home and individual patients, she began to use the same strategies to manage her workload. When she started her nurse preparation course she had very clear views of what nurses did.

> People say it's different everyday and it is different with each patient, the routine is the same and everyone has similar bodies, you're washing them so it could be anyone. There's no way I'd specialise in that (care of older people) because there's not much challenge, you could easily get stuck in a rut, staying there. Once you got used to the routine and everything it's not that amazing.
> (Helen 1: year 1 term 2)   (Narrative 2)

Her experiences in the nursing homes taught her to view caring for older people as menial and routine. She learned to consider the patients as work objects rather than people with needs and interests. As a result she saw them as the sum of a number of tasks such as washing, toileting and feeding that had to be completed as quickly as possible. She anticipated a nurse's role to be more dynamic and challenging, requiring a sound technical ability as well as theoretical knowledge. By the end of her programme she had developed more sophisticated conclusions about the role of the nurse.

> Continuity of care, advocate for the patient, a carer, listener. Like the psycho-social, biological help. Biological would be helping the patient to wash and dress or doing their ECG or caring for their wound. Psychological: making them feel at ease and recognising their anxieties, talking to them and respecting their culture or whatever and social would be, as well as liaison with the Physio, O.T and social worker. Looking at their discharge plans. Planning ahead whether they go into care or how they're going to work. Working in a multidisciplinary team.
> (Helen 11: year 4 term 1)   (Narrative 3)

Learning to manage her feelings

Throughout her programme Helen seemed to be caught in a dilemma between her image of how professional nurses behaved (stoical in the face of all human adversity) and how she actually felt as a person. This had been experienced first when she worked in a nursing home after she had discovered a favourite patient of hers had died. She saw her colleagues as being indifferent to the loss and this increased her sense of isolation and bewilderment. Helen was concerned that she might become like them, which she interpreted as being hard. At 16, it was difficult to come to terms with the death of an endearing resident and the staff seemed unable to offer her any consolation, leaving her alone to manage her own feelings and to find a way of coping.

> I felt like crying and then I thought I'm here to work, I can't cry when I'm here and everyone accepts it. You think it's the best for quite a few of them (the residents). After the shift I told my parents.
> (Helen 1: year 1 term 2)   (Narrative 4)

She wanted to find a way of being authentic when facing circumstances that were poignant or disturbing. She was haunted by stereotypical images of hard faced nurses ploughing on with their work regardless of any joys or tragedies surrounding them and found them both influential and worrying.

> The maternity placement [was the most meaningful experience] because it was something completely new to me. And although it's natural it was new and frightening because of the labour and it was frightening too because I thought the baby was dead and I couldn't contain my emotions. So what they must feel like . . . I had loads of tears running down my face and I couldn't stop it. It was really embarrassing. There was a resusc. team there and doctors and everything and they were all *professionals*. Doctors don't cry, they're probably

slightly more hardened to it. There was a student midwife there and she was all right as well. But the husband cried.
(Helen 5: year 2 term 3)   (Narrative 5)

Learning to acknowledge and to cope with her inner life was difficult and often painful. As this narrative indicates, in her efforts to appear professional, Helen was uncomfortable about expressing her emotions in public. And yet there did not appear to be time or a place to do it in private because of the unremitting workload. For her, it seemed that only lay people displayed emotion whilst professionals used different strategies to cope with disturbing or painful experiences.

The sight of blood and death

Helen's sensitivity to the political stage of becoming a nurse and the importance of impression management was even more acute as her account of working in the accident and emergency department indicated:

> On my first shift, I saw a cut finger that my mentor was meant to be looking at and it was bobbly on top and I just felt really faint. It was horrible. It was quite embarrassing. Goodness knows what my mentor thought of me because it was the first day she'd met me. Then I decided that I should tell her that I shouldn't be here doing A&E and I shouldn't be a nurse if I can't even cope with a cut finger. What use am I if I'm going to feel faint at that? It's ridiculous. I've been a nursing student for three years and I haven't really seen blood and guts in that way. So she made me sit down and the next few I saw was someone's arm being stitched up and after that I was fine. So in that way my mentor saw a physical improvement in me, not fainting all over the place.
> (Helen 9: year 3 term 3)   (Narrative 6)

On several similar occasions Helen chastised herself for not meeting her own expectations. In the second year of her degree course Helen was asked to sit beside a male patient whilst he was dying. As a result she developed a bond with him and his family. In coping with this painful event she seemed to be working with an image of how she believed nurses should manage their feelings. That was to contain or compartmentalise her feelings until a suitable opportunity arose to express them.

> . . . the patient who died and I was really upset about that, but I kept back my feelings until I'd left the ward that evening. . . . It was just like any death, you're really upset. But I was with them quite a lot, with them every day, but I wasn't there when he died. It's easy to read in books that you shouldn't get too emotional, but everyone does now and then. I had my mentor and the other nurses to support me, . . . and my mentor realised I was going to be affected by it because I'd been with them a lot of the time, so I was given support by them, so it was completely different. I think he made me feel that I'd done something worthwhile and had contributed to helping the family in their last few days.
> (Helen 4: year 2 term 3)   (Narrative 7)

In this situation the ward team members were sensitive to her needs and were willing to give her emotional support. As a result she felt valued and her self-confidence increased with the knowledge that she had contributed to the patient's care and the work of the team. Despite this support from the staff she still found it difficult to fully express her feelings. As on earlier occasions she bottled them up and waited until she was away from the ward. Her friends found her crying as she was cycling home after duty.

> I told them (my housemates) all about the guy I was looking after. It was the other day and I was really upset. I was cycling home and two of my friends, one of my housemates and my old housemate. They saw me crying in the road and they just shoved me in a car and we chatted for ages.
> (Helen 4: year 2 term 3)   (Narrative 8)

Having this support and being encouraged to acknowledge her feelings helped Helen to gain a new perspective on the behaviour of the nursing home staff. It also gave her the opportunity to lose some of her anxiety about caring for a dying patient. Somehow Helen had not begun to value her insights as indicative of her sensitivity to her patients' needs and instead she persisted in feeling concerned that she was becoming stereotypically hardened. Her relief at finding that she could express the wellspring of emotion that was so deeply buried was reassuring.

Accepting herself

During her placements Helen was confronted with the task of developing relationships with people facing distressing or life-threatening experiences sometimes as a consequence of a moment's misfortune or carelessness. Their plight was clearly moving, as well as shocking, and her task was to help contribute to the long programme of rehabilitation back to the world outside the unit. Sometimes she seemed self-conscious, almost guilty, about her own health and to feel that she was confronting her sick patients with it.

> At first I talked to them all and I'd hear all the horrible stories of how it happened, but it didn't affect me and I was almost worried that it hadn't affected me because I thought I was getting a bit hard. But then in the middle of term I was really happy for some reason and then I just thought about all the people in Head Injuries (unit). I'd really enjoyed it, but because I got to know quite a lot of them really well I cried all night thinking about them. Then after that I felt better that I'd showed emotions. I knew I wasn't hard. I don't know whether you're supposed to show emotions, but I wanted to be able to put myself in their position.
> (Helen 7: year 3 term 1)   (Narrative 9)

Her experiences of working with these young people and her feelings were profoundly sincere and compassionate and reflected a deep sense of commitment to their welfare despite the hurdles some patients created to daunt the insecure and self-conscious student. Helen's sensitivity and ability to reflect on her own experiences were both an impediment and a help when she was giving intimate care to her patients.

Talking to patients

Knowing what to say to patients, particularly people who are hard of hearing or who are mentally frail is difficult. When Helen was working in the nursing homes she became aware of how she would like to communicate better with her patients and admired the staff who seemed to enjoy so much confidence.

> I'm still not as good at communicating with them as I should be. It just depends upon your character. Some of the nurses waltz into people's rooms chatting away and they're really friendly, whereas I'm sort of, and other nurses will walk in and not, not really say anything, and maybe talk to them a bit. But I know I don't speak to the patients as much as I should. It's not that I don't want to it's because I'm sort of shy, and I just feel really silly. If patients see the nurses rushing around, then they'll feel more ill at ease and feel that they're wasting the (nurse's) time and that doesn't seem right really. I guess you just listen to the other nurses too, and that's how you learn how to communicate with them, so I know what to say.
> (Helen 0: year 1 term 2)   (Narrative 10)

Helen's thoughtful and sensitive observations helped her to recognise the subtext of some of the communications enacted by different staff. From this she constructed a model for her own behaviour that led her to feel comfortable about talking to the elderly. However, knowing how to communicate with younger adults or with her contemporaries in hospital seemed a greater challenge. She also worried about how she would be able to communicate with young children who also seemed a source of potential embarrassment. In her learning contract for the children's placement she recorded her concerns.

> Having not worked with children in this situation before, it took a while for me to be able to relax and start up conversation with patients, especially if their parents are there. I felt that if I was not doing anything 'practical', e.g. taking obs, I would feel a bit silly going and talking to patients. Although I know that it is necessary and beneficial to the nurse–patient relationship to be able to talk to patients without having a 'task orientated reason'.
> (Helen: LC: year 2 term 2)   (Narrative 11)

Having a task as a mediator

To help overcome her shyness, Helen found having a task to do for the patient gave her a means of initiating conversation rather than have to work out an introduction which might sound artificial. The patients collaborated with her and helped her to do some of the tasks that she was finding difficult.

> I found it difficult when I first went on the ward because I didn't know what I'd say to all the patients. Then you just realise that they just want to be treated normally and talk about the weather and their children or whatever. Sometimes they want to talk about their illness and sometimes they just want to block it out. Some of them have faced up to the fact that they're going to die and have accepted it. . . . Partly I would be worried in case someone came out directly and said to you 'Am I going to die?' and supposing you did know, you wouldn't know whether it was your place to tell them or not. Just talking to someone you don't know how much they know about their illness. Even if it's a cancer ward some people may not even acknowledge that it's cancer they've got and you might put your foot in it. When you

get there and are actually talking to them it seemed less likely to happen. . . . It's easier to go up to someone and say 'Can I do your obs' rather than just say 'Hello, I'm a student nurse.' It all depends on the person though. As well as being a good nurse you have to be quite confident, and I'm learning to do that better.
(Helen 4: year 2 term 3)   (Narrative 12)

As Helen highlighted, learning to talk to adults was less problematic than she had feared and her patients were only too pleased to have her with them to relieve the monotony of being in hospital. Throughout her second year, Helen seemed to have struggled with her self-consciousness and feelings of inhibition of talking to people of her own age. Her experiences of working with the elderly seemed to have been discounted, perhaps because as she implied earlier, the fear of their criticism did not seem to be as great as that of younger people. In her third year she was allocated to a rehabilitation unit (mainly) for young people suffering from serious disabilities due to major trauma. Inevitably she approached the placement with some concern which was greatly alleviated by a helpful seminar discussion which, although it did not provide any answers, gave her some ideas on how to operate:

> I was really worried at first because most of them are my age and I thought they'd look at me and I'm normal and they're in a wheelchair. . . . This 16 year-old girl was one of the worst – she was in a wheelchair, couldn't speak properly, only in a whisper, and she had spastic arms. I was asked to go and look after her with my mentor and then my mentor left me on my own with her. I just talked to her and realised she was quite sarcastic and it was quite easy to talk to her. . . . I didn't feel sorry for her so much. It wasn't patronising as a relationship. I could talk to her like I could talk to most people. Just by being her age, talking about boys she liked and because I was her age, she's 16 but quite mature, we just had a laugh.
> (Helen 7: year 3 term 1)   (Narrative 13)

By the end of her placement she felt pleased that her efforts had been recognised and valued by her mentor. This was expressed in her picture depicting how she felt about herself at the end of term (see Figure 3.1c).

> I started off by drawing two chairs and I put a hat on one and that's supposed to be me as a nurse. Basically my placement involved counselling people, or so it seemed. I was told I made a good little counsellor.
> (Helen 7: year 3 term 1)   (Narrative 14)

The encouragement from her mentor who permitted Helen to collaborate and watch what she was doing, gave her confidence to work on her own and try out some of the techniques she had learned. In a few clinical placements, Helen experienced this amount of involvement and as a result came to appreciate some of the issues beyond the day-to-day practical care needs of patients.

Social support

Influential in making sense of her experiences and in providing support, were her clinical colleagues and peer group, some of whom were nursing students and others were pursuing degrees in other parts of the university.

Mentor support

For the majority of her placements Helen did not seem to spend a great deal of time with mentors and this seems to have influenced her self-confidence and sense of identity. Where she was attached to an enthusiastic mentor willing to have her work alongside her, Helen also became enthusiastic and worked hard. Being able to debrief from practical experiences with her mentor was enormously helpful to make sense of her observations and experiences and it was a valuable part of her learning that guided her with her assignments. On other occasions she was concerned by her mentor's attitudes and questioned her influence. When I went to observe Helen working, it was clear that the nurse acting as her mentor had misjudged her needs and was unconcerned about the implications for her professional development. As a result Helen was left to carry out activities that were more appropriate for a more junior student. This had the consequence of leaving her feeling under-confident and doubtful about her ability to become a nurse. By contrast the support that she received from her peers was stimulating and enlightening.

Peer support

Attending university often provides lifelong friendships developed through hours of debating and discussing issues that are close to the heart. Travelling to and from home to distant clinical placements offered students opportunities to discuss work and to compare their experiences.

> It's one of the most useful things if you've been feeling difficult about something and they might say 'Yes, I felt like that as well'. So we're all in the same boat in a way and it brings you a lot closer. It's helpful in a different way because I might talk to my mentor and she'll tell me something I can put in my learning contract. My mentor actually gives me facts and information that are useful for my skill, writing it down in theory. Whereas when I'm talking to friends, some of the discussions we've had I suppose I could write down as objectives, but it's not actually written down. I might remember it more easily because it was an interesting talk.
> (Helen 2: year 2 term 1)   (Narrative 15)

Being able to debrief their experiences in a supportive and understanding climate and to engage in story-telling, exchanging experiences and ideas in a private, safe and entertaining manner was a vital aspect of learning to nurse. Their conversations perhaps included an element of competition that lightened the tragedy and seriousness surrounding their clinical experiences. Debriefing opportunities with peers became more important as Helen progressed through the course. Responses from her non-nursing housemates contrasted sharply with those of her nursing colleagues. Not being faced with life and death situations made it difficult for them to share her concerns and they frequently misunderstood Helen's responses to traumatic experiences.

> Last year I could talk to some of the people in the house, but they only know a vague outline of what nursing is about and have a certain idea of what I'm like. I remember coming back

from the ward and said 'This guy has just died on the ward of cardiac arrest'. And a house-mate that I don't know that well said 'God, how can you come home and say that and be so blasé?' and it really made me feel awful, I was really upset at the time but couldn't be both-ered to explain it. So they probably think I'm really hard. Some people don't particularly want me to go into details about it. I don't know, because you're not really supposed to talk about patients are you?

(Helen 11: year 4 term 1)   (Narrative 16)

Living in university accommodation or cheap housing with non-nurses Helen inevitably became part of their more relaxed social scene. In contrast to these students, nursing students were constrained by academic and clinical demands, often requiring considerable travelling time. Sharing a house with non-nursing students influenced Helen's feelings about her career choice. Her housemates had values and intentions that appeared very different from those of her nursing col-leagues. When they completed their degrees after three years, Helen still had one more year to complete, leaving her behind. As a consequence, Helen's self-image as a nurse was somewhat flimsy and she frequently questioned her assumptions about becoming a nurse. In her final painting of feeling like a nurse, Helen illus-trated this experience as a road junction with the inviting green grass in front her and a choice of routes to take (see Figure 3.1e).

The picture is diagonally cut in half with a road running from one diagonal to the other. A huge amount of grass on the left hand side and there's a road joining the main road with traffic lights and all of them are on. I'm on a bicycle. . . . The grass is greener on the other side in a way, [which symbolises being] just free to do what I want, not to have to do any more studying and not having to do nursing or whatever. . . . Also, because I'm coming up to red it's like I'm coming to a different stage in my life, where I've got to accept the fact that everyone else is leaving. I've got another year and everyone else either has a job . . . I could turn round and leave the course now, but that would be a bit stupid. But there's no point chucking in the degree now and I'd probably regret it. I probably will be a nurse at the end of it.

(Helen 9: year 3 term 3)   (Narrative 17)

Helen's accounts illustrate the dilemmas she faced throughout her degree course. She was exposed to a range of conflicting messages about student life from her chosen peers, as well as different expectations about how women behave when facing stressful experiences and sights. These expectations amplified her own doubts and concerns of becoming hardened if she remained in nursing. They also contrasted with her clinical experiences of how healthcare practitioners func-tioned when faced with daily exposure to distressing situations. Such situations are normally beyond the everyday life experiences of most lay people and yet are often commonplace for many healthcare practitioners. Because many face such situations daily it may be vital to their mental health and survival to learn differ-ent ways of responding to traumatic events. This is a common finding around the world where cultural norms influence definitions of emotional events and also influence what is a culturally acceptable response (Stearns 1995). In different professions where daily work brings practitioners into contact with emotionally draining events such as experienced by social workers, the police or people working in religious ministries, different coping strategies are learned and developed. Inevitably responding to an emotionally stressful experience will trigger different responses and even dissonance when exhibited in a different culture. By moving between the culture of university student life and the culture of busy clinical settings, Helen was experiencing this kind of dissonance.

3.1b Learning to give nursing care

A change in perspective

Starting the degree course with a lengthy experience of working in nursing homes behind her encouraged Helen to feel that she would be able work independently quite quickly. In her second year she started her first hospital placement in a unit concerned with the care and rehabilitation of older people. Care of older people in this setting was recognised to be a sophisticated and demanding specialty and the unit attracted many well-educated and committed nurses.

Helen was shocked by the unit's welcoming remarks. These communicated the belief that Helen's earlier experiences would hinder, rather than help her progress and she would need to make major adjustments if she was to be successful. Over the subsequent ten weeks and 22 days of working on the unit she came to recognise the truth in this unexpected judgement and the discrepancy with her earlier experiences.

Her first and perhaps most difficult lesson was to learn how to function as a nursing student rather than as a care assistant in a nursing home. Seeing how members of staff treated patients in the unit helped Helen to appreciate the differences in approach. She experienced a significant transformation in perspective, whilst also experiencing a dilemma. If she wanted to earn money to supplement her grant or gain additional nursing experience by working in the nursing home during her vacations she could not return to their (old) ways of working without experiencing a conflict in values. Helen's perspective transformation was partly due to her willingness to undergo a considerable re-assessment of her working practices and beliefs. Instrumental in this process was the conscientious support of her mentor, which for Helen as it later turned out, was exceptional.

> I realise that all the work I learnt in the nursing home had to be re-learnt. I found that a lot in my attitudes. I was trying to work like in the nursing home . . . just doing task orientated things all day. Then gradually I realised what my role was. The first few weeks I just thought everything was so detailed and they wrote down how they held the spoon and lifted them. As I got used to it I realised when I was in the nursing home I was lifting the wrong way, although I was bending my knees when I could. It could have been injurious to my back though. . . . I think I've realised, just from talking to people how much power nurses really have. A lot has come out of our seminars. Like the way you feed them and whether you let them help themselves. Some patients in the nursing home I'm sure, could dress themselves if they were given time and a bit of help, but because of lack of time we used to just dress them.
> (Helen 2: year 2 term 1)   (Narrative 18)

The change in Helen's understanding of how she could care for patients was quite dramatic and profound. Not only was the change concerned with her relationship with the patients but also with the manner in which she carried out the nursing tasks. This realisation was partly stimulated by working with the high quality registered nurses and partly by her course materials and the assessment strategy. They urged her to explore practice experiences using her knowledge base.

Learning from others

Working with registered nurses, both her mentor, other practitioners and her peers gave Helen unique opportunities to learn by participating, observing and talking about the care being given. In talking about Helen's learning process, an artificial division has been made in this book to make the nuances explicit. In this section the focus is concerned with the day-to-day activities of providing care, rather than specific technical knowledge or understanding of the nursing role. On her first ward experience, Helen described how she developed a great deal of confidence in her newfound knowledge which she attributed to her mentor and other members of the nursing team.

> My mentor really helps as well and it makes a big difference. It's like having a personal tutor there all the time. If you need something you can just go and ask her and she talks about it. Also, the other people in her team, the associate nurse is really helpful to me . . . I was more listening to her [the mentor's] instructions and helping her, but I didn't feel under pressure at all because she was showing me how to do it. When she's going through it she reflects on things that you might think in your head but wouldn't necessarily say. I felt at ease with her because she was helping me, as opposed to watching and criticising me.
> (Helen 2: year 2 term 1)   (Narrative 19)

Helen's account of this placement was almost unique throughout her programme. Very few of her narratives described such a close and formative working relationship. More often she described spending much of her time on her own, doing unstructured activities – her mentor had been busy on other clinical tasks, but it might have been very beneficial for Helen to participate in these also, if only her mentor had realised. Throughout the course Helen always expressed concern not to impose on her mentors but at the same time relied upon their support.

> I think I've improved since I've been there this term, just in clinical skills that maybe I've could have done ages ago. Things like doing drips. But I've never really done them on my own before. And I was really worried because I didn't understand the drip and I now I'm perfectly happy to go and change someone's drip if I check. . . . I don't mind asking anyone. Also it's better to ask not just your mentor. Otherwise you can feel, I don't want to put a strain on her and go and find her all the time and hassle her if she's got her own worries.
> (Helen 14: year 4 term 3)   (Narrative 20)

Helen's first placement was both enjoyable and stimulating and she received support and guidance from all members of the ward team. She arrived at her second placement having made a significant transition from her old nursing home practices. Instead of considering patients as a collection of tasks to be accomplished, she now recognised the importance of promoting patients' independence and of holistically implementing their meticulously planned care. Her second placement contrasted radically from the first. Rather than being taken under her mentor's wing and engaged in some of his holistic nursing activities she was given small repetitive tasks such as taking observations which fragmented her view of the patients' care.

> I helped set up drips and helped my mentor. I did loads of obs., which has been brilliant practice. I'm still probably not that good, but when I first went on the ward I think I'd only done one blood pressure and I didn't feel at all confident. . . . If I wasn't talking to somebody, or if he was busy, then I'd go and read up on someone's notes and he'd come up and he'd explain so many of the different terminologies and illnesses . . . and then later on he'd leave me to it, which was quite good. If I wasn't sure about something he would come and check it and other times when I showed him the results and that I was happy with them, then he would take my word for it. I felt that was quite a good thing. When he did check them he said 9 out of 10, I was right, anyway, so he gave me confidence, which was really good.
> (Helen 4: year 2 term 3)   (Narrative 21)

This different approach to supporting Helen was in some respects successful in providing opportunities to do tasks repetitively and so she was able to become more competent in the unfamiliar tasks she had been given. She also had a sense of not bothering or draining her mentor and so inconveniencing him. Being delegated small tasks meant she was unable to see how patient care was planned and delivered. Given such a fragmented role she could not develop a comprehensive image of how to nurse patients in the setting. As a result she became dependent on her mentor for guidance towards the next task, imposing the kinds of strain on her mentor and other staff members that everyone was wanting to avoid. She did not seem to have an identity within the unit, either as an assistant to her mentor or as a student able to care for specific patients on her own. She seemed isolated from the rest of the team and their everyday nursing practice and as a result the quality of her learning suffered.

3.1c Developing technical skills

Developing technical skills not only involves the psychomotor dexterity to manipulate instruments, or equipment, or bodies (one's own and those of patients). Helen also needed to learn how to perform these skills effectively and appropriately within a package of care. On her first clinical placement, she had spent some time working alongside her mentor, watching what she did and then trying to copy her actions, first under direct supervision and then on her own. She also observed how the other staff operated and was able to recognise when they carried out procedures successfully. Because she gained a sense of security, she felt sufficiently self-confident to act appropriately. On her third and final second year placement, a children's ward, Helen's mentor was even less supportive and she was left to manage on her own. To Helen, who had no prior experience of caring for babies or young children undertaking simple techniques that are part of every parent's repertoire of childcare, such as handling a baby, feeding it or changing its nappy were a nerve-wracking challenge. These fears were even greater when she was confronted by a fragile baby suffering from a severe medical disorder, or when anxious parents were watching. Fortunately Helen encountered an associate nurse who was willing to share her expertise and this helped her gain the confidence to look after her patient, a particularly delicate child.

> I was able to look after this four month old premature baby who was absolutely tiny and had water on the brain. I watched dressings being put on. The named nurse said how to hold the baby and his reflexes weren't very good because he was a prem., I watched her feed him first. You think it's so easy to do, but it's all nursing and you have to do it the right way. It was so tiny as well. I watched her change the nappy and then I did it. I think she trusted me with him as well, which was really nice.
> (Helen 5: year 2 term 3)   (Narrative 22)

Helen's growth in confidence and enthusiasm for this experience was striking and indicated the value she gained from working alongside such a skilful practitioner. Having had little teaching from her clinical mentors, Helen moved into her third-year clinical placement, a busy surgical ward, filled with trepidation. She felt conscious that she should be more knowledgeable and technically competent. The nurses on her surgical ward were keen that she should work alongside them and were good at sharing their craft knowledge. This support helped Helen to develop a variety of valuable nursing techniques. Amongst them was learning to give an intramuscular injection, a technique that many nursing students consider to be the most significant milestone in their career.

> Injections came up and [my mentor] said I could observe and I said I would prefer doing it if she could tell me what to do. It was an upper outer quadrant and I put the needle in and that was fine and then I got the shakes really badly, . . . and my mentor had to hold the needle. I didn't feel I'd done a proper injection at all. I did another one the same day because I was quite annoyed with myself not doing it well and I did it OK without shaking. I noticed for the first few weeks that every time my mentor had an injection to do she would say 'We'll just do this and then give an injection,' and I'd always have it in the back of my mind. I did get quite het up about it and worry that my hands would be sweaty or something. Towards the end I didn't even think about it though. But later when I was doing injections I'd take my time, rather than worrying about the patient and how long I had the needle in. My mentor told me how to change my technique. So it was just practice. Also I did a couple of injections with two other nurses, one who is a real stickler and a really good nurse. But she said my technique was really good.
> (Helen 8: year 3 term 2)   (Narrative 23)

3.1d Bundling tasks together and managing care

By the end of her fourth year Helen was under pressure to participate in the ward in the same way as the other (qualified) nurses and she was worried about her management skills and her ability to care for a patient caseload. Her education throughout the course had taught her to recognise patients as individuals with carefully devised plans of care that needed to be implemented thoughtfully. Now she was being confronted with a seeming demand to return to the practices of her nursing-home days in order to prove that she was ready to function as a qualified nurse.

> If they're not dependent then it's OK, but if they're all dependent and it's the day shift and you've got all the drugs to do and everything, there's no way I'd be able to deal with seven patients and give them the care and attention they needed. . . . My LP had a word with my mentor and I had three, and she said 'You really need to push yourself and start taking four'. I think her point is that you need, even if there isn't much care, have in your mind that you've got to juggle having five patients, whereas having three you can relax a bit more . . . . Like this week I'll have done three [patients] and last week I think I did two, but the week before that was five and the week before that was three.
> (Helen 14: year 4 term 3)   (Narrative 24)

As Helen says, it is the volume of care that patients needed which influenced the quality of care she was able to give particularly if she had a number of high dependency patients. Learning how to care for such a caseload was through watching others and talking with her mentor. But there is a sense that getting through the workload and being seen to be able to cope was important. For Helen and her colleagues, numbers of patients mattered and as a result patients were being reduced to work objects by the need to get the work completed.

Knowing how to communicate with her patients was one of the key areas that always concerned Helen and as in most situations, she used a combination of observation and theory from the literature to help formulate her own strategy.

3.1e A personal philosophy for practice

Working with desperately ill patients, presents students with many ethical and moral dilemmas that require some form of nursing strategy. Being exposed to the ways in which medical and nursing colleagues managed these dilemmas was thought-provoking.

> That was a patient I'd worked with earlier on and she'd come back in and she had about a couple of years to live and they didn't tell her. I really felt that they should have told her. . . . A friend of mine said 'Didn't you tell someone that you were put in that situation when you were sitting talking to her?' It wasn't my place to say anything, but at the same time I thought 'Here am I knowing something that's so important to you and you don't even know it'. . . . But then I didn't want to make it too blatant by saying 'You should definitely go and do everything you want'. She might turn round and ask why I thought that. It would have been really hard.
> (Helen 12: year 4 term 2)   (Narrative 25)

It was clear that Helen had been torn between the medical decision and her knowledge of the patient. Finding a solution to manage such situations is difficult and Helen drew on conversations with her nursing friends to come to an understanding of how she could respond. Part of any response must include awareness of her specific role as a student and that required a professional image.

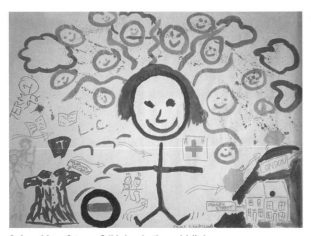

3.1a Year 3 term 2 'Helen in the middle'.

3.1b Year 2 term 3 'Sunshine and rain'.

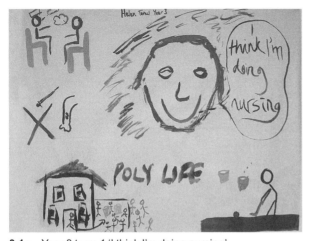

3.1c Year 3 term 1 'I think I'm doing nursing'.

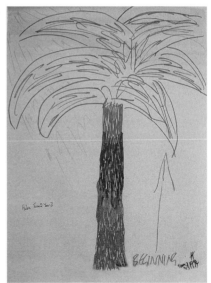

3.1d Year 3 term 2 'The palm tree'.

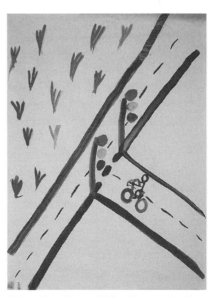

3.1e Year 3 term 2 'Junction choices'.

Figure 3.1 Helen.

Career choice and uncertainty

For most of her placements Helen never gave the impression of really feeling settled or that she felt well-supported by an experienced and committed mentor, able to facilitate her learning. Settling into her clinical placements seems to have been influenced by the amount of care she was allowed to undertake and thus her contribution to the work of the team as a whole, and to her self-confidence. The more she felt able to participate in the clinical work the greater her self-confidence and enthusiasm. An important factor may have been Helen's reliance on her mentor for motivation rather than having the locus of control in herself. At various points in her progress through the course, Helen indicated a nagging uncertainty as to her commitment to nursing as a career. Having chosen to become a nurse at an early age made it difficult for her to contemplate an alternative career. Throughout the first two or so years of her programme she was able to enjoy the relative freedom of student life. Her clinical experience made few major demands on her social life and possibly provided a certain air of martyrdom that raised her status in the eyes of her non-nursing peers. The curriculum required frequent changes of placement and perhaps this unsettled existence and not feeling that she belonged to any community of practice, caused her to doubt her career choice. As a result Helen suffered from a profound lack of self-confidence in her ability to function effectively as a nurse.

The illuminative art-work (Figure 3.1) expressing her first three years as a nursing student is dominated by symbols of parties, fun and journeys away from the university to her home and friends – images of university life rather than involvement with her nursing. Her awareness and growing concern about her career choice was heightened by a crises in the middle of her third year when her commitment to nursing was challenged by her mentor and co-mentor of the surgical ward. Helen was forced to come to terms with the discipline of her chosen future and not surprisingly, it was something of a shock. In this clinical setting it was compensated by her enjoyment of being a member of the team, and her sense of achievement of successfully giving care to people in need of her newfound skills.

Looking forward to the beginning of her fourth year she emerged from the experience feeling more confident. But her enthusiasm and self-confidence were not to last. Her doubts were exacerbated by the contrasting images of professional nurses that she encountered and would soon be associated with. The busy surgical ward nurses were highly dedicated and professional, but seemed overly conscientious and remote. In strong contrast were the medical ward nurses whom she perceived to behave inappropriately with their flirtatious friendliness. Neither group of nurses appealed to her as suitable role models.

3.1f Helen's professional development

Helen seems to present a most thought provoking profile because of the complexity of her experiences. She was deeply concerned about her relationships with patients and also about her development of nursing skills. Yet throughout the course she seemed to be distancing herself from the process. Perhaps this can be attributed to her natural reticence and inability to commit herself whole-heartedly to her intended career. Alternatively, it may be accounted for her by concern not to become indifferent to people's suffering, which was the way in which she initially perceived how nurses' responded. She seemed to have been overwhelmed by the attractiveness of student life and had difficulty in investing all her energies in meeting the heavy demands of clinical practice and the theoretical aspects of the nursing degree. Perhaps that would be a reasonable expectation of younger people entering nursing through the portals of higher education, where they identify strongly with their peers and where the student culture contrasts so dramatically. It is difficult to know to what extent Helen's attitude was precipitated by a sense of isolation from the busy clinical world of her mentors who only rarely engaged her in their work and failed to recognise her need for strong support and the opportunity to work alongside them. As a result, at the end of her final year, Helen's narratives lacked the air of self-confidence and determination that characterised those of her peers. Despite this, her clinical assessments and her academic work were good and she gained a 2:2 classification in her Honours degree and seven years later she is still practising as a nurse in an intensive care unit.

There seem to be several major themes that dominated Helen's experience, some of which she shared with members of the group. Those that are particularly her own were Helen's concern to know how to talk to patients (a reflection of her self-consciousness), her sense of isolation that resulted in a lack of confidence and her worry of becoming hardened, through losing her ability to care and to feel.

3.2 Marie

Marie started the course at 19 with nine GCSE subjects and long experience of caring for the younger members of her family. She is the fifth of seven children and was the first in her family to undertake preparation for a profession or to study at university. Her parents, who arrived in England some years ago, are very proud of this achievement. She knows that their main concern is for her happiness but she felt under pressure and was anxious not to let her mother down by failing or wanting to leave the course.

3.2a Marie's images of nursing

During much of her childhood Marie was a patient in a London hospital. Her mental images of nursing are drawn from these experiences which are remembered with affection. She describes how friendly the nurses and doctors were and how clearly she can remember their names and the way they made her feel like a member of their own family. Marie's decision to become a children's nurse was also influenced by her experiences of baby-sitting for her two older sisters and caring for her grandmother when she was suffering from cancer. Both her mother and her grandmother had encouraged her to consider nursing as a career.

> I didn't want to be stuck in an office. I have to communicate with people and doing nursing is a good way to do that. I just love being in contact with people all the time, which is one of the reasons. I know it sounds as though I like caring, but I do. That's one thing that I think I'd be good at and it's what I want to do, try and help them get over their illnesses and try and help their families. . . . Recognising that they're individuals and need different things out of life. Their needs may not be the same as yours. . . . I suppose when I used to go to the hospital, I used to spend a lot of time with the nurses. I suppose I wasn't thinking at age 7 that they were doing a worthwhile job. . . . My mum has always been right in whatever she's said and my Nan was quite a good judge of character. They only want what's best for you and if you don't do it you normally live to regret not doing it. She probably just made me think about it a bit quicker than I would have done.
> (Marie 1: year 2 term 1)   (Narrative 1)

Marie saw nursing as primarily the development of personal relationships between patients and their carers, to the extent that the nurse takes a key role in the patient's life, sharing their joys and sadnesses. Her images of nursing were concerned with providing comfort and a form of professional mothering. She knew that being a nurse meant high standards of integrity as well as having a sound understanding of practice, which carried heavy responsibilities in order to protect vulnerable patients. She saw nurse–patient relationships without this kind of closeness as insincere. She believed this approach could be emotionally painful, but was the hallmark of a caring professional. Between leaving school and starting her programme, Marie did voluntary work over the summer with people who had both physical and learning disabilities.

3.2b Being at university

Moving away from home and starting at university is a major transition for many young people. Embarking on a nursing career at the same time means they are exposed to caring for sick strangers, people who are dying and people who live with different values and have different beliefs and lifestyles. All of which can be shocking and can raise questions about whether nursing is the right career choice. Living in student accommodation, Marie was able to chat with fellow nursing students and compare expectations and experiences of their programme with those of students from different disciplines within the university. She considered the standards expected in nursing to be higher and less flexible than those required by other courses. Initially this seemed unfair. Marie reasoned this would be useful preparation for her future professional role.

During her first year she found it difficult to balance the various demands of academic work and clinical visits. In particular she needed to find her way around an unfamiliar city and its suburbs and try to get to clinical visits in remote places on time. All this work meant she had little time for the traditional student lifestyle that she saw her friends enjoy and that she had anticipated experiencing. Living in university residences put her in touch with her neighbour, another nursing student with whom she shared personal and academic experiences; having spent their evenings studying they would meet up and go out to have a break at the local pub for last orders. Their friendship was to become one of the most stable and valuable aspects of Marie's life at university. Managing on a student grant was another important consideration. In the second and third years of her course she shared rented accommodation and supplemented her grant with a waitressing job. She enjoyed this as it meant she got out in the evenings and met different people. She often worked two evenings a week and twelve-hour shifts over the weekend.

> I've been working solidly and the only escape I've had was going to work at the hotel because I haven't been out a lot. I only do two nights a week (waitressing), some weeks one night. My manager is really good because I do him favours and I can easily say no to that (working different or long shifts). I've just got a pay raise so I'm really chuffed. I don't think it makes it (the grant) more comfortable, but it makes me not worry about money so much. My parents are offering me money, so there's no problem. If I want something I'll ask them for it. And they offer it. But each time they offer it I say no because I don't think it is their responsibility to support me.
> (Marie 10: year 3 term 2)   (Narrative 2)

3.2c Learning to nurse – the social aspects

One of Marie's very first experiences of nursing was in the community and through this she began to understand how different members of society live.

Culture shock

Going out into the community to observe how people maintained healthy living was the key aspect of her placements in the first year and involved her meeting community nurses and health visitors. Students were allocated to a health visitor and then to a family within the practice. Marie found these experiences both challenging and thought-provoking and they brought home to her the reality of some of her patients' social circumstances.

> Well it does make you see things in a different light. I knew there was people worse off than me in the community living in caravans but when you go into the situation and you see it, it does hit you, and you think 'God, how can I live here?' I think it will change my whole outlook permanently. . . . when I've been on the wards, 'cos I'm on children's wards, it's made me think, 'Well I wonder if they're in the same home situation. I wonder if they've got a nice house.' It's given you an insight to the background of everybody, of where they're coming from. Although it's only a bit of insight, [that] they have got a family outside hospital, they have got schools to go to, and everything else.
> (Marie 0: year 1 term 2)   (Narrative 3)

Having visited clients in their homes inevitably led Marie to compare her own life experiences with those of her clients and potential patients. She used this ability to relate personal knowledge to her practical experiences as an important strategy to gaining insight and understanding in her learning.

Entering a clinical setting

Marie's first module in her second year consisted of two different clinical placements. These were concerned with the needs of adult patients in mental health and acute physical care units. Her first ward placement was in a mental health unit. She recalled her initial anxiety and worry about how she would be able to cope with patients and whether the ward staff would be receptive to her as a degree course nurse. She reports in her learning contract that the film *One Flew Over a Cuckoo's Nest* had also affected her feelings of anxiety. In her interview three days after starting on the ward she appeared less anxious about the placement:

> Never having gone on a mental ward before, I was very nervous and apprehensive. I was really quiet and I'm not normally quiet, I didn't know what to say. By the end of it I felt calm and comfortable. The patients weren't that bad. I must have had some really bad preconceived ideas of what it was going to be like and it wasn't like that at all. If you saw all the patients in the high street you'd just think they were normal because they look so normal. . . . I'm enjoying it and I didn't think I would. The patients are really nice and friendly. . . . When the patients ask who I am and ask if I'm a student nurse, I say 'Yes, I'm only a student nurse', and I do feel as though they treat me like a member of staff. The staff are all so nice and are interested in what you're doing. They're quite a bit older than me and they say how the training has changed since their day. I hope my next ward is as good. But because it's such a relaxed ward I think maybe that helps. You can learn a lot and it's really interesting. I love them, I'm really enjoying it.
> (Marie 1: year 2 term 1)   (Narrative 4)

Marie seemed to have been able to settle into the ward very quickly because of the welcoming and interested attitude of her mentor who was also willing to involve her in his activities. Part of this feeling at ease may be due to her mentor's desire to know about her learning needs and to offer help. It was also due to the general atmosphere of the ward and the staff, who were giving her the freedom to approach them at any time if she had any problems and invited her to question everything. Over her ten days of clinical experience, Marie had come to feel that she was contributing to the work of the ward team and that she was a welcome and accepted member of the ward community. Her feelings of social and psychological ease in that environment gave her confidence to share her anxieties about making mistakes. Leaving the ward for a new placement, in an unfamiliar ward and different type of clinical experience inevitably created anxieties. Throughout her programme Marie wanted to feel part of the clinical team and to be able to help out or reciprocate the kind of support good mentors gave her. Their role was crucial, particularly when she was finding her feet in unfamiliar surroundings and learning how to be a nurse. The mentor–student relationship was instrumental to her successful transition from being an outsider to being accepted by other members of the clinical team and thus being in a better position to learn. The quality of this mentorship support varied over her programme as the following extract illustrates. In her second hospital placement her mentor was away ill for the first two days and Marie was left on her own.

> Oh at first I felt as though I wasn't wanted there because my mentor was ill, and everyone was going, 'Well who's going to have the student?' 'Well I can't have her because I've got this, this and this to do'. And I just felt like going home and in the end the only reason I didn't was because I'd got up at 6 o'clock to get there! But when my mentor was there, it was really good, and she knew what I wanted to know.
> (Marie 3: year 2 term 1)   (Narrative 5)

A useful member of the team

Working with a mentor who was welcoming and facilitative, enabled Marie to feel part of the team and learn how to care for patients suffering from specific disorders on a one-to-one basis. Having found a 'safe haven' with her mentor she was able to relax, to look around and consider ways in which she could participate more 'adventurously' within the ward community as a whole. Initially, part of her concern was to give a good impression of her willingness and keenness to learn, but gradually she felt that it was not necessary to make a 'staged' effort of impression management:

> I wanted to make, like, not a good impression, but I wanted to show I was interested. Then I realised that if you're interested then it comes through anyway. Like in the work that you do, how much you're prepared to do.
> (Marie 3: year 2 term 1)   (Narrative 6)

However not all placements were as well prepared and some mentors were unaware of their role. As a result Marie felt disenfranchised and alienated from the other members of the ward team with the consequence that her self-esteem and her learning suffered.

> But when you're actually getting your hands into the muck so to speak, and getting doing things, you feel as though you're of more use. Because otherwise if you're not doing anything you feel you're wasting your time and their, the ward's time, and you shouldn't really – you know, what's the point of you being there? It's simple things like answering the phone in the office and that. It's just so frustrating that you can't answer the phone. You were sitting right next to the phone, 'Why didn't you answer it?' I'm not saying that is what they're thinking but that's how you feel because you're not being of any use. Say it was, I don't know, someone phoning up to see how someone's operation went or something, but I didn't know the answer, that is part of my learning, recognising that I need to ask questions, and going to you or whoever and saying, 'It's so and so, and they've had an operation', or whatever, and then I'd also learn from you saying 'Well, this happened', or 'That happened' and then I could say to you afterwards, 'Well, why did this happen or that happen?' It's part of the learning process, to recognise your own limits.
> (Marie 5: year 2 term 2)   (Narrative 7)

On this ward the telephone became an important symbol of the barrier between her and the staff. She had been forbidden to answer the phone by her mentor. She felt she was being denied access or entry to the ward community and its activities. As a result Marie was unable to participate in care-giving activities, with inevitable consequences to her professional development. She was worried she would be seen as unhelpful and uninterested in nursing. This had consequences on her ability to write her assignment and the effect on her module grade (with which the mentor was involved).

Mentor relationships

What Marie seemed to be describing throughout her conversations over the whole of her programme, is the importance of a close relationship with her mentor. Her enthusiasm and motivation to learn was stimulated by this early contact. As a result she came to feel like a member of the clinical community. Feeling like an insider encouraged her to work actively to seek out learning opportunities and to develop her professional practice and self-image as a nurse. Without this kind of good support she was unable to engage in the full range of activities characteristic of the clinical placement and thus develop a wider appreciation of her nursing role. As she progressed into her fourth year, Marie found it easier to settle into her clinical placements following initial bonding with her mentor, but without the need for constant support from her mentor. She had accumulated sufficient understanding to identify a role for herself. She felt more able to work independently and then to go to any member of the ward team if she needed help.

> It's been great because people rely on you for your support and at the end of the day when they say 'Thanks, you did a really good job'. It's really nice to go off the ward with someone appreciating what you've done. Just taking your own patients, deciding on their care, assessing their needs, re-evaluating their care plans, evaluating their care and the whole situation. I'm in there and doing it and at the end of the day if I make a decision I'd like to think that it was to the benefit of the child and team. Just by what I do I think I'm accepted by the team. I'm not trying to do anything to impress upon the team, I'm doing things for my own benefit and learning experience. [My mentor is] maybe not as important as in the past. . . . So it's almost like a child being tied to the apron strings and the strings are gradually getting longer and I'm letting go. I have the confidence to go up to someone and say 'Excuse me, I don't know how to do this'. Everyone is just so helpful on that ward. You're a lot more independent, but it's nice to know that you've the support there if you need it as backup. At the end of the day if there's a crisis you can go to your mentor and say something.
> (Marie 15: year 4 term 2)   (Narrative 8)

In the next section of Marie's case study we shall consider how she developed the skills that helped her to develop this role in which she came to feel so comfortable and confident.

3.2d Learning to give nursing care

In clinical learning environments where she felt happy and secure, Marie was excited by her experiences and motivated to invest an enormous amount of effort studying the literature in order to develop her theoretical knowledge, to the point that she was oblivious to external assessment of her achievements. She was to experience this particularly towards the end of her third year and during a period of working in the same clinical area over two terms. Her growth in motivation and enthusiasm was made possible by the support of her mentors and other members of the clinical team and is related to her observations of how they worked and the coaching they gave her. Another important aspect of her learning was the need to talk through her experiences with a sympathetic friend who understood the trials and tribulations of learning to nurse and who could understand what she was trying to make sense of. Supporting her development was Marie's striking ability to relate her personal knowledge, derived from family experiences such as caring for her nephews and nieces and to put herself in the place of her patients.

Learning from others

On her first ward, which was concerned with mental illness, Marie expressed anxiety about the patients she would be meeting. Her mentor allayed these fears and took her around with him for her first four shifts. As a result she was able to feel confident and to take notice of her environment and what was happening to the patients; to watch staff working with the patients and to learn how to behave.

> On my first couple of days I was feeling a bit nervous and I didn't know what to say to them. I was just observing what the other members of staff were doing and didn't really talk to the patients. But by the Sunday I had started talking to them and finding out about their backgrounds, that they'd got jobs. My cousin went through a bad phase and she comes from seven children and is young. So thinking about her and the things that had happened in the past, I started to realise that they must all have families. Seeing the staff and patients talk is good for you because you can start thinking 'Right, he's avoided that question because it could have led to this' or 'He's answered that question very well. He's gone around it in some way'. You can learn how to relate to the patients yourself. It's quite interesting.
> (Marie 1: year 2 term 1)   (Narrative 9)

From her accounts, Marie seems to have good powers of observation and be able to recognise practices that were congruent with her own beliefs and to try them out. After a very few days of working in this first ward, Marie seemed to have adapted sufficiently to work effectively as a member of the team. By overcoming her initial fears of the patients, she learnt to recognise the signs of their disease and to respond effectively.

Learning technical knowledge through participating in care

Having expert help to develop skill is an important part of the learning process and the coaching activities of the mentor or other members of the nursing staff were highly valued. Marie was fortunate in having many mentors who were prepared to share their knowledge. In some situations it was the theoretical aspects of care that were required, in others she needed to be taken through the unfamiliar technical procedures and to be given the rationale behind them.

> My mentor Sarah, would say, well I'm doing this now because of this, and she explained like, a couple of the operations and that for me. . . . I'd follow a patient through, which was really interesting. All she had was a metatarsal osteotomy, which is quite a simple operation, and Sarah explained it to me and drew pictures and showed me what was happening.
> (Marie 3: year 2 term 1)   (Narrative 10)

These teaching strategies used by Sarah the mentor, were very important to Marie and helped her to feel both useful to the clinical unit and that she was sufficiently worthy to be taught by someone whose skills she valued. She was also very conscious that if her technique was wrong that she could experience public humiliation, despite the respect and trust she had for her mentor. A secure bond of trust was important enabling Marie to undertake difficult techniques in the presence of her mentor. The mentor's principal strategies of (1) creating a trusting relationship; (2) sharing her knowledge whilst engaged in practice; (3) discussing the medical aspects of the patient's condition; and (4) supervising the student's practice seemed fundamental to Marie's development. Later on in her programme Marie spent some time working in the community and encountered a different range of opportunities which were concerned with taking her own caseload of patients. She found this exhilarating and it motivated her to study in order to be sure that she gave her clients the right information. As a result her confidence grew. On her return to the hospital wards she was supported by an excellent mentor who understood her learning needs and helped by involving Marie in all her own work and by coaching her as she went along. This resulted in a rapid escalation in Marie's level of confidence and competence.

> I said to her basically that I didn't have a clue what I was doing and I needed a lot of help and she was always there. She was a really good mentor because she told me 'They've got this wrong, which means this is wrong, which means you should be doing this and if this happens it means they're getting worse or better'; sort of thing, which was really good. . . . She was quite happy to let me get on with what I was doing, I think because she knew I would go to her and ask how to do things. So it was a partnership. It wasn't you student, me mentor and you do what I tell you to.
> (Marie 11: year 3 term 3)   (Narrative 11)

As a result of the support she received Marie was able to function effectively with her own caseload of patients to the point that she no longer needed the close support of her mentor but was able to operate independently.

Learning to work with parents

An important aspect of caring for children in hospitals is a nurse's relationship with the parents. Many children in hospital for any length of time receive sophisticated treatment for uncommon and often frightening disorders. Parents are encouraged to spend as much time as possible with the child and to be the principal care-givers, where possible. It requires a great deal of confidence to respect the parents' knowledge and to work in partnership together with them, especially when the child is desperately ill. Marie clearly felt comfortable with this partnership and had learned to respect and value their knowledge.

> I think with all the parents that I've come into contact with, they know their child better than anyone else. Like this child has been fighting temperatures yesterday and today and last night mum said 'I think he's getting a bit hot'. He didn't feel particularly hot to the hand but mum thought he was getting a bit hot and sure as hell he was 39.2°, so he was quite hot. So they know when their child is going downhill. They know the child better than you're ever going to know it. They don't want you to take over and if you take over all the care and they go home with these medicines, then they're going to have to learn so much in such a short space of time. You need to be able to inform the parents, teach and educate and promote their child's health. Sometimes I feel I can't do that, but I know I can go to my mentor. Or I know that I can go to the respiratory nurse or the cystic fibrosis nurse or whatever. All the nurses on the ward have their own little specialities and I know I can say 'This child wants to know about their diabetes and I really don't understand it. Could you explain it?'.
> (Marie 12: year 4 term 1)   (Narrative 12)

This example seems to indicate that Marie had developed a theoretical knowledge base to her nursing care. The involvement of parents was common to the clinical unit and clearly Marie, although very much aware of her limitations, was sufficiently confident to check out her understanding by discussing her thoughts and conclusions with whoever was available or suitable.

3.2e Linking theory with practical experiences

Marie was thrilled to have a caseload of her own. As a result she felt she could really fulfil her early aspirations and images of nursing. Her contact with patients provided profound insights to their social and personal experiences as well as motivating her to want to know more and was a frequent topic of her descriptions of learning to nurse. In her third year, Marie spent a lot of time in the community either observing children or working as an associate to her mentor, a paediatric community nurse. She spent her placement visiting children and their families in their homes, working independently after her mentor had introduced her to the families and shown her the ropes. At the end of her time she described this experience with enthusiasm.

> It was the first module I've really enjoyed in the whole of the three years. It's the first one I've really got into. Because in the third week, I was going out by myself with my own patients and feeding back to my mentor what had happened and what I thought should happen and seeing the doctors and referring to dieticians, going to see the consultants with them. It was really good and I had a good rapport with most of them. In the end they were telling me things that I fed back to Marcia [mentor]. I was linking things from my psychology in my first year and the first term this year and relating in my science and exploring lots of issues. I really felt it was good.
> (Marie 10: year 3 term 2)   (Narrative 13)

She came to use the library and the literature as an automatic response to understand her clients' conditions. Towards the end of the course Marie was conscious of her need to make the most of every opportunity to learn.

> Last night I was on a late, so there were seven children and I read up on all the conditions and I could quite happily nurse one of those children today. Just looking up as many different books as I can to get a complete picture, because I know one book's not going to be enough. And just using the BNF when I get home to look up different drugs if I've not heard of them before. It's because I've got to my fourth and final year and I'm thinking 'My God, I'm going to be a staff nurse this time next year.' And it's really frightening, because I feel I know nothing. I must have learned something because people will ask me a question and I'll answer it, but I still haven't learned enough to be a staff nurse yet.
> (Marie 12: year 4 term 1)   (Narrative 14)

Marie's excitement lead her to read widely and increase her knowledge. Such enthusiasm was made possible by the trusting environment and a manageable caseload that did not leave her exhausted at the end of each shift.

3.2f Peer support in sense-making

Having a peer group to share ideas and think through experiences was an important part of Marie's learning activities. Curiously even as early in the programme as her second year, she forgets her own lay perspectives whilst sharing her experiences. As a result she is able to develop alternative perspectives, or have her thinking challenged by her non-nursing housemates. She felt this helped to see the world through her patients' eyes.

> One of them [house mates] turned round and said they might as well be doing a nursing degree. It's like me going home and talking to my mum about it. I can talk to her about my maternity experience but she'd only be able to relate to them in terms of the childbirth she's had. So it's different. They can't say 'I've had a patient who's had this'. But they can turn round and say 'How do you think the family felt when their father died?' or whatever. And you could think about it more. Knowing how the family or patient might feel if they've been a patient. You just think about them and if what they've said will help you in your work or you find out about what they've said, then all well and good.
> (Marie 4: year 2 term 3)   (Narrative 15)

On other occasions Marie found it helpful to share experiences and sources of information with nursing colleagues. Through discussing their daily experiences Marie and her friends were able to find alternative ways in which to frame their experiences and to develop a collective understanding. By this it is suggested that the story-teller is able to develop new insights to the situation arising from the suggestions and sense making activities of her friends. Those of the group who have not participated in the same nursing activity can gain a vicarious learning experience that helps them formulate suitable actions when they have to face the same sort of situation in the future. Marie's chief ally in this activity was Penny. They had been room neighbours when they first arrived and subsequently they shared a house with two other non-nursing students.

[I talk to her all the time since] . . . my first year. We support each other through our course. I think you need that sort of support from someone and we talk to each other about patients we've looked after. We have a laugh at some of the things children do and adults, and we have a cry together, or whatever, but we listen to each other and say we can't remember how to say things and it's really nice. I get to learn about things I wouldn't otherwise learn about and so does she. It's nice to have the difference. It was nice to have someone who understood . . . nice to have someone to be supportive of your feelings and not to say you're stupid to be upset. None of the rest of my flat are doing nursing, but I wouldn't be able to talk to them the way I talk to Penny, probably because I've known her for so long and we know how we tick. She's my best friend. We've supported each other in our personal problems as well as professional too. You need someone there and I'm lucky to have her and that we've got on with each other. We've got on since the first year and we're doing the same thing.
(Marie 12: year 3 term 3)   (Narrative 16)

Having a special confidant who understood the nursing experience was distinctively different from any other informal discussions that Marie used to frame her experience and develop understanding. This was particularly true when she was wrestling with the personal and ethical dilemmas that she encountered.

3.2g Learning to respond to seriously ill children

During her fourth year Marie seems to be less concerned about her practical skills and less preoccupied with her role at an early stage. She appeared relatively secure in knowing how to function within the clinical area. Her self-confidence seemed to free her to consider other aspects of her role as a nurse and to consider the wider implications of healthcare practice. This may have been triggered when she first experienced the death of a child. On the first occasion she was extremely distressed even though she had not been present. She was concerned about how to respond to the parents of any other child needing the same kind of care or that she might lose control of her emotions if she attended the same procedure that led to the child's death. Her mentor and the other ward staff were supportive of her actions. To help her come to terms with the experience Marie spent a lot of energy reading about the condition and about death in childhood. This helped her considerably when later in the term one of the children that she had cared for in the community was admitted as an emergency and died within 24 hours. Marie felt sufficiently confident to talk to the little girl who had shared the same bay on the ward about the child's death and chose to join the family in their grief at her funeral.

I knew a child was going to die at some point in my career, and I'm glad it's happened now when I can learn a lot more and spend a lot more time learning from the situation. I was really well supported. It was really easy to speak to Julia because she knew her [the child who died], but I don't think I'd have been able to talk to anyone on the ward as well as I spoke to her and it was just such a personal experience and it had such an impact on my whole life. It had such an impact that I went away the following weekend and I started wondering where I wanted to go in life. . . . Maybe it's because of my own personal beliefs

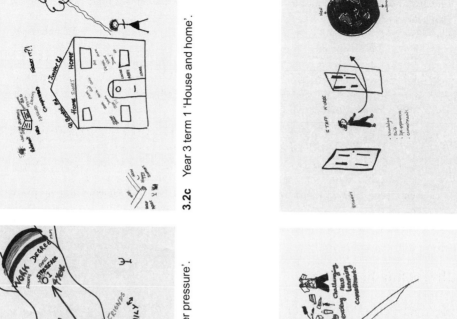

3.2c   Year 3 term 1 'House and home'.

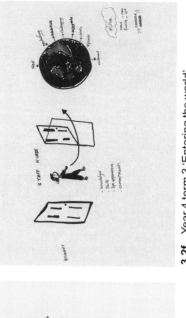

3.2f   Year 4 term 3 'Entering the world'.

3.2b   Year 2 term 3 'Working under pressure'.

3.2e   Year 4 term 1 'At slope end'.

3.2a   Year 1 term 1 'Tensions'.

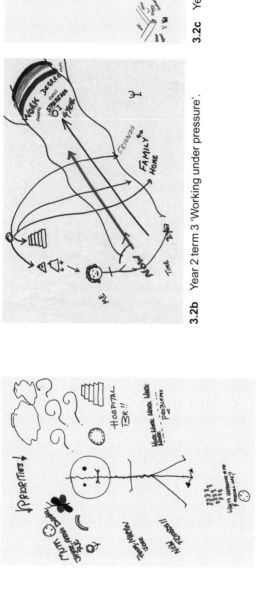

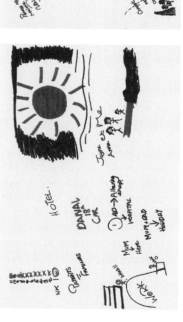

3.2d   Year 3 term 2 'Black mountains and sunshine'.

Figure 3.2   Marie.

but I think she's in a better place now anyway. It's the parents I feel sad for more than anything else and her brothers and sisters. I just see death as a positive experience personally, but it's the people she leaves behind.
(Marie 14: year 4 term 1)   (Narrative 17)

Later in the subsequent term Marie spent five days working in an intensive care unit and participated in caring for a seriously ill child receiving heroic medical treatment. This experience raised a number of questions about the provision of medical care and her future role.

It's not the nursing I like anyway because it's not team nursing. Less communicating with the child. I'd say that's equally important. It's not what I want to do at the end of the day though. I think it's the whole idea, that it's not working as part of a team. I enjoy and thrive working as part of a team and that's not like that. It's not relying on people, just having the contact with other people, and if you are rushed off your feet and someone comes up and asks if you need help, that is fine, but there's none of that on there.
(Marie 15: year 4 term 2)   (Narrative 18)

3.2h Feeling like a nurse

Interestingly, throughout the first three years of her programme Marie struggled with her choice of career. Her illuminative art and the images she created were of her home, holidays, friends and family. Of the four pictures she made over this time none pictured her as a nurse or made reference to her nursing. When discussing these pictures (Figure 3.2) at the start of her fourth year, Marie was startled to find this but verified that they reflected her ambivalence towards nursing and the course. Her feelings persisted until the end of her third year. By the end of this time Marie had been allocated to a clinical area with an excellent mentor. This helped her to feel settled in her practice placements and to see that she was functioning as an effective team member. This nourished and strengthened her identity as a nurse. This gave her the motivation to learn and helped her to conceptualise the area of paediatric nursing in which she would like to practice when qualified. In the first term of her fourth year, for the first time her illuminative artwork started representing her feelings of being like a nurse (see *Figure 3.2e*).

It's the reality of nursing now, getting in there. Realising it and don't hide away and it's quite a challenge and really exciting. Because I am learning new things all the time and I love it. But I think it takes up a lot of commitment because I think you've got to be dedicated to it. Getting up and working at unsocial hours. All the other (university) students seem to have such a great time and I seem to be working every day this term. If it's not at the lectures it's in the hospital and if I'm not in the hospital I'm in the library. So it takes as hell of a lot of commitment. I think I'm really committed now. The term has made me committed because of all the learning of new things. I had my doubts at the beginning and I think I've become committed this term as opposed to the others . . . I definitely see me as a nurse more now. I'm doing so many things. Not necessarily practical skills like hands on, but skills with communicating to people and phoning down to sort things out. I seem to be in there. I might not

> be taking blood pressures or giving injections or getting my hands dirty so to speak, but I'm in there and involved. It's really good. I really enjoy it. It seems to be right for me now, but I don't know if it's what I had anticipated.
> (Marie 14: year 4 term 1)   (Narrative 19)

During her final term Marie gave mentorship support to a second year nursing student undertaking her paediatric experience on the ward. Marie found this an enlightening and startling experience as she came to realise how much she had learned.

> It was a confidence boost because it made me realise that I do know something and that I've got good skills with children, because I don't think she had very good skills with younger children and their parents as well.
> (Marie 16: year 4 term 3)   (Narrative 20)

Throughout the last term of her course Marie continued to enjoy the autonomy of working with the distant support of her mentor and other members of the clinical team. She had developed a strong self image as a children's nurse and had made the transition from being a student.

> [I feel] Like a children's nurse I suppose. I mean I still had the badge to hide behind if I wanted it. But I suppose I was more like a nurse because the doctors would come up and talk and ask me all sorts of things [discussing care with them, changes in care plan] . . . I was in control of the care for a patient and making decisions and that. So I did feel like a nurse.
> (Marie 16: year 4 term 3)   (Narrative 21)

Marie's transition to feeling like a children's nurse was promoted by her practising all the activities she saw her qualified colleagues undertake, which included discussing patient care with the doctors. Coming to the end of her course her illuminative image represented this transition and her excitement of the future (see *Figure 3.2 f*).

> There are two doors. The subject is me now or how I see myself now. One of the doors is supposed to be open and the other closed, and the closed one is the student behind there which I am now leaving, I hope. I'm in the middle of them and there's me in the blue uniform of me as a staff nurse. There's all my commitment to nursing going with me through the door into the big wide world. I'm going to take all these skills and knowledge with me and that's what I'm going to offer the world. The world has to offer me excitement, friends, variety, it will be enjoyable, challenging, an adventure, rewarding and it will be me. And then there's my future, a very little thing because I can't see very far into the future at the moment . . . I think I will continue learning, I know nursing is a continuous learning profession . . . I'm looking forward to it, but at the same time I'm really apprehensive.
> (Marie 16: year 4 term 3)   (Narrative 22)

3.2i Marie's professional development

Throughout the conversations with Marie, several important themes have emerged. Perhaps the most dominant has been concerned with the significance of the mentor–student relationship in helping her to develop an identity within the team and this helped her to develop an identity as a nurse. Once an effective and close relationship had been established she had the confidence to undertake a variety of complex and demanding nursing activities that increased her confidence to work on her own and challenged her beliefs about becoming a nurse. Such challenges seem to have developed on a continuum. Starting with the social influences of joining a new team of practitioners and settling into their environment before being able to develop practical-technical skills. Once she felt secure and able to participate in care-giving, her knowledge development began to increase significantly. This led to an emotional maturity that allowed her to adopt an objective perspective on her nursing practice and protect her from some of the painful experiences of nursing. From this point she was then able to formulate a philosophy for her own practice. Other consistent themes have been her enjoyment in sharing her successes and exploring her confusion with colleagues and peers and her ability to relate experiences from her family life to her patients and her nursing practice.

Marie's illuminative art about being a nursing student had been of home and friends and travelling away from the course rather than doing nursing or giving patient care. It wasn't until the middle of her third year that she began to recount experiences of patients she had cared for or the challenges they caused and in the beginning of her fourth year, her artwork reflected this transition. This change could be related to an extended period of social stability whilst working in the same clinical area. At this time Marie's confidence, motivation and nursing skills increased rapidly and profoundly with a concurrent realisation of her future role as a nurse.

3.3 Nicola

Nicola is the only participant who enrolled for the mental health branch of a nursing and midwifery degree course and is one of five students in her year undertaking this branch of nursing. Her case study reflects Nicola's personality and approach to nursing as much as possible, and also reflects the ethos of mental health nursing, where care is communicated through relationships built with words and images rather than technical procedures and physical contact, Nicola's own words are used to describe her experiences. Her narrative is built in three stages. The introduction explores her reasons for choosing nursing and is taken from conversations during focus group discussions and her first interview during her first year. The key elements of her professional development as a nurse are then described using data from fifteen interviews conducted throughout the rest of her programme. These are concerned with her preconceptions about becoming a mental health nurse; learning to be a mental health nurse; and her illuminative images which describe what it felt like to undertake this learning. Throughout her narratives Nicola demonstrates her reflective nature, her awareness of others and her conscious self-development through talking to others about her experiences. These narratives illustrate Nicola's growth in professional competence and the influence of support provided by her colleagues and peers.

This approach to presenting Nicola's story is influenced by the work of Ellis and Flaherty (Ellis & Flaherty 1992). To give you a sense of Nicola's development each section of narrative has been indexed in the same manner as the other students with her name, the interview number, term and year followed by the narrative number in the case study.

3.3a Choosing a nursing career

I didn't do as well as I had expected in my 'A'-levels, and at the time last summer, there was such a curfuffle, I really decided that I'd just go and do something as near to Occupational Therapy (OT) as I could. I had thought of nursing before OT, and so I got into (this course) through 'Clearing'. I've never actually, sort of, sat down, and thought well, this is what I think nursing is, and this is why I want to do it. I mean I've always sort of, somehow, I either just said, 'Yea I want to be a nurse', because it just sort of keeps everyone quiet, when they say 'What do you gonna to do?' But, I dunno why, I chose nursing as opposed to one of the other, like, side careers. I think it probably was because I just wanted to do anything, and just get a place anywhere, rather than having to retake. And the only places available was either mental handicap nursing or mental illness nursing. So I just decided I'd go for the psychiatric, because I'd talked to quite a few people. Last term I was quite apprehensive, whether that was the actual field that I wanted to diversify into, but you can actually sort of change your course. Last term when I went on a placement, just three days to the hospital, it really scared me. I've thought about it more this term, a lot more, and I just think it will be more of a challenge somehow.

I'm quite interested in the mind, I find it fascinating. I was watching all the Jonathan Miller programmes that he did. I'm not quite sure what it will entail. I think my best bet, at the moment is to just go along with an open mind and not have any preconceived ideas because I could either be really disappointed, or, surprised. So, I think I'll just see what happens. And if it's not for me, then I have got my degree. And I can get another job, I don't know what, but sort of wait and see what happens at the other end really. I'm not sure that you can ever be completely sure about what you want to do for the rest of your life, but I think it can be quite a challenge to work in that field. I think it's quite scary as well, because it scared me. I've always associated illness with, I suppose subconsciously, with the physical. Either a bandage or something like that and to actually see these people, who are obviously very, very ill, but there were no physical signs, it was quite, quite scary really. It really did completely freak me out. It was very strange. I know that I would like to specialise in drug abuse, alcohol abuse, and anorexia. I mean those are the areas that I find quite interesting. As regards to, I think probably, a lot of talking and group therapy and obviously there'd be a certain amount of physical work involved. But that's the area that I think I'd find interesting. I think that would be quite a large part of the job, as well, work as a team. (Nicola 1: year 1 term 2)   (Narrative 1)

3.3b Images of being a nurse

What sort of nurse I will be? I really don't know. I would hope, I would like to be, sort of respected I suppose. I'd like to think people could actually communicate well. I'd like to be honest and open with people. For them to know that I'm all there, for them to talk to really. I don't know what other sort of qualities I would need to have. Whether I've got those. I've never, touch wood, been in hospital for anything, except for being born. So I've actually had very little contact with nursing as such. My aunt's a paediatric doctor, and my cousin is a doctor, and my godmother is like, a health visitor. All of them are very gentle, and unassuming. And I think that's quite important as well in a nurse. I mean, they're always prepared to sit down and listen to what you have to say and I think they sort of treat everyone as a whole individual, not sort of, be prejudiced against anyone or anything really.

I don't know whether it was just sort of, the type of person I am. But I mean it really helps me, when I have a problem, or a worry, or had an experience, to actually go and talk it through with someone. And you suddenly realise that it's not the be all and end all, or whatever. So I just feel that talking about things, sharing things, I think it's quite important. I think it sort of helps you grow, spiritually and I think it gives you a broader perspective on life as well and helps you not to be so narrow minded. And it's nice to be able to do the same for somebody else as well, not be a talker all the time but be a listener as well. Obviously to actually say, or to try and clarify what you're feeling is half the battle. I think you do need some sort of feedback from someone else, to actually put it in perspective. I've always been able to go home and talk about things, with my Mum and my Dad and my sister, and close friends at home.
(Nicola 1: year 1 term 2)   (Narrative 2)

3.3c Understanding the nature of the mental health nurse role

You have to push yourself to go and talk to the clients and it's not as scary as I thought it would be. They are normal people first and foremost, but then they have a psychiatric illness. Perhaps if I'm able to establish relationships with the clients the conversations may become deeper, but they tend to be talking about the weather and where I've been on holiday. I'm actually enjoying it, but it's going to take a bit of getting used to. I think it will be a very good experience for me, especially since I hope to be a psychiatric nurse. I actually think I probably could be one and I'll discover by the end of this module whether I actually want to be one. I can perceive myself enjoying this rather more laid back, relaxed attitude and focusing more on the actual communication. The relationship that builds up between nurse and patient is so warm and it seems really genuine. There's obviously been a lot put in to build those relationships. It's quite exciting.
(Nicola 2: year 2 term 1, first clinical experience
of working with mental illness)   (Narrative 3)

I just think it's fascinating working with the brain. There's so much that's unknown about it and there are so many different fields within that. You have all the fields within that field. The pregnant mums with mental problems, the elderly, the adolescents, children, babies with the mothers, [the] community side of it, schools, hospitals, hostels probably, working with the homeless, so there are lots you can do. It's quite a challenge. I think it's very scary still, but not as scary. You have to accept the fact that the likelihood of being mentally ill yourself because you've been working with these people is a risk; but it's a risk walking across the road. I'm not so scared.
(Nicola 4: year 2 term 3)   (Narrative 4)

On the wards there's a great mixture and it's quite nice really. I feel more self-contained this term and quite content with everything. Suddenly it's all coming together. It could just be the

fact that we're now third years and we're going into fields we supposedly wanted to do. That could be making the difference. I don't know.
(Nicola 8: year 3 term 1)   (Narrative 5)

I feel quite excited now about the prospect of doing psychiatric nursing and I want more responsibilities now and take on more caseloads. I suppose I would like to be very much nurtured, but I would also like to start taking on a bit more interaction perhaps, start going onto that side a bit more. Feeling that on the horizon, as opposed to being an unreachable dream, it's becoming a reality I hope. It's a long way off and there's a lot of work that needs to be done, but I'm beginning to think I can do it and it feels great.
(Nicola 9: year 3 term 1)   (Narrative 6)

By the end of the course I'd like to have a respect for each client. Not try and categorise them all, patronise them. I'd like to be quite confident about my practice and I'd still like to be able to go and use people as resources and I'd like to work well within the team and be assertive about what I want and my needs within that team. I'd quite like to see the results of my work and I'd just like an even wider knowledge base.
(Nicola 11: year 3 term 3)   (Narrative 7)

I think you have to have a professional role, otherwise you're fucked up basically. You'd just do your head in. At the end of the day you're not superwoman, you're nothing special. You're just a human being who is a nurse and you've learned some skills. There's a side of you that wants to work with people, but to protect yourself you really have to be professional about it because it's a job. It's a job that [means] you're in touch with yourself, so you need to be aware of what's going on for you so that you can go and seek help when things get really stressful. But thinking about me as a nursing student and me as Nicola a lot of them overlap, but definitely the way you talk to people is different from the way you do at home, and that's healthy and good. You have to be professional about it and do your job. I'm not trying to sound callous, but you've got to be very careful to make some boundaries and keep them separate, otherwise you just take everything home with you and that's not good. It's not good for the client either. You're not doing them any favours. . . . But some of the skills you've learned being a nurse might be of benefit outside where you communicate with people. It might help. I'm trying to get more in touch with my feelings, like 'Hell, I found that really hard'. So therefore I need to take some time out for a few minutes just to get my head round it. I've got to know that that's work and then I've got an outside of my nursing life and that nursing isn't always first and foremost. Most of the time it's top of my list, but I want to be me before anything else.
(Nicola 13: year 4 term 1)   (Narrative 8)

I know at the beginning of the first year I was very apprehensive about a mental health placement. To actually go in there, but then you realise they're not all scary or murderers, they're just normal people with problems: mental as opposed to physical problems. I've seen a shift in my thinking over the four years and I still find it strange when people say 'You're so brave' and that's crap because a lot of people could be psychiatric nurses and I think there's a certain sort of person who becomes a nurse anyway. But the psychiatric nurse does a bit of everything. A bit of the psychotherapist's job, [a bit of the] psychiatrist's job. You have all these specialists who take it one step further and I suppose the other nurses do a bit of counselling, but they're doing medical procedures as well, taking stitches out and actual hands-on nursing, which there is very little of in psychiatry. You approach the patient dif-

ferently as different people, so you can't generalise. So you can hide behind it [the procedure] almost. You can't do that in psychiatric nursing really.
(Nicola 14: year 4 term 1)   (Narrative 9)

3.3d Learning how to be a mental health nurse

Coping with personal dilemmas

I did write about pride and dignity and sexuality in my learning contract (LC) because I thought they were interesting issues. I learned a lot through writing my LC, watching my mentor and through developing my own skills of empathy. I suppose I have quite a good grasp of that now. Not completely, because it's such an ongoing process and there are still things my mentor did and I thought 'Why didn't I do that?' I closed the door and drew the curtains round when the lady was there, but then I wondered about the main curtains across the window. I should have done that, why didn't I think about it? But if a similar situation arose I know I'd draw the other curtains as well now. Everything concerning dignity and pride has to be input from the nursing staff. Perhaps that's the nurse's job so perhaps it's not a big deal, but it's quite hard really. I talked it over with my mentor.

I found it very difficult at one point because one of his care plans was to observe one elderly gentleman's inappropriate behaviour, which was almost of a sexual nature and it obviously was inappropriate. When that first happened I found that a bit hard, but at the end of the placement I didn't have a problem with it at all. I did deal with it through dealing with my mentor. And talking to other nursing students and housemates. My way of coping with it was to get embarrassed really, and I did, but I suppose I talked about it quite a lot as well. How to deal with it really. Just to say 'I really would prefer if you didn't do that because I feel uncomfortable when you do that. Please don't do it'. In some ways we are social role models for a lot of these people and if they went outside and did that in the community they'd be had up for indecent assault or something similar. My mentor, he said 'How would you deal with it if one of your male friends came onto you [in a way] that you found inappropriate?' and I said I'd tell them to fuck off. He said 'How about dealing with it this way?' and I did.
(Nicola 6: year 2 term 3)   (Narrative 10)

I accept that I have a role to play and to be happy playing that role. You do have to keep a distance from patients on the wards as well. When I'm at home with my friends I'm not really distanced from them, but I am from the real core of their problems, but there's a bigger distance on the wards. I think that's right because I couldn't function any other way. I think your personal life probably goes into your professional life as well. If it's all going well in your personal life, which for me it is at the moment but that scares me as well, because I don't want my new-found confidence and acceptance of myself . . . it's not a bed of roses all the time. Perhaps that's where it goes back to coping mechanisms and strategies and support systems.
(Nicola 8: year 3 term 1)   (Narrative 11)

3.3e Learning from a mentor

I think she's such a good nurse [my mentor]. I don't know what it is about her. I just admire the way she nurses. I think she's a very strong personality, but she's also very perceptive and

it's a partnership almost that I have with her. I've now got to the stage where I recognise the fact that she's a very busy lady, but I know I've got the confidence now to say that I need to talk to her and that she'd say 'OK, let's go and talk'. So I use her when I want to and we have good discussions as well, when I need her. She's a very strong personality, so sometimes she's daunting to people, but she's really straight and open with you as well and I like that. We're working together. I haven't actually been following her round the ward so much at all. We link up to discuss what I'm doing and what I'd like to do and most of my time has been spent working with the patient and sometimes going off the ward or linking up with her if there's something different happening. The lady I'd been working with had done quite a lot of self-harm as well: she's done some horrendous damage to herself. I was amazed because she comes over as a really gentle, timid, meek woman. She's about 30 but looks about 22. So it was quite hard to link the woman who smashed her fists through glass doors with the woman who I was working with. The only problem I had with all of it really was that I came off one shift a bit bemused about my role as a nursing student. I talked this over with Melissa [mentor] later and we discovered it was to do with the patient herself. She has this effect on a lot of people. So it was a bit of a conflict for me and my role. I wouldn't classify myself as a friend of hers, well I am, but a professional friendship somehow. But I was glad to have sorted that one out. Sorted out my role and making more sense of it. I don't know whether professional friend is the right phrase to use, but I can't think of anything else. I'm not her primary therapist and I don't counsel her or I'm not a psychotherapist. I'm not really a good buddy of hers because friends do all sorts of things together. . . . Basically it's what my mentor and her are working towards. It's gradually got better and she's progressed. I think working so closely with J. and actually being needed by her (are the most significant things this term). And being able to contribute something positive to her healing process. I accept that I have a role to play and to be happy playing that role.
(Nicola 8: year 3 term 1)   (Narrative 12)

Learning to be therapeutic and at risk

With any situation, if you take a patient off the ward, if there is a situation you've got to attend to yourself first if there's any danger that you're going to be harmed or they're going to turn round and start punching you. If a six-foot bloke on Section goes for a walk round the grounds with you, then you have to think through potential problems before you do it and I think that's something I've begun to learn this term. Thinking through my actions and possible implications of my actions before I actually do them. That's quite crucial really. I don't think I've got there by any means, but I've started down that road. I'm not going to do it right all the time. I'm going to make mistakes, but it was quite nice to have a bit of insight into that as well.

I think I would still feel very scared if someone grabbed hold of me or pulled my hair or anything like that. That would worry me. I think you should always try and take preventative action to prevent something becoming a situation and then having to deal with it. Summing up the progression, but I don't think you can be fully self-aware. I've started to become more so and less self-conscious. I still do get embarrassed, but I can handle it slightly better I think and don't feel so threatened if one of the male patients comes and talks to me. Yes, it is embarrassing, because I think a lot of the time they do pick up on non-verbal messages of 'I'm only 20 and a nursing student and I feel a bit vulnerable'. They pick up on that and if you make it known they can play with that basically and make it even worse, even if you don't verbalise it they just know (from) I imagine body language cues. I'm really not

sure. But none of it was a problem by the end of the placement, only at the beginning. They must have picked up on body language I suppose.
(Nicola 9: year 3 term 1)   (Narrative 13)

You gain respect from people. You have to be prepared to confront someone about something. If someone starts talking about really weird and strange ideas you don't just run away from it but explore why they think that. You have to be prepared perhaps to take things to a deeper level when appropriate. You have to realise that not everyone wants to analyse stuff all the time.
(Nicola 11: year 3 term 3)   (Narrative 14)

The nurses on there who I thought was really good were the ones who treated the children with respect and didn't patronise them, they let them know what was going on and tried to reflect back to them why their behaviour pattern wasn't appropriate. They just had respect for the children as well I suppose and they were very warm and friendly, but had enough confidence in themselves to actually make the children respect them, so that when they threatened to do something they carried it out, they didn't pussyfoot around. That's another important thing working with children's behavioural problems, sticking to boundaries and being very rigid about those boundaries. The nurses I admired were the ones who were able to do that and able to deal with the crisis situation swiftly and without undue alarm to anyone else. There are a lot of different techniques there. A lot of the children who came to the unit had behavioural problems acting out very aggressive or verbally aggressive, kicking, punching or running around setting off fire extinguishers, that sort of thing, uncontrollable behaviour. They would restrain the child physically if it got to a crisis situation, but it was almost as if some of the children wanted that because that's what they've lacked in their life – having physical contact and being told when no means no. So it was really important for them and the child would be restrained for five minutes, so there were no double messages. I tried to [practise these skills as well] but the only way you can learn is through getting it wrong, which I did. Not getting it wrong, but I think children have an uncanny way of knowing if you're not confident about something, so they push you about basically. There were loads of instances.
(Nicola 14: year 4 term 1)   (Narrative 15)

3.3f Making sense of practice

Peer support

We talk about nursing because one is an ex-nurse who started doing the course and now he's changed to psychology. It's such a hard course that you need to be able to offload onto people. Another friend who is a nursing student, one of her worries about moving into a house next year is that she's not living with any other nursing students, but you get repeatedly the same message 'I couldn't stand living in a house with all nurses'. That just seems to be the way it is with all my friends on this course. They need someone else, but would go potty if there was a whole houseful, perhaps because it's just too intense and far too analytical. Nursing students together just end up talking nursing most of the time. Perhaps it's the same as any group or perhaps it's just nursing. It's so nice to be able to pour it all out. It helps put it into perspective because there are very few opportunities to have verbal diarrhoea. I think I've got it slightly sussed, but not completely. Keeping it in perspective as well,

and realising that nothing that ever happens to you is the be all and end all. I don't doubt that I don't have the ability to do the job. I'm quite excited about it all and I do want to do psychiatric nursing. It's just a struggle, but a fun struggle and that's the main thing. I can cope because I'm lucky as I've got a wide variety of people I can talk it over with. So I'm alright. But it's quite scary really. I've no intention of giving up.
(Nicola 6: year 2 term 3)   (Narrative 16)

3.3g Integrating theory and practice

You learn about people like Freud. This term we're doing therapy stuff, psychoanalysis, Klein, you have a little sprinkling and you know a bit about them and you think that's brilliant, I like the way this person thinks. But you read up a bit more about it and begin to use some of their ideas for your practice and you think about it a bit more. When you're working you begin to hypothesise about why people might be where they are and what might have caused them to be like that. So you start thinking more why questions.
(Nicola 11: year 3 term 3)   (Narrative 17)

Personal growth through self-analysis

You should come to the pub and hear the nurses talk. You can't help analysing. It's great because you're so much more in touch and it's reflected by everyone being open, and you communicate better. I know myself more and you talk more and that's a good thing. You have to get in touch with yourself. You have to because part of the job is working with yourself in there. So you have to know what you're about. Childhood, things that happened. You can't help discovering about yourself. Good training [is] really discovering yourself, because it's reflected in the clients. Makes you think 'That's me' or, 'That's my childhood'. There's something of you there. You hide behind a role being a psychiatric nurse I think.
(Nicola 13: year 4 term 1)   (Narrative 18)

3.3h Being part of a team

This is such a crucial module, that if you don't have the support of a good mentor, and a mentor who'll take you one stage further than you've already achieved, then it would be quite demoralising really. Psychiatry is busy and there are lots of very difficult situations that arise and the stress level has been quite high this term. I've been doing things that you don't usually do if you're an E grade, which is coordinating and doing it properly and being respected for it. To do it properly you need support throughout that. [My mentor] she has just facilitated me somehow to improve on my knowledge and capabilities by just pushing me I suppose. But not pushing and abandoning me. Just cajoling, or rather encouraging. I think being very honest with me as well. She told me when I'd done something really well or what I could do to do something differently. But it's not just her that has been good. It's the whole team. That makes a difference. I'm the sort of person who really thrives having someone pat me on the back. I think I thrive more on positive input than negative. So if someone does something nice for me I think 'Well they've been really great. I want to show them how good I am'. So that works for me.
   It's giving you the freedom to really push yourself, but having the security to fall back on it all. And you get more involved with the whole ward, doing the ward rounds and things. So you're very much more responsible for what you do. I took on her patients as well because we decided that if I took my own patients on at the beginning they would actually

be the more boring ones, whereas my mentor's were people on Section 3, higher obs, more difficult patients. But when I had a less exciting caseload I was doing other things like co-ordinating and I ended up being associate nurse to a couple of people as well. Some of the time I observed what everyone else was doing and somehow at other times I'd chat about it with my mentor and other times it felt like the right thing to do really. You're developing quite sophisticated communication skills and my awareness of what didn't feel safe. I was very acutely aware of not putting myself in danger with these patients and making myself aware or just thinking of what I would do if the situation got out of hand, or just being aware of where the alarms were. Just something you get used to really.
(Nicola 15: year 4 term 3)   (Narrative 19)

3.3i Illuminative images of becoming a nurse

Adjusting to university life and being a nursing student

I've drawn a picture of myself in the centre of the page (see *Figure 3.3a*). I haven't actually got a face, just a symbol on my head and it's the Yin and the Yang symbol. It means different things to different people, but I think I want it to symbolise light and dark, good and bad. Then I'm juggling three balls in the air. One of them is me as a poly (university) student, one is me as a nursing student and one is my home. Inside the three balls are different words, which I associate with these different aspects of my life. When I'm a poly student *work* is very important and all the words are spiralling inwards. As a nursing student *responsibility* I feel is quite important in that role and then in the home circle I'm posing the question *Where is my home now? Is it at home or is home now here?* I've just put squiggles all over my body and I suppose I just wanted to symbolise chaos and non-conformity, not of myself but just that everyone's life is so different. I drew stars because it made it more colourful I think. I wouldn't say my life was magical or I was magical. I think the main message I wanted to get across were the different roles and the conflict within the roles. It's quite scary sometimes being so young and having so much going on and happening so fast.
(Nicola 3: year 2 term 2)   (Narrative 20)

Adjusting and living through the ups and downs

I've drawn an old tree, it might be an oak tree, with a big trunk and there's lots of grass and flowers at the bottom and it's beginning to get a few leaves on it (see *Figure 3.3b*). There's a leaf falling off the left-hand side. What I think I'm trying to get over is that I'm beginning to blossom a bit. Perhaps the tree is me and the leaf is me beginning to make sense of it all. But I think the fact that the leaf is falling off, even though it's one leaf, is showing that things don't always go smoothly. There's scope for having a bad time. I wanted to draw a more positive picture because I feel I've made sense of this term and having seen you last week suddenly everything has fitted into place and I feel quite positive and calm about what's going to happen to me in the future. I don't know whether it's a true portrayal of this term because it's been up and down. [The solid dark part in the centre] it's supposed to be a knot or a hole in the wood, and maybe it just depicts the flaw or the insecurity or showing that the person isn't a whole, solid structure all the time. They are flawed. Perhaps it's meant to show that you can have a flaw in a person but it doesn't stop the whole process of being bigger and better.
(Nicola 7: year 2 term 3)   (Narrative 21)

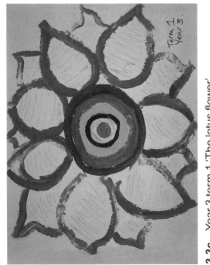

3.3c   Year 3 term 1 'The lotus flower'.

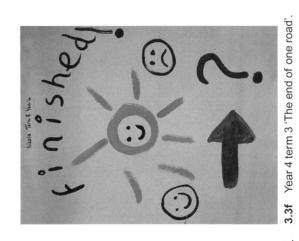

3.3f   Year 4 term 3 'The end of one road'.

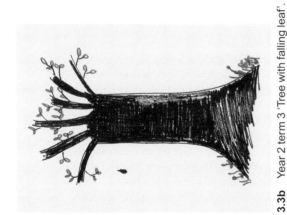

3.3b   Year 2 term 3 'Tree with falling leaf'.

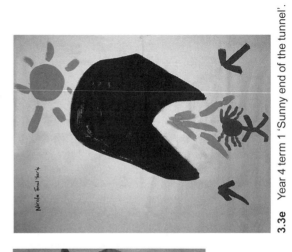

3.3e   Year 4 term 1 'Sunny end of the tunnel'.

3.3a   Year 2 term 1 'The juggler'.

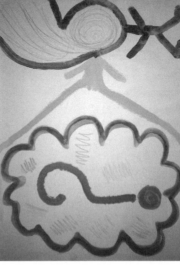

3.3d   Year 3 term 3 'Clouds of confusion'.

I've used the whole piece of paper and very bold colours and it's basically trying to depict a flower that's open and there are a lot of petals round the outside (see *Figure 3.3c*). Very vibrant colours at the core of the flower – all primary colours and I have a black ring in there as well, but it's basically very bold and positive. I think I'm just trying to depict what's happening to me this term, the fact that it's been a very positive one and I feel quite confident at the moment and quite happy within myself. I want to get the effect of the opening out and blossoming of the flower. Me, blossoming really and the term, because that's what has happened this term. I think the black ring – because it's been a really good term and an excellent placement and LC – but things at my (shared) house have been quite [pause] a lot has happened this term and it's not very good at the moment really and that's quite near to my inner self, so the black ring is quite near the middle, but not completely. Basically I don't know what to do. I think I need to talk about this first because it's a bit confused at my house and I don't quite know how to handle it all at the moment. It's been a very strange relationship between the four of us (in the house) this term anyway.

(Nicola 9: year 3 term 1)   (Narrative 22)

Making sense of becoming a nurse

I've used the entire piece of paper (see *Figure 3.3d*). On the left-hand side I've drawn a dark cloud. But it's got a big red question mark in it and it's got wiggles of colour. And I've done a great big yellow arrow pointing towards what I see as the future and then a sort of person going towards the future. And they've got swirls of colour, but it's encased in a big thick black outline and the head, or whatever, is open and flowing again. I think what I've drawn is that this is the now. I do feel a bit confused and it hasn't been a brilliant term, so that depicts this term, but it's still positive because it's got squiggles of colour in, but the squiggles are a bit frustrated and aggressive angry squiggles. But on the whole it's all going forward as opposed to looking backwards. That I can take this term and build on it and go forward and progress. There's a bit of apprehension about that, slightly scary. On the whole positive I think, but a bit of confusion and unsure, insecurity. I'm still only 21 and it seems incredibly young to be embarking on a lifelong career really. I'll get there, I think.

(Nicola 12: year 3 term 3)   (Narrative 23)

It's a big sun, a tunnel and me standing at one end of the tunnel and the sun at the other (see *Figure 3.3e*). There are two big green eyes and it's my light at the end of the tunnel. I can see the end of my four years and that's really hit home this term; that it's all coming to an end and it doesn't feel too bad. It's OK. There's a bright sun, so it feels alright. It's bright and cheerful I suppose. I feel alright about being a nursing student. I think I will always have periods of being up and then it will hit me with a big rush, but that's alright as long as everyone else around you can deal with you being crabby for a week. That seems to be the way I deal with it. My boyfriend and my mum and dad are lovely and Julie. Everyone is lovely on this course. Or my good friends are. So we all seem to use each other. I get on very well with everyone who does the mental health. We all bumble along really from crisis to crisis. Just knowing you can go and talk to someone and they'll give you a big hug or talk it through with you rationally.

It's not an easy course by any means. You're doing two things. You're being a nursing student which demands from you responsibility and being where you said you're going to be and being responsible on the wards and actually getting the academic side of things done as well. Some of it can be quite traumatic, what you come across. It's fairly mind-boggling

really and so it's fairly stressful, and trying to be a normal person having a life outside nursing is terribly important. You really find out where you're strong and weak. It's been good. I think everything just piles up on top of you and makes you feel you're in a big tunnel. You do need to reflect because it's the only way you become self-aware and that is so important, particularly in psychiatric nursing. You really need to know what you're all about before you can begin to work with anyone else. So you're not subconsciously putting all your feelings about something onto them or anything. So reflection is important, but it's very difficult and tiring.
(Nicola 14: year 4 term 1)   (Narrative 24)

Completing the course

I've written in big black letters across the top FINISHED with a huge exclamation mark (see *Figure 3.3f*). Then a great big yellow sun with a happy face in the middle and then a happy blue face and then a big brown arrow and a big green question mark. All bold colours. It's about the future really, that it is unknown. I don't know how it's going to be, but I've done green and red because it's quite bright colours. It feels OK and I'm really pleased I've finished. There are parts of me that are happy, and other bits that are really sad. It's like when you're in the 5th Form [at school] and you think 'I'm going to do A-levels' and you do them and finish school. And think 'I'll go to university' and you do that. And then now I'm at the complete end of the road as far as expectations of what's going to happen next or knowing what's going to happen next. Now I know I'm going to be a nurse, but it's not the same, it's for real. The unknown. Not being a student any more. It's a whole identity and culture really. The fun things that students do I'm not going to stop doing. It's just having to learn a different identity really, getting used to being called a staff nurse as opposed to student. But I think it will be fun. I feel more positive about it now than I did at the beginning of this year actually. I was very worried at the beginning of the year, but now it's OK. I think the beginning of the year was really strange in lots of ways because it was the beginning of my fourth year and lots of big changes. But now it's just like I've got a job, the people who are my friends, most of them are staying and Julie, my housemate and best buddy.

So I think it's going to be tough, but I feel quite positive and now that I know I'm going to Knight [ward], I think it's a good choice for me. I hope [I'll get for my degree] a 2.2 which is quite good. My average has been about 55%. I think there's far more to me having done this degree. I've learned so much about myself and just grown up really. I hope I won't stop learning, and I don't think I will. I think I'll be one of those nurses who'll rush off and do courses about things that interest me, given half the chance. I think that will be something to look forward to, but I think it's important for the next 5/6 months really just to be a staff nurse and get used to the idea.
(Nicola 15: year 4 term 3)   (Narrative 25)

3.3j Nicola's professional development

Perhaps inevitably, running parallel with Nicola's professional development, is evidence of her personal growth and transition from self-consciousness to self-awareness. Her sense of immaturity was a constant theme in all her pictures and it seemed that she worked successfully to explore her self-consciousness, by confronting and managing her discomfort and thus heightening her self-awareness.

This was achieved through an increased understanding of her own emotions and growth in confidence in her professional relationships with patients. In the process she appeared to have reconceptualised her perspective of the patients, shifting from a detached, impersonal biological view, through to one of 'I–Thou' dimensions, in which she saw patients almost as an extension of herself, differentiated only by social circumstances. Alongside her self-awareness was an appreciation that patients were able to read her body language and would exploit her feelings of vulnerability.

In comparison with adult nursing students Nicola seems to have been able to settle quickly into each clinical allocation and was supported by mentors willing to share their workload and their knowledge freely. The other members of the ward team had also been willing to support her and to talk about their practice so that she was never left feeling isolated or vulnerable from lack of support. Finding the confidence to ask questions and to assert her needs was difficult in the first two years of the course but through persistence and practice she was able to find her voice and be heard.

To manage therapeutic relationships with patients successfully, Nicola realised that she needed to develop three particular strategies. In particular her ability to manage her presentation of self through portrayal of a strong image. Being able to think through her actions and their possible implications before embarking on seemingly innocent activities with patients. Being able to develop a distancing mechanism, an emotional membrane, that would protect her from the pain of her patients' illnesses whilst allowing her to retain authenticity as a caring person. Her early family experience of using conversation to make sense of her observations and activities was a valuable aid, both for her own learning and for her therapeutic role. Her identity as a mental health nurse seemed to have evolved in peaks and troughs of seemingly painful heart-searching reflection and self-evaluation, supported and consoled by her clinical practice mentors, her special friend, peers and family. More evident than with the other students in this study, Nicola relied on the social support of her housemates and peers to make sense of her experiences. Another dimension of the peer support that Nicola created, was the apparent mirror image of her professional development. It seemed that for a time she felt the burden of her professional role in her social life and sensed a tacit obligation to develop meaningful (therapeutic) relationships with those peers closest to her. She became hurt that they were unwilling to see her in such a role and this dissonance gave her the strength to develop a new and more useful perspective on her relationship with patients which enriched and accelerated her professional development as a psychiatric nurse.

3.4 Jack

Jack is one of six male students who entered the adult branch of the nursing degree course in 1991. He was also one of the few students who already possessed a professional registration as a mental health nurse having completed his course two years earlier. He had left his home town and travelled across England specifically to study for this nursing programme. His parents supported his decision to nurse even though it did not fit into his mother's expectations.

Jack had a strong personal philosophy of respect and valuing individual rights and freedom. This was influenced by his membership of the scout movement of which he had been a member until he started nursing. His grandfather, who had lived in the family home, provided an influential role model in forming Jack's ideas about a future career. Even in old age his grandfather had been a vigorous person with a happy social life. He was a skilled craftsman and a good shot, as well as being effective in providing relief from muscular tension through massage. Jack had a profound respect and admiration for him. When Jack discovered that he had the same therapeutic skills he decided to apply to become a physiotherapist.

> If my Mum had a tension headache or something, I could give a massage and when I did it to people one minute they were in pain and then after you'd done it they felt better and were pain free. It was brilliant. It was something positive you could do. It felt natural because my Granddad did it. It was something I had grown up with and I assumed everyone did it. I could do it and do it well, so it seemed natural for me to do.
> (Jack 1: year 2 term 1)   (Narrative 1)

During his dying grandfather's hospitalisation Jack was distressed by the quality of nursing care he received and this probably influenced his decision to become a general nurse. He realised that he needed some preliminary practical experience to help affirm this decision and being unable to work in the local hospital, he spent the summer vacation working with a group of physically and mentally handicapped people. When he left school Jack went to the local further education college to do a pre-nursing course but was persuaded to use his 12 good O-level and GCSE results to take an A-level course of maths and science. During this time he successfully applied to do nursing at several schools including a university, if he got his A-levels; when his local school of nursing offered him an earlier place on their general nursing course he accepted.

3.4a Initial career experiences

In 1985, just before his nineteenth birthday, Jack commenced nurse training for the general part of the professional register. After nine weeks on the course he realised there was a significant gulf between his own attitudes and values about patients and the care they should receive and the values of the ward nurses he was working alongside.

> I think it wasn't what I'd expected, it was a big culture shock really. I think I expected people to support people more, a bit more friendly . . . 'If this is what nursing is' I thought I didn't really want to do it. I think I decided 'Bugger it'. I think it was because I turned everything else down. I'd turned Leeds, Bradford, whatever down, so this was the one place I'd chosen and I suppose it was a case of 'If I leave now I'll burn my bridges. What do I do?' I think

that's why I stuck it out. I suppose I expected people to be quite caring and understanding and support each other. OK, have differences, but at the end of the day it's the patient in the bed who's the one who needs looking after.

(Jack 13: year 4 term 1)   (Narrative 2)

Having invested so much in attending this particular school of nursing he decided to make a go of it with the view that in three years he would be qualified and could move away. An abiding aspect of being a nurse was the importance of talking to patients and finding out their worries and needs. This approach, Jack found, was much appreciated by his patients, who enjoyed chatting with him and talked about him to their relatives. By contrast, his ward colleagues expected him to share in the mundane housekeeping activities and expressed their dissatisfaction about his involvement with the patients.

> [I was] criticised for sitting and talking to people rather than finding things to do, like putting laundry away. It was boring putting the laundry away and cleaning the sluice. It was much more interesting to sit and talk to people and get to know their fears and anxieties, just getting to know them . . . I got on really well with the people who came in and out. I went to the male medical ward and that was very much the same. I didn't really enjoy that. But I did my elderly placement, which is where the lady said I was too popular. I remember one of the enrolled nurses said 'You never tell them your name, otherwise they'll shout it out'. I'd prefer them to call me Jack rather than 'Nurse' because it's this strange, mythical thing that I wasn't yet. I was training to be one.
>
> (Jack 1: year 2 term 1)   (Narrative 3)

Jack's narrative indicates that he had a realistic appreciation of his abilities and the boundaries between the practice of a student and a qualified nurse. His reporting of this incident seven years after it took place indicates his strong need to defend his beliefs about the patient–nurse relationship; beliefs that seemed so dissonant from those of his professional colleagues. His approach took courage, as it ran the risk of social and educational penalties of which he became increasingly aware. His membership of the clinical staff community was an important part of becoming a successful nurse which depended upon his good relations with them. In his clinical placements Jack became increasingly isolated socially and this eventually contributed to his departure. He lost his motivation to study and his academic work declined. As a consequence he failed the theory parts of his course and because he was not accepted by his clinical supervisors, his practice was considered to be below standard. He eventually found a bridge out of his predicament by negotiating with the Head of School of Nursing to work as a care assistant in the local psychiatric hospital with a view to starting mental health nurse training the following year.

> I started [psychiatric training] in February 1987 and it was just a complete transformation. The staff were wanting to know about you and were interested in what you suggested. At handover you were encouraged to speak up. In a general [nursing] placement you spent all the time writing things down. If you did ask questions they'd look at you and say 'Why are you asking that?' Where as now if you didn't understand they would actively encourage you to ask; which was a complete change around.
>
> (Jack 1: year 2 term 1)   (Narrative 4)

Jack qualified as a registered mental nurse in 1990 and after a period working as a staff nurse in a mental hospital, began to feel that he should finish off his general training. With the transition of nurse education to a diploma in higher education in the Project 2000 programme, few institutions were offering shortened pre-registration (or conversion) courses to nurses already registered. Eventually, Jack decided to undertake a degree programme without any remission of time for his earlier qualification and experience.

3.4b Commencing a nursing degree as a male nurse

He started the course leading to a BA (Hons) in Adult Nursing and entry to Part 12 of the professional register.

> Why did I choose this course? I suppose I felt more confident after doing my RMN training. I could deal with what I didn't like about my general training. It wasn't that I didn't like general . . . After a year of being qualified I thought there was still niggly doubts about the general training and knowing that I was good at what I was doing and could finish it off. I started to apply for the 18 month shortened courses. I must have written 70–80 letters to Scotland, England, Northern Ireland (Wales don't do it). I'd either got replies saying they didn't do the course any more or it was suspended for the time being or just no reply at all . . . I turned up here last September, not really knowing what to expect, but knowing that I was determined I was going to make a success of it, come what may. There was nothing to go back to. I'd given up my job and sold my house and that was it really. It was quite a big commitment on my part. I go back to home occasionally to see friends and my Mum and Dad.
>
> (Jack 1: year 2 term 1)   (Narrative 5)

Throughout the course Jack's energy and enthusiasm were enduring. It was striking how quickly and effectively he made use of all the opportunities available to him. He became a valued student representative for his intake; he studied for a counselling qualification and to become a mentor/assessor. To supplement his student grant, he also undertook agency nursing as a mental health nurse and had several escort trips overseas with patients. Over his course experience there are five central themes that dominated his experience. These were:

- working as a team member (and with his mentor)
- being supernumerary
- working alone
- clinical skills development
- academic performance

Not surprisingly, his prime concern after working as a qualified nurse was his ability to adjust to supernumerary status and to fit in with the clinical team. Instrumental to his learning was the support that he received from his mentor and other members of the clinical team. Memories of his earlier experiences of general nursing created a sense of unease and concern whenever he felt close to having to compromise his humanistic philosophy towards patients. Interestingly, he appeared unconcerned about being older than many of his peers or one of the few male nurses on the course. Unlike many male nursing students (Streubert 1994) he did not appear to have any major concerns about giving practical care. It may be that when he first started general nursing in 1985, he made the necessary adjustments to coping with activities that are normally taboo for men to undertake. Apart from the emotional and technical difficulties presented by caregiving, working as a male nurse raises a number of ethical and social challenges when caring for female patients, which Jack recognised.

> In one of the seminars last year I was asked 'What's it like being a male nurse, Jack?' And I said 'I don't know because I'd been doing it for so long that being the novelty item, because you stand out, no longer bothered me'. It no longer bothered me being the only man on the ward . . . I suppose I had thought about it and rationalised it. It's not what I am, male or female, it's what I do as a nurse that is important, not what sex I am.
> (Jack 2: year 2 term 1)   (Narrative 6)

This suggests that coming to terms with working as a nurse created some initial challenges of being the only male member in a team of females. He was also sensitive to the patient's perspective when talking about his clinical experiences.

> People are used to seeing male nurses. Nobody actually said I don't want Jack to do anything. I think one old lady said she didn't want a man, but that's fine, that's her choice. My mentor was trying to make sure I wasn't offended but I didn't mind. I thought it was great that she could say what she wanted.
> (Jack 3: year 2 term 2)   (Narrative 7)

Jack's past experiences gave him a sound preparation for undertaking many clinical activities, it had also influenced his attitudes and learning needs on the degree course and despite his optimism, memories often came to the surface.

3.4c Studying adult nursing – the degree course

> It's the beginning of what I wanted to do. I'm looking forward to it. I think it's going to be quite a positive thing. The negative vibes from L. [his first nurse training school] have gone, through meeting the lecturer–practitioner and the mentor. I think this is going to be positive and I have a more realistic attitude. The first time I came with quite a naive attitude to what I expected it to be.
> (Jack 2: year 2 term 1)   (Narrative 8)

Adjusting to being supernumerary

Jack's background indicated that he might have to make some considerable adjustments in order to settle into the course. His (pre-diploma) nurse training placements had been designed to last ten weeks with students working as members of staff. If students were allocated to a ward setting, they often made up the majority of ward staff. As a result they were expected to be fully functional from the moment they started. Since completing his mental health qualification he had spent nearly two years practising autonomously as a registered nurse. The structure of this nurse preparation programme was radically different and was reflected in the duration and nature of students' placements. Students were supernumerary to the normal workforce of the area and this freed them up to work alongside their mentor or take part in peripheral but legitimate nursing activities. As they progressed through different clinical settings they were expected to develop competence in an increasingly complex range of professional skills. Being used to the old system, Jack frequently found the short placements of eight, ten or twenty days frustrating; particularly as in his second year when they were fragmented by external visits with different healthcare professionals or to other departments. In the early part of his programme he complained of these differences and he was clearly finding adjustment difficult. At the beginning of his second year Jack was able to describe his experiences through a pictorial image of his feelings as a nursing student, using the metaphor of a maze (see Figure 3.4a Jack : The maze):

> The course, it just seems a bit of a maze at the time sometimes. I suppose I work on the wards this term. One of the problems has been that you only work 2 or 3 days a week and I feel that I was just getting comfortable on the ward and getting confident in being a general nurse and suddenly I've left and I'm going somewhere else. With my RMN training we had about 10–12 weeks and you were there for 5 days a week. You could spend a couple of weeks sussing out the placement and getting to know what you were supposed to be doing and not doing and you could relax and enjoy yourself and get involved in things. In this supernumerary status it's nice because you can go off and do other things. But sometimes I think I like to spend time on the ward and you feel a bit of a spare part because you don't really know what's going on and you have to keep asking people. It's just now over the past couple of weeks that my mentor gave me my own client or two to look after, which is quite nice . . . It's just as if you are up and running and know where everything is and the placement ends.
> (Jack 3: year 2 term 1)   (Narrative 9)

Working in a supernumerary capacity required a different attitude and approach to work to which he was accustomed, either as a qualified nurse or as a student. It was a challenge that took some time for him to overcome as the course progressed.

> I didn't think I was very good at the beginning of the year. If the shift started at 8:00 am and it finished at 4:00 pm, I'd stay until 4:00 pm. I'm getting more selfish in a way. I found it difficult saying 'Can I go and spend the rest of the afternoon in the library?' Even now I sometimes feel it's a bit difficult asking to leave, but I'm getting better.
> (Jack 7: year 2 term 3)   (Narrative 10)

A member of a clinical team

Feeling accepted by the clinical staff was important to his ability to settle-in and learn. Confirmation of his acceptance came from the clinical team of an area that he visited as a relief mental health nurse.

During the summer I was working at the Knight [mental health] hospital and that was a new area. I did six or seven shifts at the Knight hospital for a week and the Nurse Manager there said 'I've been discussing you with the rest of the staff, Jack'. And I thought 'Oh God!'. And she said 'This week you've felt more like a part-time member of the team rather than a bank nurse'. And I thought: 'YES!' I can go somewhere that I don't know. Where I haven't got much experience and I may not confess to know everything, but at least I can fit in. That did wonders for my ego and made me realise I could make a go of the General bit, because I was a bit unsure about it.
(Jack 1: year 2 term 1)   (Narrative 11)

Receiving mentor support was varied from placement to placement. The quality of support and the attitude of staff also influenced his decisions about future employment. In some placements it was the companionship and support of his mentor that enabled him to survive a busy or hostile clinical environment.

I suppose the general moan has been that it's been a really nice placement and I've enjoyed it but it's too short. This is only my third Tuesday with P [mentor], but my fifth/sixth shift. It's coming to an end almost. You're stopping almost as you're getting going, which I find very frustrating. It's like starting a new job every three or four weeks. Even more so this one.
(Jack 7: year 2 term 3)   (Narrative 12)

The only continuity I had last term was my mentor. It was laughing in the face of adversity basically because neither of us were enjoying CTU. They didn't want me there. They told me that the very first week. We were talking about things and doing things and I was learning from her. It didn't stop us from caring for people. In fact I think I've learned quite a lot but I wouldn't want to work there.
(Jack 9: year 3 term 1)   (Narrative 13)

As he progressed through to his third year, Jack began to feel more settled and his confidence grew. His end of term illuminative artwork reflected this with his image of a human figure in the centre of a range of healthcare practitioners representing not only his view of the patient being at the heart of the team but himself, as his narrative indicates (see Figure 3.4c).

The doctor would come in and say 'What are we doing with this person? What do you want? What do you think is advisable?' Several times, even ward rounds when people come, I'd chip in if I didn't agree with what was being said. People would respect what you said and take it on board. You felt you were being listened to, be it just as a student or a nurse.
(Jack 10: year 3 term 2)   (Narrative 14)

Being able to participate in the care planning of his assigned patients boosted Jack's confidence considerably and from that placement onwards he talked less about his role within the team and more about his clinical practice and the learning experiences. This sense of membership with the clinical team indicates how important a secure environment was to his learning. It is also possible that he had found a strategy to help him adjust quickly to an unfamiliar clinical area and become an accepted team member.

I think I felt part of the team towards the end. In a way it was quite difficult because I only had 60 hours to do and they work 12-hour shifts, I could have done five 12-hour shifts and that would have been it and I would probably have learned bugger all basically. Probably enough to write my essay, but I felt it was important to go back and do a few more shifts, to do three or four shifts on the trot. . . . Turning up on time. If they started at 7:45 am I was there then, staying until the night staff came on. The only times I used to go early were on a Thursday when I said 'I need to be at the Freeman for 6:30, so is it OK if I go at 6:00 pm?' And they'd say 'Give yourself a break Jack and go at 5:00 pm'. So that was fine. But that was the only time I'd go early.

(Jack 14: year 4 term 1)   (Narrative 15)

Early in the second year of his course, Jack was impatient to work on his own and practice some of his clinical and management skills. This may have been impatience with spending so much time watching rather than working alongside his mentors. Alternatively his experiences of working independently as a student in earlier programmes and subsequently as a registered nurse perhaps gave him a sense of frustration with this new way of supporting students. He needed opportunities to practice his newly learnt skills under the distant supervision of his mentor or what he called being able to 'fly free' or 'fly solo'.

Developing professional craft knowledge

Jack had a strong self-image as a nurse derived from his previous experiences of nursing. As with Grace he felt an underlying anxiety that he was not functioning as proficiently as he should. This anxiety and desire to prove himself may have been made worse by the short clinical placements and the consequent lack of opportunity to give care on his own. In his previous training programmes Jack had been able to develop technical procedural skills such as giving an injection or washing a patient and had developed confidence in his ability. These training programmes had been worker-orientated and as a result Jack had undertaken a hierarchy of tasks repetitively. The benefit of opportunities to undertake repetitive tasks is reflected here.

If you do it once you think maybe it's just the one off, but to do it 20 times and for everyone to say 'Have you finished? Oh that didn't hurt'. Then you realise that you can do it. I sometimes think that's what's missing. That's what I was thinking last week.

(Jack 1: year 2 term 1)   (Narrative 16)

However he was conscious that there was much for him still to learn.

I did one dressing on a Friday. The lady I did had been in almost as long as I had been there, about three weeks and she was being discharged on Saturday and I did the dressing on the Friday. I'd seen it being done a couple of times. The last dressing I did with someone watching over me before this was when I did my general placement in the psychiatric training which would be the beginning of 1988. So I know the principles and the general technique but things have been brought into the market since then, so it's quite difficult to know what to do for the best really. . . . Again its having the confidence to do it.

(Jack 3: year 2 term 1)   (Narrative 17)

Jack's approach to patient care was influenced by his personal beliefs and values and with his established confidence in performing a number of competencies, he was able to practice at a more advanced level of practice than his colleagues.

When being observed giving care, Jack appeared confident and competent in the procedural aspects of essential skills. As a result he had the intellectual and social energy to develop a sensitive and profound relationship with his patient. This contrasts with less experienced students who were either too worried about technical procedures to have the mental energy to interact with their patients, or too preoccupied with making their patient socially at ease and the techniques they were using to notice anything else. Jack's level of skill was commensurate with Dreyfus' (Dreyfus 1986) level of a competent and even perhaps of a proficient practitioner, which is beyond the normal expectation of a newly qualified nurse (Benner 1982).

> He has Parkinson's and quite limited ability in his arms. Usually in the morning they're shaped quite badly and he only manages to wash his hands and face and clean his teeth and I give him a razor to shave. That's about all he can do. His wife usually does everything else. Sometimes he manages buttons, sometimes not. This morning he managed quite well but then you have to take his jacket and dressing gown off and sometimes he likes to shower. He prefers that to a bath because it's what he's got at home. So this morning he wanted a bowl of water. The shower takes quite a bit out of him because he has to stand there for quite a while. He had a bowl of water and washed his hands and face himself. I washed his front and back and then had to get him dressed . . . I just try and do it with dignity and keep some of his pride. By doing little bits and asking if he's dry, rather than just drying him. If he's not dry I'll have to rub a bit harder or whatever, so he's got some control over it. I may be able to see where he's wet, but if it's damp you can't see properly. He may feel it rather than me see it. It's easy to rub hard on yourself because you've got some internal feedback, but by asking them if they're dry you get some feedback on whether you're doing it right. It's hard for him. Whether that's right or not I don't know. Nobody has complained it's too hard. Some have said it's too soft.
> (Jack 4: term 2 year 2)   (Narrative 18)

Jack's narrative also indicates a sound understanding of underlying theories concerning patient care as well as an ability to be involved in the patient at an emotional level. Jack seems to be learning from his patient whilst subtly adjusting the care to meet his needs. Tasks like these are not always pleasant and may involve feelings of embarrassment and disgust. During this procedure and all the others that I either observed or overheard during the several visits made to see Jack at work, there was always a sincere and genuine intention to be responsive and professional towards his patients whilst undertaking intimate tasks. Such behaviour requires great tact and sensitivity as well as fortitude. His commitment to caring for people was evident from his accounts of learning to cope with some of the routine nursing tasks.

> I've worked in various places, private nursing homes, general hospitals and psychogeriatric wards as well, and in a way it's rewarding if someone is incontinent or is uncomfortable, to clean them up and refresh them. It's like a sense of achievement in a way that you've done something for them that they were unable to do for themselves. Or giving someone a bed bath when they're hot and sticky and horrible. If they say 'Oh, that feels better' then it's those few words or phrases that make it all worthwhile in a way. I suppose it's something I've just got used to over time.

> I know at first I was quite frightened that I had to do something. But it gets easier as you get used to it. Like I don't like the smell of vomit, but if someone is vomiting I have to do something, so I'm usually so busy and absorbed in making sure that they're OK, that I haven't time to think that either I want to vomit or don't feel well. I wouldn't want the patient to think that they're so bad that it makes the nurses want to throw up as well.
>
> Some people might find it easier than others. I found it quite difficult at first because I was feeling nervous and anxious and scared that I didn't know what to do. You think you usually avoid that sort of situation, but suddenly you're confronted by a situation where someone is throwing up and suddenly you realise that you have a responsibility to do something and you're being paid to look after them . . . If you want to be a nurse you have to put up with the unpleasant and difficult and trying, as well as the good. The agony and (the) ecstasy in a way. Once I'd made that conscious decision it was easy. Once I'd faced up to it, probably towards the end of the second placement it was getting easier.
> (Jack 2: year 2 term 1)   (Narrative 19)

Jack describes the emotional membrane that he needed to develop to cope with personally distressing situations whilst at the same time maintaining his concern for the patient and a façade of indifference to the unpleasant aspect of a task. He called this the *'agony and the ecstasy'* of wanting to learn to become a nurse whilst giving care that is distressing for him. It is the most difficult aspect of nursing that students have to face as it challenges their commitment to live out their values and beliefs of what it is to be a good nurse. Jack (and indeed the others) had to face up to his own discomfort and make a conscious decision that it was more important for him to become a nurse. He also had to come to terms that as a nurse he had a responsibility to provide unconditional care and help to his patients if he was going to be effective. As a result he took the first conscious personal transformation which could lead him towards his goal.

3.4d Mentor support

Through his contact with experienced nurses Jack was able to increase and adapt his repertoire of nursing skills. One of the most challenging problems for nursing students to explore is concerned with finding what are acceptable and unacceptable risks. Discussing his third year experiences of working Jack provides examples of how he benefited from his mentor's expertise.

> My mentor was probably the best one I've had almost because she was very experienced in what she did. She was really good with patients and knew what she was doing all the time and was always quite focused and relaxed as well and able to assess each situation with merits and bend the treatment or plan accordingly . . . She was really good when a chap came in who was dying and he was being a pain and quite arrogant and offensive. Maybe it was his insecurities coming out, but she was really good with the relatives and spent a lot of time with them afterwards. I stayed there all the time and she was looking after the relatives in the patient's interests.
> (Jack 11: year 3 term 3)   (Narrative 20)

In such incidences, Jack could work collaboratively with his mentor and then discuss his observations with her afterwards. In other situations Jack came to recognise the value of a particular technique used by his mentor as a means of relieving tension for clients who were struggling to maintain their dignity: their use of humour. This is a delicate tool that can be beneficial as Åstedt-Kurki and Liukkonen describe (Åstedt-Kurki 1994). Nearly 50% of the professional nurses in their study used humour intuitively and in a way that was directed at helping their patients overcome particular difficulties. They found that male patients were more likely to use humour to relieve stress. In the following example, Jack writes how he observed and considered the actions of his mentor before he tried using humour in his repertoire of nursing skills.

> At first it sometimes seemed inappropriate but it broke the ice and the clients seemed to like it. So I said nothing and waited to see. The jokes were aimed at getting the clients to laugh, not laugh at the clients. Humour is seen by King et al. (1983) as an important part of interpersonal skills and should be encouraged. I had not thought of humour as an interpersonal skill except for a comedian. Rogers (1961) states that the counsellor should be honest in the relationship so if they feel humour is an honest feeling then it is fine. It comes down to the nurse knowing their clients and what they would find funny and what not. There is no substitute for knowing your clients. I found myself after talking to the trainer from C [the mental health unit] using humour myself. But I was careful when using it. It seemed to work especially with Peter who was a wheelchair user and has a similar sense of humour to myself. It helped to find someone with the same sense of humour as me and I feel I would use the humour in similar positions in the future if I felt that would help.
> (Jack: LC 12/13: year 3 term 2)   (Narrative 21)

From this entry in his learning contract Jack has clearly fretted about how best to use humour and whether it was a professional way to behave. His characteristic sensitivity and awareness of the complexity of the activity is evident. It would also appear that he was making use of a range of literature to explore his concerns which suggests an attempt to use theory to underpin and explain practice. The anthropologist Goody (Goody 1978) describes using jokey behaviour as a strategy to establish face-saving relationships. Jack spoke enthusiastically about the good support his mentors gave him, and their enthusiasm and knowledge of their clinical speciality was especially invaluable when they worked together. Another helpful approach they used was when they challenged him and helped him to integrate theory with practice.

> I think it was important for them to draw out the theory and tie it with the practice. A lot of the time it was 'What's happening now, Jack?' and it was just to draw out what I'd done in science and relate physical symptoms to the patient's experience . . . The other mentors would have a talk afterwards or towards the end of the shift or during a quiet period and they'd say: 'Why do we give oxygen to people with chest pains?' I had to give the rationale about that and the effects of GTN and what you should look for. All the things I knew, but she was making sure I knew it and tying it all together to make sure I fully understood. It was good. It was just to keep you on your toes really, to know why you were doing what you were doing and to rehearse it so that you know what you're going to do next time round. And that was good.
> (Jack 14: year 4 term 1)   (Narrative 22)

Shortly after this placement experience Jack took a professional course preparing practitioners to become assessors and mentors (English National Board Course 998: Teaching and Assessing).

> I suppose I amalgamated all the mentors that I'd had in the past and looked at the good and bad points of all of them and did what I thought had helped me or would help him. At the end of every shift I tried if not once every shift perhaps once or twice after every second shift. If I hadn't done it the day before I would definitely make a special effort the following shift; to sit down with him and go through his concerns and see where he was up to and what he was doing and what he planned to do and his caseload as it were. I really enjoyed that and it was interesting. Before I came on the course I really enjoyed teaching students.
> (Jack 15: year 4 term 3)   (Narrative 23)

As with the incident of using humour, Jack was drawing from his own experiences as if using an index file to sort through those that he found beneficial and then used them to develop his own of practice, so developing a repertoire of experiences to inform his nursing practice.

Reading through Jack's learning contracts and our conversations, there was a strong sense of his commitment to giving professional care to his patients whilst maintaining a sense of being ordinary and at one with them, which is described as the most therapeutic kind of care (Taylor 1992). This type of activity was central to Jack's philosophy of nursing care, and the one that had caused him so much pain in his first attempt to undertake general nurse training. It seemed that at last he was able to operate in a manner that was truly congruent with his beliefs: a style of working that is advocated by nursing theory and made possible by the support of his mentor and a manageable workload. These beliefs about what constituted good nursing care sustained him throughout his early, bumpier experiences.

3.4e Managing a caseload

Towards the end of the course and when he was working on a busy medical ward, Jack became very disillusioned. Not only because he was unable to fulfil his ideal methods of practice, but also because he felt he was failing to function at the level expected of a registered nurse.

> At the moment I'm having a tough time on [the medical ward]. It's really busy and I seem not to be able to get everything done in the time. It's quite difficult. I don't know if it's just me, but I think a lot of the full-time staff have to stay late as well. I had a really bad day yesterday and my mentor said 'I only did two things for you, Jack. I didn't think you had a tough day and you seemed to be coping OK'. I suppose it's me just setting up high standards again and knowing I'm not achieving them and I suppose it's a bit frustrating as well because I've got lots of things to do, having to check drugs with someone and if my mentor is busy, it takes longer . . . They're [patients] quite dependent . . . I suppose it was just bringing back memories of my old general training and why I didn't like general nursing and why I gave it up. I suppose it's frustrating because I'm wanting to do the best for it and I'm failing

miserably. This is the last management placement and should turn you into a staff nurse. This is when you should be functioning as a staff nurse.

(Jack 15: year 4 term 3)   (Narrative 24)

Despite his more experienced qualified colleagues encountering a similar work-load difficulties Jack's despair is palpable. Yet the caseload that he was taking was intended to help him develop organisational and management skills. It was antic-ipated that such experiences would equip him to survive in the busy environment of a general medical ward as a registered nurse. It is possible that such expecta-tions were unrealistic and that they only served to diminish self-confidence. The social environment of the ward was supportive and despite these workload pressures, Jack began to regain his self-confidence. However, he was sensitive that he was taking longer with his patient workload than was 'normal' and he was willing to invest extra time to achieve a good standard of care, as indicated earlier, by working many more hours than required by his programme.

3.4f Jack's academic struggle

During his course the learning contract was the central academic vehicle for developing and demonstrating his knowledge. Despite having such a good acad-emic school record, writing up his clinical experiences for the assessment was one of Jack's most challenging encounters. Perhaps he was spending too much time in clinical practice leaving him less time to spend on academic work. Some of Jack's frustration with the learning contracts was his inability to express himself adequately in his writing, which was subsequently diagnosed as dyslexia. His other frustration was concerned with what he viewed as inappropriate con-straints imposed by his mentors on what he should write about. His expressive difficulty was acknowledged by a perceptive lecturer practitioner who suggested that he could be experiencing dyslexia.

> I think I was having a tough time then because I was struggling with my English and then suddenly an explanation was found out as to why. I'd had a preliminary test to find out whether I was dyslexic or not. If you got nine or more of these questions with the answer yes, then it suggested that you had dyslexia. I think I got about 17 yeses or possibles and they said they thought I was dyslexic. I remember coming home and I sat on my bed and started crying. It wasn't just feeling sorry for myself. There was a reason . . . I thought it was just me and how people write . . . I suppose I knew I was pretty good at looking after the patients and I could tie in the theory with the knowledge, but the problem I had was stick-ing what I knew on paper. Many a time it was a case of 'Your LC doesn't reflect what you're like in practice, Jack'.
>
> (Jack 14: year 4)   (Narrative 25)

Having been diagnosed as dyslexic was clearly a great relief. With the help of the university student services Jack embarked upon a study programme to help him reduce his difficulties. This helped him improve his writing and his grades. It is possible that bound up with his anxiety about his written work was the ghost from his earlier training experiences, not only causing anxieties about his academic work but also his ability to meet his own expectations (as a qualified nurse) to complete the course.

Jack's frustration with writing his learning contract (LC) was the struggle to integrate clinical experiences with course requirements and relevant theory.

> My LC this time, there were lots of things I would have liked to have written, but trying to tie it in with a competency, because a lot were just observation, was a bit dodgy. Also, what care plans do you use? Well she doesn't (use a care plan). There's not a lot of written things. I think that's what really frustrates me about the LC. Trying to reflect on what you're doing and doing well . . . Sometimes you think 'Perhaps I've gone on the way to learning that and maybe I need to do a bit more work on that' . . . It's this one thing that is very adult and learning oriented and the other thing is sort of school child oriented and it's trying to marry the two together and it doesn't always work. Sometimes it works really well and others it doesn't.
> (Jack 6: year 2 term 3)   (Narrative 26)

Jack was frustrated by his perception of the academic contortions to discuss his practice because they limited the scope of his writing. In some respects the learning contracts became a straitjacket rather than a tracksuit. Despite his frustrations with writing for the learning contracts and the seeming conflicts between the course philosophy and the how clinical and teaching staff were using it, Jack seems to have been able to use his writing to explore and understand his practice more fully, as some of his learning contract work extracts indicate. At the end of the course he graduated with a 2:2 classification and an average mark of 57%.

3.4g Jack's professional development

From his interviews and observation of his practice, it is clear that Jack is highly committed to seeing the world from his patients' perspective and to finding ways of making their hospitalisation more comfortable and perhaps more bearable. His narratives indicate how throughout the programme he was able to develop this ability and that support from his mentors was important. Unlike the other students who relied on peer support, Jack only once talks about letting off steam to friends. Perhaps he had completed a lot of his sense making about giving care and becoming a nurse in his earlier training programmes. Alternatively his course in counselling skills provided a place to vent his feelings. This may have freed him to think more widely about issues affecting his patients and his nursing practice at an earlier point in the programme. At the end of term 1 of his fourth year he saw himself approaching the end of a tunnel (see Figure 3.4d).

> It's supposed to be a tunnel and train tracks and a light at the end of the tunnel, with the train tracks going that way and green fields and coming to the end of the tunnel. The black is the tunnel and there's the light. There were these images of coming to an end and something dawning. I suppose that's what it's been like this term – a dawning, starting to pull everything together that you've learned and practising it. And knowing that physiology and anatomy is being used to your advantage really. It's having the confidence to pull it all

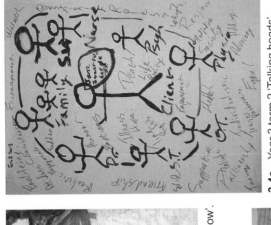

3.4c Year 3 term 2 'Talking heads'.

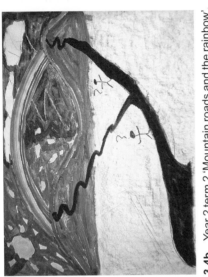

3.4a Year 2 term 1 'The maze'.

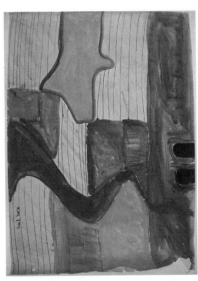

3.4b Year 2 term 2 'Mountain roads and the rainbow'.

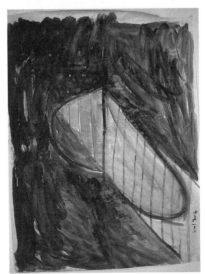

3.4e Year 4 term 3 'On peak top'.

3.4d Year 4 term 1 'Light at the end of the tunnel'.

Figure 3.4 Jack.

together. You don't know everything, but you should be starting to stand on your own feet now. So that's what it's trying to sum up.
(Jack 14: year 4 term 1)   (Narrative 27)

Jack's narrative seems to suggest that he had achieved some form of transition whereby the theoretical and practical elements of his programme could be integrated and where he began to feel part of the clinical team. His earlier experiences of (general) nurse training had a profound and detrimental effect on his self-esteem. Despite this, Jack demonstrated enormous courage and motivation, perhaps fuelled by his sense of injustice, to succeed in his second attempt to become an adult (general) nurse.

> I suppose we all have handicaps holding us back, some more than others. I suppose that's how I looked at it . . . I suppose a lot of people there have done what I've done, which is to turn the anger against whatever . . . and I suppose in that way it's what I've done with this course somehow, starting my general training again, I was that determined to show them . . . but in some ways it's better than getting depressed about it.
> (Jack 16: year 4 term 3)   (Narrative 28)

By the end of the course Jack was feeling optimistic and proud about his achievement, as well as thrilled that he had been able to secure a job in his chosen area of general nursing where he could also use his mental nursing skills. Throughout his programme Jack's unfailing conviction of how to provide good care never seemed to desert him and as his understanding of nursing theory grew, so he came to feel that his views were endorsed by the literature. His final picture reflected this profound satisfaction and sense of achievement (see Figure 3.4e).

> I had two visions in my head. One was of the earlier painting I did with two mountains and the maze in between and the other one was a feeling of coming through a tunnel to the end and the relief of coming through and achieving something. I remember there was a mountain at this side and a mountain at that side of the paper and I had to get from one side to the other. So this is the view from the top of the hill looking from the other side of the hill. The maze is this side and I've achieved the hill and this is the future. I have this feeling of just achieving what I wanted to achieve and feeling I suppose on top of the world and a bit apprehensive and nervous about where and what I'm going to do next. I suppose I feel I've spent ten years to get to that point and it's been a lot of hard work. In some ways it reminds me of the times which were the happiest, hiking in the Lake District. You'd spend a long time hiking up a hill or a mountain and the view at the top is breathtaking and wonderful and it's the feeling that it's been a lot of hard work getting to the top of this mountain . . . I need to think of what I want to do next really and how I'm going to achieve what I want next.
> (Jack 16, year 4 term 3)   (Narrative 29)

Jack seems to have developed his clinical skills through a combination of factors. Central to his success was feeling an accepted member of each clinical team. Part of his self-image was influenced by the social isolation he had experienced when he first started training to be a general nurse. A second influence was his earlier and concurrent experience of working autonomously as a mental health nurse. Following successful negotiation of his place in a clinical team, he could then relax sufficiently to learn. When working with patients, he used his gifts of talking, listening and learning from his patients in order to develop a more profound understanding of their needs. He enjoyed a similar partnership with his mentors, gaining enormously from observing their work and discussing what they had done together or he had done on his own. Engaging in a similar dialectic with the literature also helped him to develop his knowledge and understanding of his care. Throughout Jack's story there is evidence of a profound commitment and tenacity of purpose, coupled with an ability to question and critique his observations. His illuminative images suggest a gradual evolution and integration of the different strands of the course to his practice, leading to his ultimate success.

3.5 Grace

Coming into a nursing degree course at the age of 27, Grace was fulfilling a long ambition to become a qualified nurse. Like Helen, she had started on her career pathway at young age but hers was complicated by a range of factors that were to influence her life as a nursing student. She had started nursing at the age of 15, working as a care assistant and then tried a range of other jobs, before embarking on enrolled nurse training. She left that after six months and subsequently enrolled for a BSc in a nursing (adult) programme after successfully completing an access course at her local college of further education.

> Satisfaction. You know, I've done other jobs, I've worked in an office and I've worked in a cake shop. But it, I wasn't getting any satisfaction out of working there. OK you were dealing with people, but it's not, I didn't feel as if I was really achieving anything. Whereas when I worked on a ward, even being an auxiliary nurse, even making someone's bed, or helping them to wash themselves, or clean their teeth, I felt as if, I'd go home at the end of the day, and I'd think, yea I've really achieved something today. I've helped Mrs Jones, who's had a, I don't know, she's had a hip replacement. I'll think, I've helped her, she's got up for the first day today, and I worked with the occupational therapist, and we went up and down the ward with her, after a lot of rehabilitation, she's gonna be able to walk by herself. I saw somebody getting better, and going home, that's the main idea, isn't it? Getting better and going home. That's what I mean. If I hadn't had any nursing experience before, then I wouldn't know what to expect. But it's by actually doing it, even as an auxiliary nurse. You just feel as if you are achieving something. The access course was easy, compared to this. I haven't done that much.
>
> I did 6 months in a hospital in London [as a pupil nurse], and I worked for a year as an auxiliary nurse. So I've got some nursing background . . . We did a bit of A&P. And then after the four weeks we went onto the wards. And I was, the only ward I actually worked on was a medical ward. And I stayed on there until Christmas time. And that was really interesting. And I gave injections, I even I went on a drug round, so I gave out drugs. I learnt about how to do dressings, but I'd already learnt that (when I was working as a healthcare assistant) by watching the other nurses, but I hadn't actually done any dressings. . . .
>
> This course is more theory. It's more knowledge based, to begin with, and then you go on to the wards. Well I knew it was going to be different to State Enrolled Nurse training, the

old training. I didn't realise it was going to be that different. I didn't know that we're gonna have to learn about lots of science, and things like that. Even though I did that on the access course; and I didn't know that we'd have to do nursing research! I knew we had to do health and health care, and things like that. I didn't really, sort of realise, how much work I'd sort of have to put into it. How much written work. I found it difficult at first, as you know, when I came to you and said 'Oh I can't do the research! (laughing) I don't know how to do a critique!' But I just, by asking, and by really listening in the seminars and asking other people, I found I could actually manage the work. But my problem at the minute is the deadlines. I've got so many other things to do, I don't seem to get the work done on time.
(Grace 0: year 1 term 3)   (Narrative 1)

Grace's experiences of being a pupil nurse on a second-level nursing preparation programme were designed to prepare her to give patient care under the direction of a registered nurse. Enrolled nurses were not expected to take responsibility for the management of clinical settings, although owing to staff shortages many in fact did. Many enrolled nurses worked in community settings where they enjoyed more autonomy. This form of training has since been discontinued and much of their role has been delegated to healthcare assistants. Conversion programmes for enrolled nurses to become first level nurses have been available to any enrolled nurse wishing to convert.

Grace's decision to take an access course at her local college of further education offered her access to a university degree programme. She could choose whether to take a degree in nursing offered by her local university, or go outside the district to take a three year diploma in higher education, nursing programme (also known as the Project 2000 course), which was supported by a bursary. Students taking the diploma in nursing spent two-thirds of their programme as supernumerary students and the final third as members of the workforce. As a degree course student she would receive a student grant that was approximately half the amount of the bursary. If Grace decided to take the better-financed diploma programme she would have to move away from the area and the support of her family. Grace's results from her access course were good enough to be accepted by the university and the professional statutory body for nursing and midwifery. These were equivalent to the minimum entry requirements for a degree (5 subjects in the GCE O-level at grade C (including English language, maths and a science) and three advanced level subjects at grade C). Being a single mother and in receipt of a student grant made her eligible for financial assistance from government agencies, such as housing benefit and income support. Despite these benefits and her grant, Grace struggled to cope with the additional financial demands of bringing up a little girl and studying for a nursing programme, where travelling around the county to clinical placements was necessary.

3.5a Beliefs about nursing

Grace's decision to become a nurse had been influenced by observing how other people cared for each other and these memories provided a model of how she wanted to be as a carer.

Watching too much television [laughing]. Watching 'Angels' I don't know, I mean, from the media, I suppose. Well you get that image, don't you. You see it on television, when you're little, a nurse on the ward, doing a really good job. And my brother lost his eye when he was younger. And by looking at the care that some of the nurses gave him. I either thought 'Yes I really want to be like that, or no I don't'. It was just this whole idea of caring for people. You know. Through out my life, I just thought, that's what I'm going to do. It's just by watching other people caring for one another. I'd see an elderly lady walking down the road, and she'd be pushing her husband in a wheelchair, or, you just see it around you, people caring for one another. I just thought, that's what, I, I know it's not a very well-paid job, but that's what I want to do.

(Grace 0: year 1 term 3)   (Narrative 2)

These images of family members being cared for provided a strong template for later impressions gained whilst she was working as a care assistant. On the wards she used to notice how different nurses cared for patients, some of them taking great trouble to meet their patients' needs and to get to know them, whilst other nurses tended to leave most of their work to students.

And I thought to myself, if, when I get qualified, I'm not going to be like that. I'm not going to just be a qualified person, sitting at the desk giving everybody orders. My idea of being a nurse to be qualified is to be more competent to do things. Not just sit there and give every-body else orders. I'm gonna be teaching the students. I'll be doing just as much work as everybody else. I wouldn't try and change in any way from when I was a student.

I think the new care that they are bringing out now, the primary nursing, I think that's really good. Whereas before you went on to a ward and every day you were allocated dif-ferent patients. So I think the new nursing is better. Because if you really get to know the patient as an individual you can give better care.

If you're a good nurse, you really get involved with the patient. You get to know them as a person, you get to know, I don't know, some nurses don't think about how a patient likes sitting if they're going to have a dressing done. Or, whether they like having a wash instead of a bath, and things like that. Before they just used to, 'Oh you're having a bath and that's it, 'cos it's your day to have a bath!'

(Grace 0: year 1 term 3)   (Narrative 3)

Grace's commitment to providing individualised care was reflected in the reality of her practice. Having so much earlier experience of nursing as a pupil nurse and an auxiliary (healthcare assistant) gave Grace the confidence to put across her strong views about how she wanted to relate to patients and their family into her practice. She generally had the advantage of feeling confident to communicate with patients and as a result could settle quickly into her clinical placements. However, this was not always the case:

Because I've looked after patients before and, I don't know, you just build it up over a period of time, don't you? I mean when I first looked after patients I was hopeless. They said I was hopeless. Well, I just didn't know how to communicate with patients properly, because I'd never, you know, had to deal with anything like this before. And of course I was really young when I first started working at 15. And you're just exploring yourself and discovering about yourself. I mean to look after, to go in from sort of seeing well people to seeing really sick people it's quite a shock. You just think to yourself 'Oh my God, this could be me, or the family'. Sometimes it was like hard to deal with, especially with the really old people who had Alzheimer's disease and things like that. It really made you think. I remember looking after a lady one day, and she'd been incontinent, . . . she had it all over her. And the nurses, like, 'Come on Grace, put on a plastic sort of like overall and we'll put her in the bath'. And the hands were waving all over the place, and I was thinking 'I really don't want to do this'. She got it all over my uniform. I was thinking 'Maybe this isn't me' . . . But now, because I'm older and I don't know, it's just become so easy to be able to communicate with patients and build up a rapport with them.

(Grace 5: year 2 term 3)   (Narrative 4)

During the first year of her programme she went on observational visits to different clinical settings to meet statutory and European Union requirements relating to different parts of the Professional Register. In her first year she visited community and adult nursing settings. In her second year she went to care for children in hospital and the community as well as maternity services. She also spent some time in a community residence for people with learning disabilities. During these placements Grace felt comfortable with the familiar environment of a hospital ward and could draw on her earlier nursing experiences. She was relieved to find she could reciprocate the time staff were spending on talking to her by helping them with various routine tasks.

The only way it made it easier, was by actually going onto the wards on my observational visits. Because, because, I knew what a ward routine was like. I could actually go onto the ward, and, instead of just sitting there and observing, I could actually help out. Which they didn't mind at all. I mean obviously, I couldn't do dressings, or give injections, because that's not part of the course at the moment. So I mean, it's helped me out in that way, but other ways, no. Because of working on the wards, I'm used to sort of like, mixing with people and talking to the patients and things like that. It's helped me, when I went out to visit my family. I could actually relate to them, because I knew how to talk to people. Because I already had interpersonal skills by working on the ward. It helped me in that way. But, erm, work wise, the actual, all the science, and all the essays, and referencing, and, and the contract and things like that, no it hasn't helped.

(Grace 0: year 1 term 3)   (Narrative 5)

Developing professional knowledge

During her community placement with a health visitor in the first year of her programme Grace visited clients in their homes. The aim of the module was to provide an understanding of different concepts of health and lifestyles. She was encouraged to develop a questionnaire based on models of health and to use this to interview her chosen family. Over a period of ten weeks she visited the family regularly and made friends with the mother.

Well if you interview someone on the ward, you know that's your job, and you've got to interview this person and, in a way you are intruding but you don't feel like you are. I don't know, the patients seem to have trust in you. They expect you to ask all these questions, they expect it of you. And that's what makes it easier. I found by just dressing in my ordinary clothes that none of the patients expected anything of me. They thought that I was a visitor.

It's community visits, so I'll have to interview people there. I don't mind. I'll be dealing with people that I like, I don't know, say an old people's home, or an old people's residential home. So it'll be much like going in to talk to people on the wards I suppose. So it'll be easier. No I don't think [I'll feel an intruder], I know it sounds mean, but, I've actually been to old people's homes and when I worked in London, you had to actually go on, visits to these residential homes and talk to people there. Because it was sort of like, a hospital setting you didn't feel like you were intruding. I think it's because the patient has come into an environment that I know. I just, thought well you went onto a ward and got on with it. And you didn't feel, you never felt like that you were intruding. But it's so different going into someone else's home, seeing them, asking them all these personal questions. While if you interview someone on the ward, you know that's your job, and you've got to interview this person and, in a way you are intruding but you don't feel like you are.

(Grace 0: year 1 term 3) (Narrative 6)

At the start of Grace's second year she went to her first hospital placement on a children's ward. This was followed by a week in maternity and then a week with a school nurse in the community. Going to so many different settings was quite disruptive, especially as Grace was fitting her visits around regular timetabled academic slots. Being a single mother with a 4-year-old daughter she had to make arrangements for child-minding to supplement the university nursery facilities.

I thought it was bad last year, but this year it's working on the wards as well as doing everything else. I'll get used to it. It's just my life basically. It's so busy. I have to be up early in the morning to take my child to school. I get up at about 7:30 am and then I get her up and give her a wash and take her to school. Then I have to pick her [up] at 3:10 pm. If I'm really busy my parents will pick her up or they'll take her to school, but I've still got the care of her at the moment. [When I am looking after her in the evening I have] only from 8:00 pm onwards [to study]. Sometimes I leave her at my mum's. Tomorrow I have to go and work with the health visitor, so she'll have to stay with my mum and dad and my dad can take her to school in the morning. But by the time I've seen to all her care and got her ready for bed and read a story, then she goes to bed about 7:30 pm and by the time I've walked home that's 8:00 pm, so it's getting quite late. During the day I have to go out and get books and research things. Or like today, I've come to see you. I've finished on the wards now. When I was on the wards I wasn't getting any days off at all. I went for about 17 days without a day off because one week I would work a weekend and then Monday, Tuesday, went to college Wednesday and Thursday and Friday went to work.

(Grace 1: year 2 term 1) (Narrative 7)

3.5b Learning technical skills

Even though Grace had spent sometime working as a healthcare assistant and learning how to give care she still felt anxious about giving technical care, especially when she was participating in caring for sick children.

It wasn't so much a practice module, more observational because I'm not going to be a children's nurse. It's just to give you some idea. I followed my mentor around and got an idea of what she did and the ward routines and then team nursing. They have a yellow and green team and the nurses are put into different teams and within that you have two or three patients to look after, so they can give more individual time. I thought that was really good. They use [a nursing] model, a care plan, so anyone can come along and look at the care plan and see what's going on. That really helped. I learnt about that and my mentor showed me how to take a temperature and do babies' respiration and their pulse. Especially babies have a really fast pulse and you listen to their heart with a stethoscope and count it that way.

Largely I didn't do anything much and in my other nursing experience all I've done is look after adults, so I was learning something different. I learned to take a temperature, axillary and orally as well, so I just applied that to the babies and popped it under their arm.

I watched Margaret [mentor] doing it and then she told me the correct way of doing it. . . . One thing I thought was funny was that I couldn't get the hang of taking their pulse to begin with. I'm used to doing it at the wrist. It was so fast. It takes a good couple of days to get it right.

Because it's all about learning. If I couldn't get it right I would say so to my mentor and she'd take it. You can't put down the wrong thing. So she took it. She found it easy with years of experience. She was really good. Even when I made mistakes she would say 'Never mind. Just remember this is the way to do it'. It's all about learning and making mistakes. But then again you wouldn't be left to do really major things.

I learnt about saturation testing. They have a special instrument which they put on the baby's fingers or toes and if the baby has a heart problem – because the ward dealt mainly with children with heart and respiratory problems – it can test the oxygen level in the blood, so I learnt about that. I learnt about basic care for someone with respiratory problems, neb- ulizers or inhalers. One little boy had a humidifier in the room because he had croup. It felt really good [doing these technical things].
(Grace 2: year 2 term 1)   (Narrative 8)

By working as a supernumerary student Grace was able to work alongside her mentor and could whilst observing her mentor, learn not only how to carry out technical tasks but also to see how she related to the children and to their parents. Having a mentor who was willing to let her experiment and to make mistakes, meant the quality of her learning was high. In her adult nursing placement she developed her technical skills further:

I know that there's a lot of room for improvement, because I mean, I've got two years to do. But I mean I feel confident in doing sort of like basic things. Because I'm not worrying about you know doing a blood pressure, because I know how to do it, and I know how to listen out. Sometimes it's difficult and I'll say, 'Oh no, can you hear this? I took this man's blood pressure and it's very faint, so I'd prefer you to come and listen to it and tell me what it is.' Sometimes I need reassurance like that, but generally I find for doing basic care, I know it's important to do things accurately. Giving somebody a wash or whatever is easy. But when it comes to things I haven't seen before or I'm not sure about, then I feel a bit nervous. So it's changed from my practice previously to now, I just feel more confident in doing things. It just comes. One day you just go onto the ward and think 'I'm not worried about giving a blood pressure, doing a blood pressure. I'm not worried about giving an injection so much now'. I just talk to my mentor. Because they do understand that even though you're mature, you're still a student. And even if you're older than they are, they're the one that's qualified, so they speak to you and help you.

. . . I took this man's stitches out, and it was like really difficult. It went inside. It was a continuous one, it's difficult to describe. And she really – well I know how to take stitches out, you know just the ordinary ones. And she went through it in a lot of detail. Why you

need to cut it close to the skin, so that I'm not dragging through sort of like . . . [the] dirty part. So if I cut it close to the skin then I'm really pulling through a minimal part, and the chances of there being anything on that . . . And how to do it, to get it out easily, and why we did it the way we did it. She was guiding me all the way how to do it. [It was] brilliant, I mean, I felt a bit guilty about sort of like talking over the patient's head, but he didn't mind either. At least he understood that I was a student and that's why we did it like that.
(Grace 5: year 2 term 3) (Narrative 9)

This form of learning from an experienced and knowledgeable practitioner is clearly enormously beneficial for Grace, as indeed it was for the other students. Grace was able to develop safe techniques as well as understand the underlying rationale. As a result she was able to make links between what she saw in her practice with what she had read or been taught. Learning from a knowledgeable practitioner was not confined to technical skills. Grace's narratives indicate how she was using her observations of the manner in which practitioners gave care. She could then decide whether she wanted to adopt their approaches and techniques.

3.5c Relating to patients

Her earlier experiences of working with sick people and their families helped Grace overcome her initial inhibitions and freed her up to concentrate on giving care. This was noticed by her colleagues:

Once you get used to talking to people . . . the communication takes a while and for some of the girls who haven't done any nursing before it's difficult. My friend was saying I was really good because I knew what to say and do, but I've been an auxiliary nurse and cared for people before, so it makes a difference. That's one thing I don't have to worry about, the communication. I can get on and learn my practical skills. I remember it's quite nerve-wracking knowing what to say to patients, especially if they're confused. Now I can sit down [and talk to them]. Ages ago I wouldn't know what to say to them and it was frustrating, but even if they ask something over and over again you can just sit and explain to them until eventually it registers. It just takes time.
(Grace 3: year 2 term 2) (Narrative 10)

She realised there was still quite a lot to learn and again through watching staff she learned to develop her own approach.

She's a little bit older than me. She's very nice and very empathetic towards the patients. She's really good. One day there was an elderly lady and she expressed to me the feeling that she didn't like taking her tablets because she thought they were responsible for her feeling tired. I said that to Sophie and when we did the drug round the lady commented on it again and I was stuck for words and said 'I'm sure they don't make you tired'. But Sophie said 'Elsie. . . .' and didn't just tell her she had to take them for all her problems, but she explained that it wasn't the tablets that were making her tired. The tablets were to help and she explained that she had one drug for her chest to make that get better, another for her heart. And so she explained really simply and she mentioned her poor circulation, which is one thing she understands. So Elsie then said 'Oh well, I suppose I should take them then'.

> She could have just given her a quick answer but didn't. She really tries to think of the
> patient as a whole.
> (Grace 3: year 2 term 2)   (Narrative 11)

Having the opportunity to watch her mentor develop this kind of rapport with
patients was an invaluable learning experience that Grace could use in her own
practice. Learning how to relate to people who are stressed because of their illness
or the circumstances in which they find themselves takes skill and understanding.

Working in a residential unit for a small community of people with learning
disabilities presented Grace with new challenges.

> First of all when I went in there they seemed like funny men. I know I shouldn't say that. You
> have to look at it realistically. They're not like everyday people because they have a learning
> disability and some have quite severe learning disabilities. You couldn't even speak to them
> and have a conversation with them. You used sign language and basic body language to
> communicate with them. They said a few words, but you couldn't have a deep conversation
> with them. First of all that was quite difficult – because how do you communicate? If
> someone can't talk on a level you're used to, it's difficult. Some of them couldn't even talk
> as well as a child. I just got to know them and what they could say and couldn't say. It just
> comes to you how to communicate by watching Pam [mentor] [and then I did it myself]. I
> tried to say 'Ooh, what's your name then?' very slowly and clearly. They'd just look at you
> with a blank expression as if you were stupid. One of the guys there – I'll call him John –
> was partially deaf and had a learning disability, but he was more able than the others and he
> looked at me, looked at Pam and made a funny expression because he thought I was screwy.
> Basically he was saying to Pam 'She's not all there, is she? She's talking to me as though I
> were stupid'. Basically. I didn't mean to, but I was talking to them like little children I
> suppose. I ended up doing it because I'm used to being round children. Basically you just
> talk to them like normal people and they understand every word you say, apart from Philip,
> because he's partially deaf. We don't know whether he lip reads or not.
> (Grace 6: year 2 term 3)   (Narrative 12)

Learning how to talk to patients who are dependent upon you changes the power
relationship between adults and Grace was conscious of this. She strived to establish partnerships with her patients, although as we have seen, she needed help to
learn how to put this in action. Responding to people who are behaving in a
manner that is unconventional is another dilemma many nurses have difficulty
with. As we read in Nicola's case study, using everyday techniques to defend
themselves against inappropriate behaviour can sometimes be helpful but on
other occasions students needed to learn ones that were more acceptable in a professional setting. This is particularly the case with people who are confused or
mentally ill. Learning how to relate to young men who have a learning disability
and behave in a provocative or socially unacceptable manner creates a number of
dilemmas.

> He just put his head in my lap. I didn't mind. That's why I think I get on so well with
> patients. I'm just myself. I don't see them as patients or clients, I see them as people that
> maybe need a bit of help in some areas. Yes, that's how it was in the house. It was their home
> and you were like friends coming into their home. We did quite a lot. Cuddled the residents
> and showed them affection, because they're like everyone else, they need that and comfort.

If they don't get it from us they're not going to get it from anyone else. Pam did have a set line where they couldn't be over-friendly, because of course they're men whether you like it or not. One of the residents kept trying to look up our tops and he'd become a bit friendly. But Pam said 'You mustn't look up Grace's top'. And he'd get annoyed or try and look up her top, but she said it wasn't acceptable and so they knew the boundaries and they just didn't cross them. He tried to get away with it with me, but Pam told him not to by saying 'Other people wouldn't look up Grace's top, so you mustn't either'.

(Grace 6: year 2 term 3)   (Narrative 13)

This demonstration of how to respond to residents provided the kind of support and guidance that taught Grace how to behave therapeutically in a way that protected both her and the men when faced with such situations. It is often a subject too difficult to deal with in classroom activities and many nursing students, especially recent school-leavers find it particularly embarrassing to raise. More experienced students may have developed their own strategies that are not necessarily appropriate in a nursing context and they too need help. Despite her wide experience of life, at the age of 29 Grace found this sort of guidance helpful.

3.5d Learning to be therapeutic

For many beginners just walking into a clinical setting can be very frightening and most have difficulty seeing or recognising the significance of what is taking place around them (Fuhrer 1993). Her earlier experiences of nursing provided Grace with a foundation of knowledge that helped her to see what was taking place. This gave her an advantage over her less experienced colleagues and she was able to use her observations to inform her practice as well as draw on materials she had learned in class.

One thing I really have to stop myself from doing is over helping, doing everything. Before it was geared to helping the patient [by doing] as much as you can. That's what I've done in the past. Almost everything. Now I have to stand back and see if Mr Jones can pull up his trousers or whatever, or Elsie can put on her dressing gown. Just to do something for themselves . . . If you take over all the hygiene needs of the patient it's not being very therapeutic. It basically means you're taking them over. If someone did everything for me I'd wonder what I was doing here. I wouldn't like it at all. But some patients have been geared into having everything done for them. They no longer feel they have any self-worth. I think they can get really uninterested in life and it's bad for them.

Doing this course (has changed my approach). Honestly. It wasn't until I came here and we're geared to learning in a different way. Thinking of being therapeutic . . . it's the school. Before I did everything because I thought I was being a really good nurse if I helped the patient as much as I could . . . Now my role is different because nursing has changed. I'm an advocate for the patient. There to assist them with their needs, not do everything for them. I think it's because I'm older as well and have a child. As she's getting older I say to her 'Why don't you wash your hands and face?' and she cleans her own teeth. It was seeing her doing it and she's five years old and doing things for herself and I wondered why we were babying the patients. We're treating them worse than five-year-olds.

(Grace 3: year 2 term 2)   (Narrative 14)

Through drawing on her course knowledge and experiences of caring for her daughter, Grace could recognise how to provide care that was more patient-centred. She still needed guidance from her mentor to make sure that her strategies were appropriate for specific patients. But she had achieved a stage of professional development when she felt sufficiently confident in many of her interpersonal and technical activities to think beyond them and to consider the context of her care delivery. Drawing on personal knowledge and experience helped her to communicate empathy when a client was in distress and thus reassure the client that he or she was in safe hands.

> The bit I remembered most was when she was having the gas and air. It made me realise how painful it was. It made me think I was exactly the same. She kept holding on to the gas and air and I could appreciate why she was doing it. When she cried because she knew she had to have stitches, I did the same thing as well. When she knew I'd gone through the same sort of thing she responded to me better. She said women who can't have children don't appreciate what she'd been through.
> (Grace 1: year 2 term 1)   (Narrative 15)

Reading through Grace's case study it might appear that she was making rapid progress and had a profound insight to her role. Certainly this was mostly the case, although she acknowledged that she did make silly mistakes and in some situations she found it difficult when faced with hurting a patient to provide the appropriate care.

> You always wonder if you're hurting the patient. One of the patients I looked after was really anxious and he said 'Not an injection again' and that puts you on edge. I gave him an injection and he complained and I thought I'd given him a really bad one, but afterwards he said 'I was just anxious. I'm fine really. You didn't hurt me'. I don't like injections either. I had to laugh. I reflected on that.
> (Grace 4: year 2 term 3)   (Narrative 16)

3.5e Being a team member

Grace was fortunate in meeting clinical practitioners who were experienced and able to juggle all the different demands on their time well enough to give her the kind of educational support and attention she needed. An important aspect of this was the induction programme that the unit lecturer practitioner organised for new students.

> In a way, yes, because everybody was friendly. Not as much as I did in [the elderly care unit], because that's more laid back and . . . I did feel as if I was part of a team and everybody was being friendly. They were helping me the whole year. If I wanted to learn anything on anything, they didn't mind. They'd take time out to tell me. You know, I wanted to stay there every day and just do my practice. This is what I would really like to do, like spend all my time, weeks on end there, do my practice, write up my evidence and reflection, and have nothing else to think about. But it's like the days are so bitty. [I did] three days a week [over] five weeks. [15 days] well, let me think, how many shifts did I do? I did 10 shifts.
> (Grace 5: year 2 term 3)   (Narrative 17)

The most important person for Grace was her designated mentor who took her along to all her nursing activities and involved her in the care she was giving. Once she had assessed that Grace was competent in different tasks she assigned her to care for particular patients. Both types of working provided learning opportunities that were invaluable.

> We did quite a few injections. I've given them quite a few. But the way Anita said to give a subcutaneous one was a bit different to how I'd normally given it, because the needle's different, the needle sizes are different. You can do it like that, I mean squeeze the thing and put it in at an angle, can't you? But with the smaller needle you can just put it straight in. So she explained that. It felt different, because I don't normally give them like that. I normally, I'm used to giving them you know at the beginning at a sort of an angle. Still, that's one thing I've learnt. And I gave an injection to this guy that's, . . . he's got stuff like bowel problems. He'd got really thin and I was worried about giving an injection to him, because of course it's more difficult if there's no muscle, because he's so thin. I just looked at the point – Anita said 'Look at the point where it went in, where the needle went in, and then just move it down a bit'. And it wasn't until I actually did that I realised, the importance of, you know when you do sort of like an intramuscular, and draw it back in case you got a blood vessel. But when I hit the blood vessel, I though 'Gosh, if I hadn't have drawn it back, then I would have injected it straight into a blood vessel'. So that really made me aware of why you do something. Until you experience it, you think, 'oh well, I know why I don't do that, I know why I sort of like pull back the plunger'. So now, when I give another injection, I'll always be thinking 'Oh, I remember when I gave Brian his injection, I hit a blood vessel'.
> (Grace 5: year 2 term 3) (Narrative 18)

These sorts of situations provided the necessary stimulus for Grace to go away and read around her practice. Sometimes her mentor's practice or the policy of a clinical setting gave Grace food for thought and combined with her course assignment requirements she was able to develop her own understanding and emerging craft knowledge as she documented in her assignment.

> It was 10 days post-op. He wasn't mobilising very well. You know, on the first occasion I walked him he was in pain, and I felt bad about it, but I knew why we had to mobilise him. Sort of like looking back on it now, I realise that his pain wasn't controlled, and it could have been controlled better. And even then when I said just that, she [my mentor] didn't think the pain chart was appropriate. And maybe it wasn't, because he was so anxious. Maybe it wasn't, maybe she's right that it wasn't. But the other option is we could have used a simple chart and then he probably would have felt that we were really trying to find out about his pain. I just said that I gave him an injection and realise now that a lot of his pain was to do with his anxiety. When we got him up and we were washing him and we walked him, and we . . . , it was so stressful for him. But of course he was, you know, he was in more pain, wasn't he? More anxious?
> (Grace 5: year 2 term 3) (Narrative 19)

3.5f Academic pressures

Writing up her clinical experiences was a challenge for Grace. This was partly because she preferred to be engaged in practical clinical activities. Finding time to get to the library and searching out all the necessary information meant she had to juggle all her other study and home commitments. Despite this she achieved good marks in the B/B+ (50–70% range). Her written work was rarely submitted on time, much to the exasperation of her tutors and mentors who were unaware of the pressures she was struggling to overcome and survive. Being in the early stages of a new programme many mentors were unfamiliar with the assessment strategy and students frequently received conflicting advice from different people (tutors, lecturer–practitioners and mentors). Grace had a strong wish to represent her practice experiences in her learning contract, but still needed to learn the academic skills of presenting this information in a style that was acceptable.

> But there was a problem. I felt under stress and when it came to the learning contract (LC), because I don't think I'm very good at writing them anyway, I felt I just couldn't write the LC the way my mentor wanted it. She gave me a lot of guidance, she was quite good and I just thought I couldn't express my practice as well as I thought I could. Because my practice is quite good. I just feel I'm letting myself down by not expressing it in the LC. I know I need to work on that [reflection] and express my practice.
>
> When I worked on the ward there was pressure for me to do this LC and learn all these things. And achieve all these competencies and have all these set objectives. Whereas when I worked in community housing, because it's different, my objective was just to look at how the care in the community differs from institutionalised care. I said I'd got all the information from my mentor or books because I didn't know. Another objective was to achieve some of the competencies I didn't achieve in the first half [of term]. There was pressure on me to do the LCs, but I felt I was able to do them because I felt relaxed in the house. I didn't feel I had to rush around and do all these things.
> (Grace 6: year 2 term 3)   (Narrative 20)

Her professional tutor was being bombarded by complaints about Grace who was not submitting work on time. She was giving the impression of being unreliable.

> Then there's my professional tutor, he's very nice. That's Frank. Maybe I haven't been that fair to him. I've been going to see him. Is everything fine? Why is your work late? WELL, some excuse and he's let it go on really. He's finally written me a letter saying 'Why didn't you tell me you had all these problems? Even though you come and see me on a regular basis you didn't discuss it'. So I think he's quite angry with me. He feels I should have been able to talk to him and I didn't. I just didn't want to unburden my problems to him really. He's my professional tutor and we talk about how I'm getting on with my college work and why my work is late, things like that. I thought the other things were separate and as a student I saw him about nursing things, not my personal life. I thought it was unprofessional to have a complicated personal life. You have to keep the two things separate really don't you? You can't keep bringing your personal life into it, but then it's spilled over into my college work. [It affects how well I'm able to function] more and more. First of all it started off really mild, but it's come to a head at the end of this year. Not being on time, being unreliable to everyone, not doing my work as well as I could do it. He knows I can do better work and that I'm not going to be an 'A' standard all the way through. I might get a few As somewhere along the line, but he knows my standard is B/B+. I think he thought I wasn't achieving and wondered why the work was late and why I didn't do my LC. I felt under pressure.
> (Grace 6: year 2 term 3)   (Narrative 21)

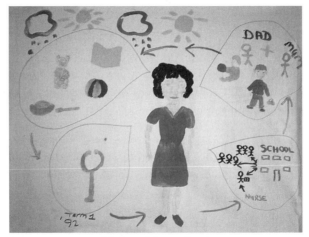

3.5a   Year 2 term 1 'Living different lives'.

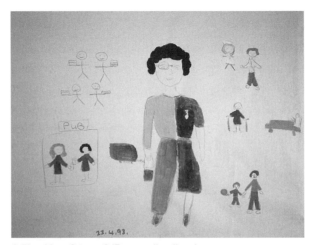

3.5b   Year 2 term 2 'Demanding lives'.

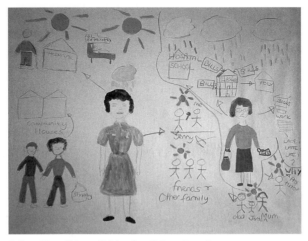

3.5c   Year 3 term 3 'Nursing living stress'.

Figure 3.5   Grace.

3.5g Being a single mother

The pressure that Grace was experiencing was her poverty and trying to juggle being a single mother and being a full-time student on a nursing course. Grace was fulfilling her lifetime ambition to become a qualified nurse. She had successfully completed an academically demanding access course that had met entry requirements for the nursing degree course. Having worked as a care assistant she had a lot of valuable experience to contribute even whilst she was a student, and this is evidenced by her narratives. Being a single mother added the already considerable pressures that nursing students experience. For Grace, the two main pressures were finances and study time, which were associated with childcare. Her illuminative artwork throughout the study was dominated by images of her family, the financial pressures and the academic pressures of her work, illustrating her preoccupations with these factors (see Figure 3.5a).

> The other week, because everything was getting on top of me, when I drew the picture that was how I felt. Basically, what I'm trying to say is that although I've had lots of problems in my personal life, nothing to do with the course, I've really enjoyed the course and I'd like to carry on. Hopefully, things in my personal life will sort themselves out.
>
> Last year I didn't say anything and just let them build up and I felt it was difficult to do the course and look after Daphne and do all the work. It looked as though I was being lazy or maybe I wasn't good enough because I just got passes for some of the work or perhaps they didn't think I was suitable. It wasn't until this year when I let things really build up and I thought I couldn't cope with it all that I talked to my lecturer–practitioner and it really helped and I found a way of solving my problems.
> (Grace 2: year 2 term 1)   (Narrative 22)

Even when she did talk about the problems, not everyone was sympathetic as her final image illustrates (see Figure 3.5c).

> That's my home, with all the bills round it. At one time I felt I couldn't go there to live. I just let the bills pile up because it was one thing I didn't want to worry about. That was pressure for me. It's a pressure leaving Daphne with my mum and dad all the time, but I've got used to that now. Not having the family life I would like and which would make my life easier. I talked to [course chair] and she said 'Oh I get lots of people with financial problems. Everyone has problems'. It was just the way she said it. It's too bad, everyone has problems but you should get on with your work. As though she didn't really understand. I felt as though she didn't understand the pressures I was under. I felt none of them did really. I know they're busy and they can't be bothered with every student's problems. They just can't be overloaded with it.
> (Grace 6: year 2 term 3)   (Narrative 23)

Financial worries

The student grant designed for young adults with no external commitments and ability to live in student accommodation or with their parents was wholly insufficient for the demands of Grace's life. Many students supplemented their grant by working in the evenings and vacation periods, or obtained help from their parents. In Grace's case, working during the vacation times, meant she had to find child-minding facilities that were expensive or seek the support of her parents. Working in the evenings to supplement her income presented similar difficulties and led to her relying on her parents to look after Daphne. Her ex-partner had since married and ceased to meet his financial obligations towards their daughter. As a result Grace relied upon her grant and any other form of benefit she could negotiate from the local department of social security offices. The university student services department provided students with information and support, and over the two years of the course Grace was able to negotiate her way through all the bureaucracy. But this took up valuable time.

> I'd be worrying about this and that, sorting this and that out, worrying about the lease on my flat because I couldn't pay the rent. And I know they seem like really silly problems . . . So, being as my brother and his girlfriend are in my flat, and they're helping me pay most of the bills, they're paying two-thirds of the bills. I've moved back in there now. They also said, if like I'm away and I can't get to pay the telephone bill or I can't get to put the money in the bank for the rent and stuff, she'll do all that, because she's always . . . so she'll sort that all out. So I don't have to worry about that. And if I am short on money, they said that sort of like they'd pay the bills and I could give them the money back. Like I've got huge water rates. I owe hundreds of pounds on the water rates. So what I'm going to do is I'm going to pay off the arrears and they're going to pay off this year's water rates completely. That's a big help. I can afford to go to the dentist. I worked last summer and I worked for the first two terms of this year, and I thought 'no, even though I need the money, no'. It's better for me to stay at home and take Daphne out more – take her on holiday if I can afford it, and have a rest during the summer, so that when I come back I'm sort of quite refreshed.
> (Grace 5: year 2 term 3)   (Narrative 24)

Childcare facilities

Daphne was nearly four when Grace started her course. She was able to use the childcare facilities provided by the local university where she was studying. But being a nursing student meant that she was spending considerable time travelling to and from clinical placements outside her home town and thus needing childcare outside their hours. Being able to fit in course work, attendance at lectures and her clinical hours meant Grace had to do her clinical placements over weekends. This meant she had to juggle her time so she could meet all the demands of being a university student and a nursing student, as well as find ways of supplementing her income. Fortunately her parents lived locally and they were willing to help look after Daphne.

> I've got my mum and dad to look after my little girl, so that if I know she's being looked after by them, I can do my work. I can't do both. Some people can. I'm quite happy that I know she's being taken to school and has her needs taken care of. I can be a more efficient person and do my work. It got to the stage where I was handing in work that wasn't very good because it was done at the last minute. Then it was late and the more you worry the worse it gets.
> 　[My mum and dad don't mind looking after my daughter] as long as it's not at the weekends, when my mum likes a break. I have her back at the weekend. I had a happy childhood

with my parents. They were really good. We didn't go on expensive holidays or have expensive things, but we just had a happy life with them. We always had nice clothes and shoes and nice Christmas presents. Even though we didn't have a great deal of money they had their own house, so we didn't have to worry about moving about. So I'm quite happy to leave Daphne with them.

. . . I'm catching the bus in the morning and there is an earlier one that gets you here about ten to [8]. It's supposed to be three days a week minimum here, but I'm not going to be able to work over the weekends and can't work Monday and Tuesday, so to compensate I'm going to work Friday, Saturday, Sunday, Monday. By doing four days in a row I'm getting a better idea of running the ward and I'm going to try and be here for report. Unfortunately on Sunday the buses don't run that well, so I have to get a later bus. My parents will look after her next Saturday and Sunday. I've accepted it now. I want to be there and help her with her reading but it's no good me staying at home with her all the time if it's not what I want to do. I'm not going to be a better mother to her by living on social security and being there all the time. If I don't achieve anything for myself or have any self-worth, how can I be of benefit to her? I'm just going to be an older woman living on income support. As my mum and dad have taken early retirement and my dad can't work again because he's had a stroke which affects his vision so he can't read properly, they look after Daphne. My dad gets tired and he says 'Now your mum's here she can put you to bed'. He's really sweet. He forgets to give me my messages, so I have to stress the importance to him. He wears glasses and tries to read large print. I think the stroke did affect his sight. He can see well enough, but it's just reading. Sometimes he can see better than others and gets lots of headaches, but I imagine his blood pressure is still high. I've told him to ask what his blood pressure is next time he goes to the doctor and I can find out whether or not it's high.

(Grace 2: year 2 term 2)   (Narrative 25)

Inevitably the pressures of caring for her family and doing her course built up and Grace reluctantly decided to follow the advice of her professional tutor and intermit from the course for a year. This would give her time to get a job as a care assistant and pay off her debts. Her daughter would be old enough to go to infant school, leaving her more time in the day. She would still need the support of her parents so she could work in the evenings and do her studying. Grace returned from her break and successfully completed her course five years later.

3.5h Grace's professional development

Grace entered the course with a wealth of practical experience. She had worked as a care assistant (auxiliary nurse) for several years and had undertaken six-months' of enrolled nurse training. She had also successfully completed a demanding access course that gave her the necessary academic qualifications to enter the degree programme. In her clinical practice she was supported by effective and knowledgeable practitioners who coached her through her initial concerns about demonstrating that she was up to the course and helped her overcome worries about learning technical and theoretical aspects of her programme. Her narratives illustrate her commitment to giving person-centred care in partnership with her patients and that she was willing and able to learn from her colleagues. Through her practice experiences she could recognise her knowledge needs and her written work provided a focus for developing her professional craft knowledge.

As with all the other students she found it difficult to juggle the academic demands of the course with the clinical demands, and her experiences of clinical practice encouraged her to spend more time attending to the latter. Probably this was largely because once she was in the placement she had no other distractions. In contrast attending to her academic work was fraught with other distractions caused by her poverty and being a single parent with a young child to look after at times which other students use to study and socialise.

Grace's accounts of her struggle to become a qualified nurse illustrate the difficulties confronting many women who are older than their contemporaries. She was one of a small minority of mature students when this study was conducted. Her teachers and mentors were mostly unfamiliar with the difficulties facing mature students. Since that time government directives have encouraged universities to offer more flexible modes of entry and more flexible programmes. However they have not resolved the problems caused by student poverty, or the discrepancy between funding students taking different vocational programmes. With demographic changes in society and the attractiveness of other more lucrative careers, fewer young men and women consider it as a career choice. In many university nursing programmes the average age of entrants is no longer 18 but closer to 35. With at least 50% of entrants to nursing tending to be mature woman with families, unless they receive strong social and financial support from their partners or alternative sources of support, it is likely that they will encounter similar difficulties.

3.6 Ruth

The decision to embark upon any professional training which is long and demanding, particularly after success in another field of employment, requires a great deal of courage and commitment. Ruth is a well-qualified 24-year-old who finished school with 11 0-Levels and 3 Science A-Levels. When she finished school Ruth had considered becoming a nurse but had rejected the idea in her wish to exert her independence. So she entered an accountant's office and successfully worked there for five years, studying at night school and gaining Parts 1 and 2 of the Certificate in Accountancy. After a while she became dissatisfied with her job, not liking the cut-throat and selfish attitudes that she saw around her. Both her parents had been career nurses and were delighted when she decided to enrol for a degree in nursing. She chose to do a degree course rather than the more common diploma course for several reasons. She believed she would be in a better position to change her mind if nursing did not live up to her expectations and having a degree could improve future employment prospects. She was aware of her parents' influence on her decision and also on her expectation of what she would be doing as a nurse.

They've always like said, 'You do what you want'. But I feel particularly with my Dad, I don't know whether it's because it's nursing or because it's a degree, but although he's never said anything I feel at last he thinks 'Gosh ! She's fulfilled, she's fulfilled her potential'.
(Ruth 0: year 1 term 2)   (Narrative 1)

3.6a Ruth's vision of nursing

Both Ruth's parents enjoyed successful careers as nurses and she had grown up hearing their nursing stories and going on Christmas visits to her parents' hospital wards. So it was inevitable that their views would have a strong influence on her perception of the sort of work she would be undertaking.

> So I could be a mum to somebody, even if he's a gentleman who's 20 years older than me. If I could still create that mumsy environment that makes me feel secure and hopefully would make someone else feel nice.
> When I saw my Dad in hospital, he was in a couple of times; and I thought, 'my Dad is my Dad', you know, 'A mega important person, and there he was with all this row of beds, with his little jim-jams on'. And he looked a different man in a way . . . I always want to keep the individual touch, 'cos that's, that's to me, what counts.
> (Ruth 1: year 1 term 2)   (Narrative 2)

Her business experiences had taught her that goodwill and dedication can be exploited by 'the system'. Her perception of her father as a caring but tough nurse supported this view and encouraged her to believe that nurses need to be confident, self aware and assertive in order to protect themselves and could be so, without losing the essence of nursing in their care. Like many students she had only a hazy view of the day-to-day interaction between nurses and other members of the healthcare team or in fact of the need for a sound academic background to her practice.

> I've never done it you see, so I don't know. I haven't seen all three shifts. I've never done night work and stuff like that, so. I realise that it could really mess you up, sleeping-wise and socially-wise. But I think that's the sort of thing you have to take on board when you take a job on.
> I think you need to know the workings of the body and the workings of drugs. It gives you a better insight as to what you're actually doing. If you know what's going wrong within them then you can be part of the team helping to sort that out. I think you also need to be taught how to do the basic things like washing and bathing, and lifting, definitely, how to do lifting, and dressings and things like that. As I say being taught to get on with people, but I think that's something that comes as you meet more and more people then you will. You can learn all the theory in the world but really, if you've got a personality type to get on with people, then that should come. They're the main things.
> (Ruth 1: year 1 term 2)   (Narrative 3)

Ruth's robust common-sense approach meant she had no illusions about the tough programme she was facing. She also had no illusions about her options if the nursing part of the degree did not end successfully. She did have concerns that perhaps by the end of the course she may become less sensitive to human suffering.

I don't know what I could turn out like at the end. I really do wonder at times – quite tough, and a lot of harder than I ever thought I would be, which I don't think is necessarily a good quality . . . I'd like to think that I would turn out a very caring person. But I'm aware that I may not be at the end. And I, I don't know whether that's good for nursing or not, I really don't. I feel you will have computer skills, you will have management skills. So I mean, if even at the end of it, you thought 'Well, I'm really not sure about this,' you wouldn't be up a gum tree as to go into other areas.

(Ruth 1: year 1 term 2)   (Narrative 4)

3.6b Adjusting to the programme

Changing careers at 24 is a challenging experience, particularly after some considerable success and effort. Ruth was used to holding a job and participating as a valued member of the organisation in which she had worked. Her day had been familiar and structured by the normal routine of office work. Starting the university course presented her with a completely different lifestyle. She had a strong sense of alienation that was compounded by her peer group being five or six years younger with different life experiences and thus they had little in common. By comparison, those people who were her age, were also her mentors and thus separated by their status in the organisation. Looking back on her experiences she wondered how she managed it.

> I've found being a student more stressful than doing the job in some ways. It was so structureless. I think the first year in college it was quite easy [easy time] when you've done full-time work. You have three lectures a week and the rest of the week is pretty much your own. I found that mind blowing. I think you had to find a routine to your week. When I worked, I studied in the evenings and studying in little bursts I can do fine. Whereas this was very much really you should or could study all the time. How am I going to deal with that? One way is avoiding it. That's what I was doing for a year of the course, running away from it. I felt I lost a lot of stability. It's only when you get to this stage that you appreciate why you've done it. But that's really hard to see.
>
> (Ruth 21: year 4 term 2)   (Narrative 5)

As Ruth's narrative reveals she had developed a very successful pattern to her life whilst in full-time employment and had passed several professional examinations. This was a considerable achievement. Transition to university life as a full-time student required a different type of discipline at a time when she was perhaps mourning the loss of a familiar and busy work routine and support of her family and friends. Her sense of loss was particularly compounded in her first year by having to engage in unfamiliar activities and without a clear role.

> The idea wasn't that you followed the health visitor, you had something to look at. I did a bit of both . . . When I was with her I asked her how she wanted me to conduct myself and she said just to watch and not to say anything . . . I was very aware on the days I shadowed that nobody spoke to me . . . But at Play Group and Mother and Toddler [Group], I was pretty much on my own which was awful at first. I just sat there wondering what the hell to do, but with children they come and play with you. So I did that . . . All I could do in any of

the situations was to introduce myself and really to my mind, to be non-threatening and just get on with people . . . Having met a group of people on two occasions I don't think I'm in any position to question them to that extent.
(Ruth 3: year 2 term 1)   (Narrative 6)

In this situation like many others, Ruth very much needed an activity and a role to help her settle into the placement and to feel the support of her mentor. With this sponsorship she then felt able to ask questions and thus learn about what she was observing, or perhaps even to *see* what was happening. From her conversations throughout her programme it became evident that social support and having a clear role were very important to her wellbeing and progress through the course.

3.6c Social support

In addition to the self-doubt caused by frequent changes of clinical placements and fractured relationships with one set of staff to be followed by having to establish new ones, Ruth was beset with the self-doubt that often accompanies moving to unfamiliar, sometimes painful and often, for the novice, frightening situations. As part of their academic assignments, students had to identify and analyse critical incidents from their clinical practice, incorporating personal insights. Working through these reflective activities inevitably raised personal doubts and insecurities from their subconscious. Students needed good emotional and social support if they were to achieve an adequate level of reflection and analysis of their practice.

Social support from family and friends

Ruth's main support and companion throughout the course was her mum. Being a practising nurse she was able to recognise Ruth's dilemmas and experiences and could give her the quality of support that encouraged her to maintain her self image without threat.

I've got certainly one friend here I feel I could talk with if I was really bothered about something. And I could always go back to Mum and Dad, particularly Mum. They know me and the nursing side. Sometimes you can't put things into words but you can say 'That really upset me what they did.' Even if it seems a really trivial thing . . . Maybe it's just important to identify a person, regardless of where that person is, whether they're uni. or family, but just knowing there's someone you can go to.
(Ruth 3: year 2 term 1)   (Narrative 7)

With the shortage of university accommodation and Ruth being a mature student meant she had to find her own accommodation which was on the outskirts of town rather than in the suburb where most students lodged. This meant she did not have the same contacts with any of her peers. She also found it hard being older than most of her peers and had difficulty empathising with their concerns that she attributed to growing up. This isolated her even further. It was not until her fourth year that she shared a house with other nurses. To develop a social circle she participated in a number of university activities including driving the women's bus one evening a week. It may be that her high self-expectations created a sense of vulnerability that was too painful to share.

> In the house I'm quite a private person and being six of us in there I often find it too much. I often go in and go straight to my room. If I want support in terms of whether I'm doing the right thing, I would look to get that from the ward staff, mentor, clinical teachers. Or a lot of it is that I want reassurance about me as a person and I can get that from my landlord or you or my mum. We get on fine in the house, but I don't want to take it any further ... Perhaps because I'd feel threatened by their practice. Two of them are qualified nurses already doing paediatrics and Liz is very good academically. She gets As every time and I think I feel intimidated a bit by it. So I know it gets the hairs on the back of my neck going if I say 'I did this' and she says 'No, maybe you should have done this, Ruth' and I feel like saying 'Bugger off'. So there's an element of me that doesn't want to discuss it when I get home. I feel comfortable talking to my mum because she's out of it. I do feel threatened by these other people because they're so good.
> (Ruth 20: year 4 term 1) (Narrative 8)

Ruth's self-criticism and high self-expectations masked her true achievements and hampered her ability to enjoy the course. Often her clinical colleagues were aware of this and sought to redress the imbalance by summarising their views in writing on her learning contract.

> Ruth states she feels as though she has been of little constructive help to the ward. Rubbish! I have found that Ruth has required minimal supervision. She has based almost her entire time on the ward with patients, building sound relationships with them. She seems to have a natural flair for interacting with people, demonstrating a genuine enthusiasm to spend time with them, showing a keen interest in the individuals with a sensitivity to their needs. Due to her confidence and her ability to use her intuition she has been valued by the nursing team on this [mental health] ward who have appreciated her efforts.
> (Mentor's comments on Ruth's Learning: year 2 term 3) (Narrative 9)

Ruth was anxious to have a role and to be useful to the ward team, to reciprocate the support they were giving her as a means of legitimising her presence. She seemed to have a good ability to relate to patients, despite some initial anxiety of working with them. Ruth's mentor was responsible for providing supervision and support throughout her placement. On some occasions this worked very well and on others Ruth found this more difficult. It is revealing that her mentor was pleased that she could manage with minimal supervision and one wonders whether she had a clear view of what and how Ruth would learn whilst allocated to the unit with out supervision.

Mentor support

Ruth was often working under the supervision of registered nurses who were younger than herself. They were probably oblivious to this but for Ruth it was important. Her ideal mentor was an older person, willing to share her feelings and thoughts. Some mentors were good at sharing their knowledge by talking her through their actions, others would sit her down at a convenient time and chat about the relevant theory or they would debrief from the day's activities. Even if the mentor was not particularly knowledgeable, the good quality of their relationship meant she was a legitimate member of the team. She was then empowered to go out and engage in practice and seek the necessary information from other members of the team.

> She was the best mentor so far. It helped me because rightly or wrongly I get on better with older people. She was perfect for me. I have had mentors my own age or younger which I find difficult. I'm aware that they're younger than me and maybe I feel threatened and maybe they feel the same . . . I was working with her and helping her. On the whole she could answer [questions] not terribly technically. There were younger staff nurses there who could probably have been a lot more technical for me, but I wasn't unduly worried about that. She was good.
> (Ruth 11: year 2 term 3)   (Narrative 10)

This mentor understood a student's need for sponsorship to her setting and was willing to offer friendship. This provided Ruth with a secure social environment to work from. Her strong desire to be helpful and to be part of the team was also fundamental to her feeling settled in the clinical area. In many respects she felt it gave her a legitimate reason for being on the unit and for seeking help, to ask questions and to learn. This was partly achieved by having a clearly identified role, which included time working alongside her mentor and also time working independently.

Team membership – sponsorship to the community

When she first started the course it was difficult to know what her role should be and without the guidance of her mentor or an obvious role to fulfil, Ruth found herself feeling isolated and useless. When asked whether she felt like a nurse or a nursing student she frequently replied during her first three years, that she felt like a care assistant. In situations where she did not receive sponsorship she felt isolated, or as her mentor wrote in her learning contract she was 'able to work with minimal supervision'.

> We're not specifically allocated anyone, so I almost feel as though I'm nudging my way in, with my elbows out. You've got the staff in a circle and the students are on the outside and you're trying to push in between and say 'Here I am, if you want me I'm here'. I find it very disheartening at times. But then again maybe the staff think that's what the degree is about. You're here to watch and observe and then go and write about it, and to some extent I feel that typifies student life. You're removed from reality, watching it all going on, theorising to the heavens about it and not doing much.
> (Ruth 8: year 2 term 3)   (Narrative 11)

Ruth equated the experience of learning to settle into each placement as being like a wooden 'puppy dog' on wheels, trundling behind her mentor where ever she went, as if she could not afford to let her mentor out of her sight. Perhaps this was a strategy to gain the type of attention she needed and to learn how to operate independently. Other factors helped her to gain a sense of being visible and of belonging.

> [I felt accepted] and valued; to the minor point that I got my name up on the board, which I've had before, but I think on the last surgical ward [when] it was my mentor /me. But in this case I was given two people.
> (Ruth 15: year 3 term 2)   (Narrative 12)

With good sponsorship she was able to develop independence from her mentor and look for help from the other members of the team. This helped her to become accustomed to the ward routine and her confidence increased. However Ruth seemed to conceptualise this time and attention as creating an indebtedness to the staff that required repayment through her undertaking tasks that were within her ability and which she was only too willing to do. Looking like or being treated like the other members of the team were other aspects of the process of social integration. When she wore the same dress as her clinical colleagues or was treated by visitors in the same manner as other members of the team, her confidence soared and allowed her to feel (almost) like a member of the ward team.

> Being a fourth year I was more than happy to help the ward out, to help the team and my mentor. That's what I was there for. To do things generally as well as my learning needs. I was happy to have a mentor otherwise you become a float for the ward don't you really? . . . You've got someone there who's on your side when you arrive on the ward and they're a facilitator, and that's true to a large extent. . . . I certainly was very at ease with my mentor, but did feel less so with other members of the team. Certainly in terms of asking them for a lift or whatever. Then it goes through your mind that you're not their student . . . I think being able to sit and have a bit of a social chat at handover. That helps . . . What made me feel part of the team? I think being kept informed generally.
> (Ruth 22: year 4 term 3)   (Narrative 13)

If students were unable to find an entrance to the social setting of the rest of the team, they seemingly became invisible which in turn inhibited opportunities to seek or receive help. For the most part of her programme learning was achieved through a number of activities concerned with observing and participating in nursing tasks with her mentor; undertaking delegated activities such as observations of vital signs. Some of her skill development evolved from her commonsense approach or by observing and learning from other members of the team.

3.6d Acquiring nursing knowledge

In the early part of her programme Ruth was assigned to mentors and it seemed that she was expected to trail them rather than to actively engage in their work alongside them. As a result Ruth longed to work independently (or in Jack's terms to 'fly solo') and learn through her own experiences. Without opportunities to work alongside practitioners she was unable to access their craft knowledge. Although as she indicated earlier, her mentors were not always able to share their knowledge. This may have been because they were intimidated by having a university student, or because they had not yet developed the language to express their actions. Ruth was a conscientious student and her illuminative artwork portrays her spending long hours in the library trying to make sense of her experiences through the literature (see Figures 3.6a and 3.6d). She was able to compensate for the lack of clinical tuition and could link her classroom learning with her clinical experiences. But her preferred approach was to participate in giving care and observe her mentor.

Learning by watching

Ruth's observations of nurses provided different images from the familiar stereotypes portrayed by the media and frequently she felt she could adopt their approach.

> I liked a lot of the staff nurses who were mellow when dealing with the people there. In no way was it 'Nurse knows best' sort of thing. It was a gently, gently approach, and I think you have to take that approach with some people. I thought they were all very considerate and they always treated people with a lot of respect, which was nice to see.
> (Ruth 6: year 2 term 2)   (Narrative 14)

During one early placement, Ruth spent ten days on a children's ward. This offered a very new experience partly because she had no younger siblings or family members but also because it was an early clinical experience where everything was new.

> I don't know anything about baby care. Using different cotton wools for each eye, watching her clean the nappy area and certain things I'd never seen before, like taking the blood pressure and temperature, using a digital thing, so I would copy her [my mentor]. I don't know how much is consciously making a note of it, but a lot of what you're doing is very similar and you wonder if it's you or her influence. It's probably more when I face the problem on my own and I wonder what she needed. Something strikes you in particular, then you might remember another time, but then again you're seeing so much and so much looks routine that you don't really make a mental note of it . . . You just get a general feel for what's going on. We didn't do an awful lot of specific techniques. I think I saw an aseptic technique once and certainly I saw them taking blood occasionally, so those things will probably stick in my mind more than a bit of baby care. They're the more unusual. You care for yourself everyday so your own common sense should tell you the sorts of things to do for care. Every now and then it went through my mind 'what would I like if this were my baby?'
> (Ruth 4: year 2 term 1)   (Narrative 15)

This seems to encapsulate a number of strategies that Ruth used throughout her programme. Some of her techniques were derived from using intuition and personal knowledge, others appeared to be remembered from her mother's teaching, other nurses or from trial and error.

Coaching

On other occasions when the task was recognised as being technically complex she received direct support and coaching from her mentor, although this could also create some tension.

> I feel I'm getting more of wound dressings now. I still feel very cack-handed obviously. But setting up the trolley and things, it sounds terribly menial in a way, but I think it's OK ... It's a case of thinking 'I wish people didn't have to watch me' because it makes it even worse ... I've not got enough experience of things going wrong probably to appreciate what damage I could do if I'm not careful ... I was very aware of how my lady was. She didn't like the look of the wound at all, which was quite reasonable, so she had her eyes closed and looked away ... I'm very aware that I must develop more talking to someone to reassure them during the process, but really at this stage I don't see I can cope with everything ... But I've got my mentor there supervising me. She would totally stop me if I was out of order. I think I'm relaxing more and hopefully getting more confident at what I'm doing. I've watched her before doing a dressing. The same one. You have to have a really good relationship with your mentor to get into the politics of how you feel when you do something. Also, it's taking criticism back from her and after the dressing she said I'd done it fine. I wasn't prepared to go into going through it step by step. I think you have to trust someone very much for that to be really effective. It's not that I don't trust her, I just don't have that bond or closeness.
>
> (Ruth 12: year 3 term 1)   (Narrative 16)

Clearly there are a number of factors affecting Ruth's concentration during this incident when she was making one of her first attempts to carry out a wound dressing without introducing infection. It is evident that she invested all her concentration on following the procedure correctly and could not afford to be distracted by attending to the emotional needs of the patient even though she recognised they existed. To achieve such an integrated performance would have required a greater ease with the technique. Paramount was her concern not to be criticised in front of the patient and this required a bond of trust and confidence between them. Fortunately in this situation, Ruth appeared to have been successful in negotiating all the obstacles and receive her mentor's affirmation. It was also evident that she was not confident that this would be the case and the relationship was not strong enough to permit a full discussion and thus extend her knowledge.

Flying solo

Perhaps as a residue from her previous career pattern, Ruth was anxious to 'pull her weight' in the clinical team and it seemed that she saw this as being able to work independently. This she found both satisfying and problematic, requiring ingenuity and perhaps a measure of good fortune to be resolved. The following example represents the unexpected complexity of a seemingly simple task and provided a useful learning experience.

I was bathing someone. I got myself in a bit of a pickle on lifting. I got her [the patient] onto a lift and into a bath, fine. She was very thin lady and she said it was really hurting her on the seat. So I said 'Right if you could raise your bottom, I'll stick a towel underneath'. It seemed a great idea to me; and of course by lifting her bottom up, which I could only just do, she flattened out and I just wasn't happy about it. I think I should have gone to get someone and we should have stood her out, but I kept on going. It was probably one of those mornings when I've thought 'Oh yes I can do that, I've done it before', and went swanning off. Maybe I should temper my enthusiasm.
(Ruth 6: year 2 term 2)   (Narrative 17)

Ruth found this a stressful experience and was concerned for her patient. Perhaps she would have benefited from more frequent opportunities to work with her mentor, so that she could have shared in the care-giving and gained from her craft knowledge. Additionally being able to debrief with her mentor following a period of working independently provides a valuable opportunity to think through unfamiliar experiences and to find alternative strategies.

She'd come in at 9:00–9:30am and she'd say 'OK you hand over your patients to me and tell me what you're doing because I don't know anything about them'; and that made me actually explain what was going on, what stage I'd got to. I basically use them for advice and say 'This is what I'm going to do'; go off and do it and then come back and say what I've done and how it went and asking them if they think I've done it right or not. Rather than being led by them or even having them supervise me by having them standing with me, unless it's something I would need supervision with.
(Ruth 21: year 4 term 2)   (Narrative 18)

During the vacation periods Ruth went home and worked either in the local hospital or nursing home. As a result she developed her confidence in some of the more routine procedures that caused new students anxiety.

That's probably one of the difficulties of working as an auxiliary. Again, you're not part of the team . . . Some people are grateful just to have the extra pair of hands. Ultimately that is the view I take. That I'm a pair of hands. But it's difficult when I'm asked to do things. In a way I don't want to do them, because sometimes I have to swallow what I've learned here and the way I want to practice as a staff nurse and fit in with what they want. This summer on the other orthopaedic ward and they had their auxiliaries doing amazing things, virtually everything bar giving out the drugs. One morning there were two staff nurses and four auxiliaries on. So staff nurse and auxiliary left side, another staff nurse and auxiliary the right side and she looked at me and said 'I want you to start on the obs'. And I'm a bank auxiliary who they've never met before and they give me the BP machine and the temperature and my job is to go round all of them up and down. That was the staff nurse asking me to do that. It was good experience for me. But don't you think that's unsafe because I'm an unknown quantity. I don't know what training auxiliaries have.
(Ruth 20: year 4 term 1)   (Narrative 19)

Experiences of this nature seemed to provide opportunities to rehearse skills and develop strategies for dealing with different patients and their individual needs. As a result Ruth encountered new problems that broadened her understanding and skill. Giving care to a small group of low dependency patients gave her the opportunity to know them well and as a result she came to see herself as their ally against the world of the institution. Such feelings may have been a reflection of her own sense of being an outsider to the established clinical team and inevitably they influenced some aspects of her learning. An example of this is reflected in her account of giving care to a patient she had befriended in order to write her assignment, a case study of a patient's hospitalisation experience.

> The one thing she did and I was very happy for her to do, was to take the catheter out . . . I wasn't prepared to ask him, I didn't want the embarrassment perhaps of having to do that for him. He was a 50-year-old man and I was still relatively young and I'm junior, a student. I've never seen a catheter come out either, so it would all have been me fumbling around and getting in a state with it. He was my case study man and I really wanted to get on well with him and that was really important . . . I went and watched the operation and then I followed him into ITU. I went back that evening to see how he was getting on and I also went back the next morning before college, just to see how he was doing. Not because I want brownie points but I wanted to see how it was all going and I did bother about him.
> (Ruth 15: year 3 term 2)   (Narrative 20)

Part of Ruth's concern about removing his urinary catheter may have been her discomfort at having to perform such an intimate task for somebody that she had become friendly with. She had not yet been able to develop a professional distance that may have protected them both from embarrassment. At that stage of her course she did not seem to have recognised such a need and perhaps this was as a result of her philosophy of solidarity with the patient.

3.6e Coping with ethical and moral dilemmas

Throughout the course Ruth demonstrated a thoughtful and in some aspects an almost rebellious attitude to her perception of much that was taken for granted by her peers and colleagues. An indication of this was illustrated by her questioning the purpose of healthcare and the ethical issues that this posed for someone who had no religious faith.

> I can see myself getting into an absolute mess with like, this ethical bit, totally. It's not that I didn't appreciate, it's just that I never have thought about it a lot before. Never really thought that as a nurse, you are invading somebody's body and what right have you got to do it. I can see me getting into a complete conundrum about issues like abortion, 'If it's what the woman wants, it's right'. And yet, even now, I can see, well is it? And I think that either I'll stay a bit grey and never really work it all out, or maybe I'll sort it all out. Personally, I do feel, people who have a spiritual or religious background, it helps them a lot more, to see the black and white. Because I don't have any religious grounding at all. I find it quite hard at times. I was talking to somebody about the issue of death, and they said well, if you know that they're going onto a better life that will help them to deal with it. Whereas you see I don't, I just don't know where, when people die I don't know where they go. I haven't got a clue. And, it doesn't worry me at the moment. But, yea it's something to think about.
> (Ruth 1: year 1 term 2)   (Narrative 21)

Having a philosophical framework to view her experiences of caring for patients and their relatives was important to Ruth. Knowing who she was and how she should behave with them also gave her much on which to reflect.

That also comes back to deciding to be on the patient's side. I'm not on the side of the hospital staff. If that makes sense. My bottom line is that I'm a person like anyone else who walks through the door. Maybe I perceive it all wrongly, but I get the impression that that's what the Health Service has done in the past and nurses have been as guilty of that as anyone else. Looking down on the naughty little patients who don't behave themselves. Whereas I think I'm just as human as anyone else. I've realised that a big part of nursing, as much as doing the dressing, etc., is your attitude and your way of being yourself. I think I've realised the impact I can make as an individual through just being myself and that's important.
(Ruth 20: year 4 term 1)   (Narrative 22)

This was a particularly important theme for Ruth and it remained with her for the majority of the course. Whilst she was caring for a small groups of patients independently she felt outside the clinical team. This perspective seemed to be influenced by her self-image as a nurse. However when it was threatened by a patient's lack of co-operation she needed the help of her team colleagues.

I also find one of the patients I'm looking after a bit difficult too, but with my mentor being very good it's OK. I was handing over to them and I said 'I just find her a bit tricky'. So we went in the side room and he asked what my problem was. I just explained all about it and didn't know if it was me. The issue is more that if I find someone tricky I tend to back down and she could almost be getting her way to her detriment. But they were fine. They took her on that evening and then I chatted with them next day when they were handing over and the male nurse did say that he found her the same. So that just made me think 'OK, I won't worry about it too much'. I always feel threatened as a student anyway, personally. I don't feel as valuable as the staff nurses, so although I don't necessarily think the patients always think that I'm not a member of staff. Again, you want to be, not popular with the ward, but I want to prove that I can fit into the team and do a job.
(Ruth 21: year 4 term 2)   (Narrative 23)

Ruth's feelings of vulnerability were important as they clearly influenced her interaction with her patient. This seemed surprising in view of her earlier assertions and perhaps indicated a transition in her social position where she was worrying about becoming a qualified nurse. Fortunately she was well supported emotionally by the staff, and it is evident that she was a sponsored member of the team. This made it possible to approach them for help and to share her experiences. Interestingly there was no evidence that the staff helped to her to see the world through the patient's eyes and thus broaden her own vision. Part of the image Ruth hoped to portray was one of efficiency and competency. It almost seemed that she saw this as a shield for ensuring patient compliance in undertaking the prescribed treatment. Perhaps because she was unsure how much she could safely allow the patient to deviate from their planned care and this reflects her isolation from the practices of expert nurses.

3.6f Presenting an image

Several of Ruth's narratives suggest her awareness of creating an image to her patients and her colleagues. She saw this as having an influence, not only on their response to her but also as a strategy to promote the patient's well-being. In her third and fourth years it became more overt and was observed during two visits to her placement. Following one observation, when she was making physical observations of an emotionally distressed patient, she was able to describe what she was thinking and feeling, not only about the impression she was trying to communicate but her thinking on how she created it.

> I thought it was important for him to talk and I didn't want it to look like I'd only come to do his temperature and blood pressure. I feel terribly sorry for all people in his position where I feel he really needs to unburden the anxiety he's carrying around. It's not that I was insincere to him at all. I'm concerned to listen and yet I can't help doing that, time is ticking away and it's part of my working hours. [I was trying to communicate that] I've got time to sit here with you and we we're on an equal level.
> (Ruth 18: year 4 term 1)   (Narrative 24)

It seemed that she was developing a fine balance between professional empathy and interest whilst shaping her patient's attention to her own agenda. This is a very complex and difficult activity when undertaken with subtlety and even more so with a disturbed patient. Ruth believed she learned to achieve this quality of performance by linking theory from the classroom activities and her reading, as well as from observing how others operate. On another occasion during an observation of her in practice, she coped with a potentially life threatening situation with confidence and reassurance and dealt with her own anxieties discretely in order to protect the patient.

> I don't think I've done neuro obs properly. I've never done neuro surgery or neuro medical before, so to some extent I was a bit out of my depth and I don't think there's any point in panicking in front of the patient. What I often do is walk out and panic in the corridor. But that's something I hope I'm good at and also the course has told us to be good at, and the staff expect it of us when we' re getting out of our depth. So by my mentor going off it wasn't a big problem because I just went and got someone.
> (Ruth 20: year 4 term 1)   (Narrative 25)

By giving the impression of being unconcerned she left the room and sought help and was subsequently taught how to carry out the procedure effectively. Essential to each aspect of these narratives was her belief that she needed to portray a particular image.

> I think it's important that I always portray a certain element of confidence to my patients, even if I don't feel so. You've got to look as though you know why you're there and what you're about and to give certain vibes to people. You should always look confident, although you don't feel it. I think my mentor would say I looked confident from day one, but obviously my confidence grew the more I got used to the ward and the staff ... I can imagine if you know you've got a bad day ahead of you, you stand at the door, take a few deep breaths and think 'OK, here I go', push the doors open and that's when it starts, the new role. I would compare it with the actor who puts on one costume, which is what you do as a nurse with your uniform – your costume, to portray this part. I like to hang onto my uniform in a way because that gives me a mask to hide behind.
> (Ruth 21: year 4 term 2)   (Narrative 26)

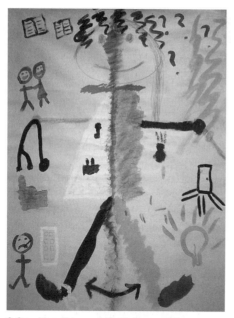

3.6a Year 2 term 1 'Split demands'.

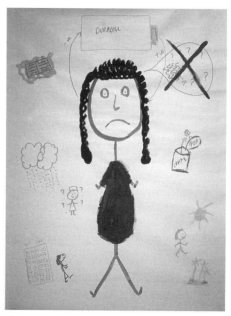

3.6b Year 2 term 2 'Duracell girl'.

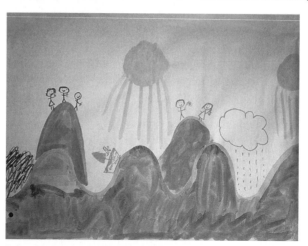

3.6c Year 2 term 3 'Good ship Ruth'.

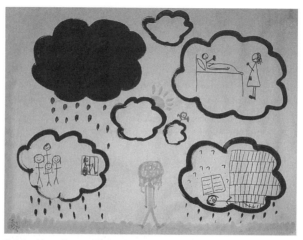

3.6d Year 3 term 2 'Shifting sands'.

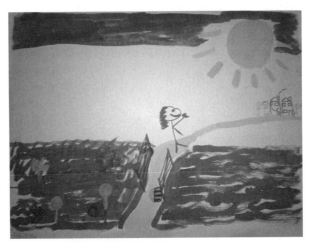

3.6e Year 3 term 3 'Green fields'.

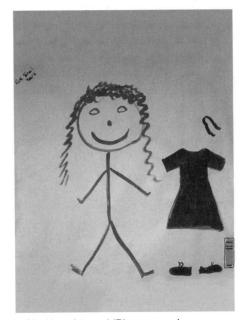

3.6f Year 4 term 1 'Pin-on nurse'.

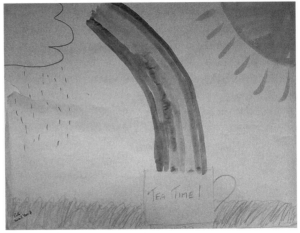

Figure 3.6 Ruth.   **3.6g** Year 4 term 3 'All in one'.

Wanting to be a nurse and to act like a nurse is a need that Ruth shared with her colleagues. Being able to create such an impression was an important part of becoming accepted by their clinical colleagues. Ruth's presentation of self as she was featured in her images which illustrated how she felt as a nursing student at the end of each term will be discussed in Chapter 5.

3.6g Ruth's professional development

Throughout her conversations, Ruth came across as a highly committed and conscientious person who frequently undervalued herself. Her pictures demonstrated the periods of self-doubt and preoccupation with the theoretical aspects of the course (see for example Figures 3.6a, 3.6b, 3.6c, and 3.6d). She resented spending so much time in the library when she would have preferred much more practical experience. Ruth always seemed to start her allocation with her learning objectives prepared and she worked consistently at developing and maintaining her learning contract as she progressed through each placement. She was exemplary amongst the students in doing so. It is possible that her science background and later attendance at evening classes for her accountancy examinations gave her this self-discipline. Despite this she found writing her assignments, the learning contracts a constant struggle because she had high expectations of her overall performance and became distressed when she did not meet them.

In her clinical placements, she occasionally talked about being alongside her mentor, actively engaged in giving care. Particularly in the early half of the programme, her main concern was with being left to trail around behind her mentor or feeling indebted to her. Rarely did she appear to feel she had a role as a member of the clinical team. This perhaps created a sense of guilt at taking her mentor or other members of the team from their own (more important) work when she needed help. As a result she wanted to reciprocate and compensate for their time by making herself useful, or by working independently. She was aware that she needed to keep in touch with her mentor and to seek help when necessary and it seems that her theoretical knowledge gave her a reasonable sense of this. The feedback she was receiving from her clinical mentors was good and she was clearly very able to rationalise her actions. She worked hard to increase her theoretical and practical understanding and knowledge about the patients she cared for, and she found the support of a small group of people invaluable in helping her to make sense of her experiences. She saw herself as being her patients' ally and working outside the team, rather than working as a member of the team working for the patient. She only developed her identity as being a team member when she felt sponsored to the community of practice and able to undertake the same activities as her qualified colleagues. Once she achieved this she developed a more objective view of her patients. It also helped her to integrate the different aspects of her life role: her personalities as Ruth the person, the student and the nurse. Her image (see Figure 3.6f) illustrates how she distinguished her role as a nurse from her everyday persona. For her at this stage in her development nursing was like stepping into the limelight and going on stage after donning her costume. It was not until her final term when she was able to feel settled into the clinical team that her identities merged as illustrated in her final picture (see Figure 3.6g). Despite her lack of self-confidence Ruth achieved a good 2:1 classification in her degree.

References

Åstedt-Kurki, P., Liukkonen, A. (1994) Humour in nursing care. *Journal of Advanced Nursing*, **20**: 183–8.

Benner, P., Wrubel, J. (1982) Skilled Clinical Knowledge: The value of perceptual awareness. *Nurse Educator* **VII** (3): 11–17.

Dreyfus., H.I., Dreyfus, S.E. (1986) *Mind over machine. The power of human intuition and expertise in the era of the computer*. Basil Blackwell, Oxford.

Ellis, C., Flaherty, M.G. (1992) *Investigating subjectivity: Researching on the lived experience*. Sage Publications Inc, Newbury Park.

Fuhrer, U. (1993) Behaviour setting analysis of situated learning: The case of newcomers. In: *Understanding practice. Perspectives on activity and context* (eds S. Chaiklin, J. Lave) Cambridge University Press, Cambridge.

Goody, E.N., ed. (1978) *Questions of Politeness: Strategies in social interaction*. Cambridge University Press, Cambridge.

Streubert, H.J. (1994) Male nursing students' perceptions of clinical experience. *Nurse Educator* **19** (5): 28–32.

Taylor, B.J. (1992) From helper to human: A reconceptualisation of the nurse as person. *Journal of Advanced Nursing* **17**: 1042–9.

Chapter 4

Being a Nurse

The six case studies illustrate each students' progress towards becoming a nurse. Linking each student is their motivation to become a nurse and images of their relationships with patients when giving care. These images appear to have been influenced by everyday observations of people, friends, family, neighbours or nurses and doctors caring for others or their own experiences of being nurtured by their family or by nurses in hospitals. Students who were unable to describe their approach to being a nurse in similar terms found that nursing was not for them. In contrast, the students who completed their programme did so because of their determination to realise their images. Somehow they sustained students' motivation to continue with their studies despite setbacks and challenges to their own identity and to their commitment.

Being a nurse and doing nursing were distinct in students' minds. The *being* aspects were concerned with affective needs; the *doing* related to tasks and technical procedures. Students' images were concerned with human aspects of nursing, such as giving emotional support, helping patients or their carers cope with illness, filling them with encouragement, being their advocate and being their ally in the face of adversity. These approaches to caring have been described by various authors as spiritual care, intimate care and emotional labour. By contrast students' understanding of the doing kinds of activities were drawn from television programmes and their views of nursing work tended to be instrumental and subservient to doctors. Inevitably as students progressed through their programme their understanding of their doing role changed from a lay to a professional perspective. But their images of how they wanted to provide care remained central to everything they did. Their concern was to learn how to give this kind of effective emotional support to their patients whilst presenting a professional demeanour. Whether they could achieve their dream in their everyday practice was very much influenced by the kinds of help and support they received from their clinical mentors and colleagues and the workload they were given. In this chapter I will explore the kinds of beliefs students in this study held when they first started as nursing students and how they learned to provide emotional care as they progressed through their programme.

4.1 Images of being a nurse

Before starting on their career the students had rejected ideas of working in an office, shop or factory as being boring. Several of them had tried it, either as a job or as a money-generating venture during their holidays or at weekends. By contrast, they equated nursing along with teaching as a worthwhile job. They viewed nursing as having job variety and they liked the idea of working with people, whom they anticipated would be grateful for their efforts. But students had no starry-eyed assumptions about the amount of stress nursing could cause them. Central to their beliefs was the emotional involvement with patients which they defined as caring. This presented a dilemma between over-involvement arising from close contact, and their personal need for the protective distancing that they believed and feared could result in hard-heartedness. They saw a fine distinction between the optimal level of each approach to caring and anticipated that team colleagues would provide a supportive network in times of stress. Their first encounters with people as clients in their first-year placements to the community came as a startling reminder of the variety of social backgrounds their patients came from. As Marie's narrative in Chapter 3.2 (Narrative 3, page 51) indicates, this was something of a culture shock.

Images of being a nurse: a guide to personal practice

When they started their course all the students carried images of how they saw themselves operating as nurses. These seemed to arise from a variety of sources, such as experiences of hospitalisation or being mothered when ill. They rarely believed that media portrayals of nurses had influenced their origination, although they acknowledged an avid interest in television programmes such as *Casualty*, which fostered their images. Individual images of nursing were concerned with the kinds of social contact they would make, talking to people and trying to make them better or being a 'mum' and acting as an advocate on their behalf. Their images influenced how they related to patients and also motivated them to continue with their course despite various setbacks and deterrents. Being supernumerary to the clinical team in their placements meant they had more time to relate to patients and to give care in the way they believed and had been taught constituted holistic, professional practice. This supernumerary status also gave them time to develop the necessary professional and clinical skills without undue workload pressures. As a result they could conserve their commitment to nursing and feel excited about extending their caring role, as so many graduate nurses have before them (Fitzpatrick 1993). Jack's strong images of how he wanted to practice, motivated him to seek an alternative path to his dream rather than modify his expectations. He held onto such images throughout his training as a psychiatric nurse and again all the way through the degree course. It was not until his final year that he began to wonder whether his efforts had been in vain. This was in his final clinical management module when he was under pressure from a workload that stressed even his qualified colleagues.

Perhaps this is what daunted so many student nurses who undertook their course without the luxury of being supernumerary and the 30% who promptly left on completion of the course. Helen knew she had always wanted to be a nurse but seemed to have difficulty articulating an image of what her ideal nurse would be like. Perhaps after so many years of working in nursing homes her original vision had become modified. Throughout the course she was uncertain whether she had made the right career decision and seemed unable to articulate what she hoped to give her patients. She found it a struggle to identify her own needs, acknowledging that she needed to be pushed by her mentors. Possibly it was part of a natural reticence or that her experiences in clinical placements had drained her enthusiasm and led to disillusionment. Despite their reservations both Helen and Jack as well as the other students continue to be in clinical practice some seven years after qualifying.

Interprofessional relationships

In stage one of the research it was evident that only Grace and Jack could draw on their earlier experiences of nursing, and so understood the complexities of different nursing roles or their relationship with other healthcare professionals. Despite protestations to the contrary, students' concepts of daily life on the wards appeared to have been derived from the media. They saw their future relationship with doctors as remote and hierarchical, with doctors prescribing treatments and care and generally functioning in a manner that was divorced from the everyday realities of patients' needs.

> *Nicola:* I think it [nursing] is the most difficult job because they have to interpret what the doctors say and it's prescribed in medical language and they have to interpret, explain in more simple terms.

> *Marie:* I think it's harder for nurses when one of their patients dies without the doctor coming. The nurse is caring for that patient. You can't not get [emotionally] involved if you are caring for someone all the time.
> (Group Interview 0/1: year 1 term 2)

Whether they came straight from school, from office work, or from nursing practice students held the same beliefs about how they would care for people. All but one research student held strong images of their relationship with patients, of *being* nurses. They had a limited concept of what they would actually be *doing*, the practical aspects of nursing other than what they had seen portrayed in the media or had actually experienced. Often their images of being a nurse had become an integral part of their personality, as if they had been formulated over a long period of time and were evident in different ways throughout their programme. Despite their limited understanding of how they would relate to other members of the healthcare team, or the detail of their day-to-day nursing role, students' images were concerned with the essence of practice and provided the rationale for all their actions and intentions as nurses. They were concerned with artistry rather than practical knowhow. Many aspects of their images relate to descriptions of holistic care as described by various authors writing about nursing intimacy (Williams 2001), spiritual care (Baldacchino 2001), or multicultural care (Holland 2001).

Students' images of caring

Three of the students had left school shortly before they started their course. They each held images of caring that were similar to those held by the older students. Marie had spent some time as a child in hospital and retained strong memories of how the nursing staff befriended her and made her feel part of a family.

> . . . thinking when I was growing up how much they [the hospital nursing staff] did for me, I suppose in a way I wanted to pay back the system . . . When I was younger I always used to take my nephews and nieces out and babysit for them. I also have two little brothers who are five and six years younger than me and so I've been brought up bringing up children and when my last nephew was born my sister couldn't look after him because she had an emergency Caesarean and she couldn't lift him. So my Mum and I looked after him. You can get used to looking after someone and you know what it feels like. I just loved it.
> (Marie 1: year 2 term 1)

These experiences of caring for her younger siblings as well her nieces and nephews encouraged her to become a children's nurse. Throughout her dialogues and indeed her observed practice, she appeared completely at ease during interactions with parents and children. They never feature as being problematic. It is as if her constructs of how to relate to children were so fully integrated into her whole personality that she never questioned her approach. Her commitment to relating to childrens' parents and meeting their needs when accompanying a daughter or son in hospital was also strong and she never appeared to be self-conscious or uncomfortable in their presence. Towards the end of the course she came to see herself as a team member and enjoyed the peer support and interaction that life on a hospital ward afforded.

> Intensive care isn't for me. That's important because before I thought I might like to work there. You don't have as much contact with parents because if they don't like seeing their child in there, and understandably some don't – some don't even like hospital let alone intensive care – you don't have as much contact with them. So it's made me realise that I like nursing on a medical ward. It's made me appreciate what my values are of nursing. As I'd like it to be team nursing, family-centred care. It's just made me look at myself more I think, and what I want out of my career. There's a buzz about being on the ward.
> (Marie 16: year 4 term 1)

It seems that whilst Marie worked in the children's intensive care unit she missed the satisfaction of developing close relationships with her patients or their parents. When entering the programme she identified the importance of being part of a ward family and the friendliness of her own hospital experiences. Creating similar kinds of relationships and environments for her patients and their families made nursing worthwhile for her. Working in intensive care was too remote from this kind of contact for her satisfaction. She was shocked when she realised that some children's wards did not permit free visiting. Her image of being a good children's nurse was to work in partnership with their parents.

The second school-leaver was Nicola who chose to take the mental health nursing programme. Early on in the programme her reasons for choosing nursing were not clearly formulated but her commitment to talking and listening to people, which is an essential part of the therapeutic role, was evident.

> Perhaps my view of general nursing, there's some stereotyping I'm sure, there's just as much basic chores in what there might be aspects of nursing as general – part of the job really. When I got back last week [from observation on a psychiatric ward] – it made me think: 'Yes I think this is what I want to do'. Sort of made it clear in my mind but I think that I do want to do it even more perhaps . . . I used to say to friends that I wanted to be a nurse. People used to say to me 'Er! What do you want to do that for?'
>
> That scares me more 'than anything else', the actual physical, injecting, taking blood pressure, rather than like sitting down and talking to people. I'm sure you can do damage talking to people but it's not like doing physical damage. I think it's horrendous . . .
>
> Perhaps the word therapy is a strong word, but I mean it is emotionally disturbing and you need to be able to talk about those things. Well, I do, I know. I do think it's very important to be able to talk about what you're going through . . . and then to keep it all in proportion. Just to tell you that you're doing all right and it's not the be-all and end-all.
>
> My mother, she was always the one who nursed me, when I had been ill at home, so I do think we do carry on that sort of, 'play the role' model. Like I think the media, programmes like *Casualty*, and Florence Nightingale images all spring to mind, when you mention nursing. I don't know how I'd nurse actually, if it was me. I think sitting down and talking about it. You can't talk about someone being sick, obviously you've got to do some practical.
> (Nicola 0: year 1 term 2)

Nicola gives the impression of viewing nursing as a physical activity that she seems to find unattractive. Her individual interview revealed her desperation to make a career decision and a need to understand mental illness better. Yet despite her uncertainty about her career choice, she held very strong views of the importance of talk as a medium for maintaining emotional health. In the early stages of her course, she found it hard to attach this belief to psychiatric nursing and yet it is an image that she pursues throughout her programme. Her second concern was her youth and need for personal development, to know herself better. Nicola's openness and willingness to share and examine her feelings were essential ingredients for her preparation and future role as a mental health nurse. She expressed this more clearly after her first experience of working in the speciality:

> . . . the majority of them you wouldn't know that they were mentally ill. Perhaps you do begin to realise when you form a relationship. Perhaps mental illness is just when you lose control completely and you just can't cope and it's your way of coping, but not coping. Or perhaps it is biological or chemical. My immediate reaction is that I want to form a friendship with them and try and draw them out that way. I'm actually quite shocked that I've said that because I didn't think I'd feel that way, but I do. I don't feel very scared that that's what I would like to do and then begin to tackle the problem by looking back over past events and trying in a different way to treat them. But then again I don't feel I know enough about it, so I hope when I qualify I will know enough about it . . . That was my worry really about the whole thing. That I could relate some of my emotions to how they feel, but actually I feel at the moment fairly self-aware. I know my strengths and weaknesses I suppose and I'm probably quite lucky that I can actually do this and can cope with it, but I haven't had many

eventful things happening on the psychiatric ward yet. It must be a big fear though that you could perceive yourself as mentally ill. There seems to be such a thin line between the two that you probably just need the strength of character to jump back to the other side of the line when you go home and knock off work. That's quite an interesting point really.
(Nicola 2: year 2 term 1)

Nicola's willingness to acknowledge her own fears perhaps gave her strength and opportunities to receive the support she needed. A stronger picture emerges of her willingness to relate to patients at a personal level and to understand their difficulties. In effect she translated her own ideals into a role definition for becoming a mental health nurse. She continued with this method of learning and developing her role as a mental health nurse throughout her programme and even at the end she was able to explore her own feelings both as a means of understanding herself and those of her patients.

I must admit that this term was the first term that I had a conflict within the team and actually could acknowledge to myself that one of the patients really pissed me off and that's quite a big thing because you're almost expected not to have these feelings about people. I wrote quite a lot about that in my LC. It was really difficult because I don't think I really handled it well or not. She was a woman who's very intrusive on staff time. If you're sitting out in the corridor doing obs on people she would always come and sit right next to you and talk at you for hours . . . You feel like saying 'Shut up and go away and leave me in peace' . . . When I went away and thought about it a bit more, I thought I'd been quite blinkered in my attitude to her because she really pissed me off badly and I couldn't see beyond those feelings to actually think about what may be making her the way she is. So I now think it's important to recognise that you feel these things about people but to feel them and then get rid of them if you can. Look beyond them to what's going on for her really.
(Nicola 15: year 4 term 3)

Through self-examination Nicola learned how to use her ideals in a constructive manner to support her role. Even though in the early stages of her programme her images of nursing work and being a nurse were unclear. Her guiding principle of talking and listening sustained her commitment and her practice. This contrasts with Natalie who started the course and then decided to leave after her fifth term. She held only vague views about her role as a nurse and her commitment to nursing was uncertain. She was more concerned with being a university student and enjoying the kind of life that it offered.

Really I think I did want to be a nurse. But I didn't want to train as a nurse because I wanted poly life. So, if I hadn't got my grades to come here to do a nursing degree, I wouldn't have gone and done nursing training, I'd have just done any degree that I could get on because I wanted to be at poly. My brother was at poly and I went up to stay with him and I knew what life was like for students and I loved it. I thought, 'I've got to go to poly or university, whatever'. So that was more important, in a way, than anything else.

But, I did want to do nursing, and so it was good, because I could get both nursing and uni. I would do everything [for the patients] I want to chat to people, I want to take temperatures and blood pressures, clean and wash them – I just want to chip in and do everything. I took this boy's temperature – it's nothing, is it? But as soon as I'd done it, the parents looked at me and said, 'Is it alright?' and I went, 'Yes, it's fine, it's normal' and I wrote it on

his chart and that was like, 'Oh, WOW! I'm a nurse.' It was such a simple thing, but it was a really good feeling.
(Natalie 1: year 2 term 1)

Natalie's decision to leave the programme was perhaps influenced by a complex range of factors. She had only a vague notion of what she would be doing as a nurse and found it difficult to describe any image of how she would be caring despite participating in the focus group sessions and hearing the other students talking about their images. She experienced a conflict between her career choice and her enthusiasm to be a university student and as result she left the programme and completed a biology degree.

Helen struggled throughout her programme to resist the conflict between being a university student and being a nurse. She had worked for five years in her vacations as a care assistant in nursing homes for the elderly. Her images of nursing were influenced by her past experiences of working as a care assistant, as a result she did not value giving essential care to her patients. She envisaged nurses as being more technical. Despite this, she clearly imagined how patients should be cared for and could recognise differences in approaches used by nurses, sometimes selfishly and sometimes as a result of external demands on their time. Her descriptions of nursing were more concerned with concrete tasks. Her concern was to balance what she perceived to be a professional demeanour (of indifference) and her fear of losing or blunting her feelings, perhaps her feminine side. Rather like Natalie, she believed that she would learn sophisticated techni-cal activities, but she also held strong images of how she would be as a nurse and this was essentially concerned with the nature of her relationship with patients. Towards the end of her programme this became more explicit when describing her concern about the different ways she saw nurses relating to patients.

> What's really been annoying me this term is the image of nursing. Like the patients thinking 'I'm alright because I've got all these lovely nurses around me' and a lot of the nurses I find invade the patient's space and I know having been a patient I don't like someone being really close to me. You can't escape if you're in bed. Just the way they joke around and flirt with the patients, I hate it. I used to think that was the image of nursing and you had to be that kind of person and now the thought of it makes me feel awful. I feel the more they do it, it's almost as though the nurses are living what they're supposed to be – their image. I don't like it. I think that's another thing that is putting me off nursing. I didn't really see it on the oncology ward or the head injuries, but perhaps that's just different circumstances. I've seen it somewhere else. I didn't feel I didn't fit in. But then the surgical ward had a very profes-sional approach and they scared the living daylights out of me. And I just thought I wanted some nurses who talked about everyday things once in a while rather than always talking about nursing.
> (Helen 10: year 4 term 1)

This suggests Helen held images of an ideal nurse who was somewhere between these two extremes and she was struggling to find her own way of relating to patients that was authentic.

The three mature students who had given up jobs and homes to start nursing were able to talk about their images of caring with greater confidence. Ruth had visited her parents' when they were on duty in their hospital wards when she was a child. She came to the course after several years in the commercial world and gave the impression of being an independent thinker. She held very strong images of how she would be working as a nurse. These were concerned with a combination of interpersonal skills and knowledge. She advocated a 'loving attitude' to promote her patients' wellbeing and cooperation; being 'mumsy' as she described it.

> If you realise what makes you feel nice, if you were in a strange bed and things like that, then that would help you to appreciate the little touches for a person, coming into a ward, so there is value in all those sort of reminders. I've always just thought a loving attitude, really, to actually, like, want to hold people's hands and I think you need an element of toughness in you too, not to be pushed around by people . . . and being, confident in yourself. Well I think you need to know the workings of the body. You can learn all the theory in the world but really you've just gotta, to get on with people. They're the main things.
> (Ruth 1: year 1 term 2)

Ruth presented a warm friendliness and respect for patients that was congruent with memories of seeing her father in hospital and feelings that she would like to be a mother. A further strong image was of wanting to make a difference to patients' hospital experiences, of imbuing a sense of spring, sunshine and optimism.

> I think it's part of just your daily being pleasant to people. At the right time have a smile on your face and always be willing to have a laugh and a joke. With all this research and educational approach to nursing I worry that we may lose some of the human touches. I think it's in my nature. It just helps me get on with people really. It helps people accept you.
> (Ruth 11: year 2 term 3)

Throughout her programme Ruth held onto these beliefs. While she was able to enjoy the privilege of being a student, she also came to see herself as an advocate for her assigned patients working outside the ward or departmental team. She was also aware of the dilemma some nursing duties create, such as doing tasks she found personally unpleasant or too intimate.

> I think part of the beauty I find of being a student is that I have time to spend with people and one would hope I can actually use this time. We do it all in theory, the therapeutic relationship and spending time with people and I'm very aware that as a qualified member of staff I won't have the time to do that, which is sad, but I think that's the way it probably is. So everyone that I admit I want to make it meaningful. I've really got this sense I suppose that someone coming into hospital is slightly the underdog and they're quite vulnerable and I don't want them to think that I'm not on their side because I am. And that's something I'll have to balance out as I become qualified and even now. There are times when I'll have to do unpleasant things with people and I'm sure part of the professionalism will be learning to marry the two. Like the parent who has to be firm, there will be times I have to do that, but maybe I can get away with it at the moment. I'm still feeling my feet, but I'm still on the balance of holding hands with them and the 'I'm on your side' type thing, rather than 'Look, I'm the nurse and you do what I say' type thing. My bottom line is to relate to them hope-

fully as a person. Have this sense of 'I know what you're going through' – I was going to say that but that's not fair because I don't. Rather 'You're not alone'.
(Ruth 15: year 3 term 2)

In trying to find a suitable image that exemplifies the kinds of activities and role she may have to assume Ruth sees herself in a paternalistic role that contradicts her other ideals. At the end of the course, in her last placement she was working as a member of a busy clinical team and under pressure to achieve a specified workload. This shifted her focus away from patients' individual needs and her contribution to meeting them and towards her contribution as a clinical team member. It suggests that by adopting a professional identity somehow her earlier ideals are suppressed. She still retained her image of caring for individual patients but this had been tempered by expediency.

> Certainly you're moving back from being totally round the one patient. You're moving away from the patient and I think my quandary is that, that is what professional nursing is all about. About a bit of distance and objectivity and in my opinion, a bit of less caring. Maybe that's what certainly my mum would say 'You're becoming a professional now'. Whereas I actually think you're losing something by becoming that professional and I suppose my quandary is, particularly in this current climate of quality: 'Is that still very high quality professional care or could professional care be better?' . . . I will probably have to rationalise that it's the best professional care I can give, given the constraints of the environment. I would see that movement away from the patient as an unfortunate side effect probably.
> (Ruth 22: year 4 term 3)

Perhaps in order to survive as a full member of a nursing team Ruth has had to sacrifice her principles of individualised care and of being central to her patients' wellbeing. She seems to have adopted a stance that frees her from guilt and allows her to cope with her workload. Her vision of being patient-centred, or 'mumsy' and an ally, was tempered by her encounters with a larger workload and consequent reduced time to relate to her patients.

Like Ruth, Jack had strong beliefs in the importance of getting to know his patients, of befriending them. Throughout his programme he maintained this view of putting patients first and several observational visits also confirmed this. Jack's images of caring included his concept of therapeutic touch and being engaged in supporting people as individuals, giving them hope, helping them make sense of their experiences and relieving both physical and emotional discomfort. He had experiences of working with disabled people that contradicted the stereotypes that his first teachers gave him and as a result he resisted categorising people, preferring to acknowledge their individuality. His images of being a nurse were powerful and sustained him through the difficult early months of his first attempt at general nursing. So strongly was he committed to this ideal that Jack left because of the conflict between treating patients as work objects and his desire to realise his vision of caring. Like Ruth he found taking on a full caseload of dependent patients limited the time that he could spend with individuals and caused him to feel despair and to wonder what he had sacrificed so much for. However he maintained his optimism and vision as he became more adept at managing his caseload

> I don't think I've essentially changed. In some ways nursing in the last ten years has come round to my way of thinking. That sounds really arrogant, but you know what I mean. The idea of talking to patients and getting to know them, which is what I wanted to do at [first training school] and was getting criticised for. It's somehow become accepted as good nursing in a way, which I felt then but couldn't articulate it. Alan Pearson's book [*Primary Nursing*], that sort of thing, that way of working, which was my philosophy I suppose. That sounds arrogant, doesn't it? Not even a philosophy, but the way I wanted to do it. I'd sit and talk to patients and does it really matter if the sluice is clean? It's been cleaned this morning, it can be cleaned again at night. But somehow this idea of sitting down talking to patients, getting to know them as individuals, not treating them as the appendix in bed 6. Not doing the back round at 3.00pm. Actually giving them the tablets when perhaps they want the tablets and not at 6.00pm when perhaps they don't need them. Giving them at 4.00pm when they've got a pain. It just seemed so sensible to me then, but I couldn't seem to reason with anyone. [Mentors here have encouraged me to use that] as a way of working and I suppose in some ways that's why I felt more comfortable doing it. Nursing has caught up with me in a way.
> (Jack 16: year 4 term 3)

Grace who had considerable experience of working in hospitals as a healthcare assistant and as a student nurse had strong feelings about giving care that met patients' personal and emotional needs.

> If you want a not, not so good [nurse] you just go there and you give the care. You really don't get involved. You just do what you're supposed to do. You give the dressings, 'Oh I'm supposed to give Mrs Jones a dressing'. You just go and do the dressing. Whereas, if you're a good nurse, you really get involved with the patient. You get to know them as a person. I don't know, some nurses don't think about how a patient likes sitting if they're going to have a dressing done. Or, whether they like having a wash instead of a bath, and things like that. Before they just used to, 'Oh you're having a bath'. And that's it. ''Cos it's your day to have a bath!'.
> (Grace 1: year 1 term 2)

These three older students joined the programme with a commitment to become registered nurses. This was not to be without considerable financial cost. Their strong images of how they anticipated relating to patients formed the central aspect to their nursing role.

4.2 Caring and intimacy

Jourard (Jourard 1971) describes nursing as a special case of loving, through an ability to be open, honest and in touch with self, which promotes self-development. Students' conceptions of their relationship with patients epitomised much of Jourard's vision. Such combinations of intimacy, reciprocity and partnership relate to Muetzel's description of therapeutic nursing (Muetzel 1988) and characterise the aesthetic dimension of nursing care described by

Carper (Carper 1978) whereby patients are seen as people experiencing life-events that are part of the student's life experience as well. Students' ability to provide technical care, to relate to patients whilst providing care and to have a sound knowledge base which informed their practice were all important components of their professional knowledge. More subtle attributes of caring and nursing were concerned with the manner in which they offered care and the ethos they created by their interactions with their patients. Being able to implement their vision of caring was promoted by students' supernumerary status. This gave them the necessary opportunities to relate to patients without any extra stress of having to get a set amount of work done within a time limit. Their course philosophy embraced the concept of reflective practice, and assessment strategies encouraged students to develop self-awareness. As we have seen from their case studies they often found this work challenging and sometimes painful, leading them to appraise and question their experiences. Perhaps Nicola was the most vulnerable of the students as she was the most conscious of using her selfhood when working with patients. As she identified among other things, she was frequently discomforted by her patients' socially inappropriate behaviour. As her case study illustrates Nicola was conscious that she needed to develop a strategy that safeguarded herself without jeopardising her therapeutic role:

> You are offering up you. You offer up part of you that's been adapted into this psychiatric nurse role. I do offer up myself, but I know that to keep myself sane I have to hide part of myself. I think you have to have a professional role, otherwise you'd just do your head in. (Nicola 13: year 4 term 1)

Nicola's strong awareness of the boundaries of her role and relationship with patients is reflected to a lesser extent in the narratives of other students as they developed their role. As they became more confident in their knowledge and technical skills, their ability to provide care which was in keeping with their images of good practice began to inform their approach more fully. Her ability to distance herself from her practice was a healthy development and perhaps saved her from suffering from burnout. Nicola's approach to caring could be seen as the essence of therapeutic care. But it can come with some cost to the practitioner unless she or he develops ways of maintaining authenticity without suffering emotional harm. Indeed some writers suggest that creating such relationships is positively harmful and defence systems such as those described by Menzies (Menzies 1966) where responsibility is passed through the organisation are effective ways of protection from burnout. Hochshild (Hochschild 1983) argues for effective preparation of practitioners engaged in emotional labour. Drawing on experience from social work Aldridge (Aldridge 1994) argues that without adequate emotional training and support, nurses face mental distress and exhaustion. In times of financial stringency, shortages of adequately trained staff, and maximum bed occupancy, nursing staff and students receive little effective support and their professional skills are more likely to become debased and devalued by incentives to get work done.

Throughout their programme students were exposed to a range of theoretical models of nursing practice, all of which advocated an holistic approach to patient care. Students' narratives illustrate how they strived to achieve this. Students' development was derived from a range of sources beyond the technical or managerial. They saw ways in which they could act out as well as try and implement their own beliefs about therapeutic practice. As they became more experienced, their workload changed and they were faced with a sense of regression when they struggled to implement prescribed care for a group of patients. Jack expresses the challenge they all experienced:

I think you're trying to give high quality care. This lady is depressed. I think I could really help her. This morning she's a lot brighter. I don't think that's anything I did because I was on yesterday morning looking after her and she was totally flat. And this morning she's totally different. Maybe it's the anti-depressants starting to work because she's been on them just under a week. But I suppose that's the thing that's lacking. You're giving her good physical care and looking after her that way, but that isn't enough, but you could spend half-an-hour just sitting chatting to her and I haven't got that time. She does need quite a lot and you wash her. I'm spending a lot of time trying to motivate her, so I am putting the psychological bit in there while I'm doing the physical bit. It's all aimed at her getting to do a wash and you're asking how she feels and she says 'I don't know, I'm fed up'. But it's just that, [it] still isn't enough in a way. I suppose it's because it's an acute medical ward.
(Jack 15: year 4 term 3)

The essence of nursing and of giving such care was students' ability to be 'present' with their patients and to see and respond to their needs effectively. Having such presence is described by Godkin (Godkin 2001) as having a healing nature and to be an essential attribute of expert nurses. Nursing students' such as these, holding the attitudes but not yet the knowledge and skills can still contribute to such therapeutic care when supported by expert practitioners. Inevitably students would be unlikely to deliver care that matched their ideals all of the time but it was evident from their dialogues that they held their images in mind and they provided great personal satisfaction, despite being difficult to articulate:

One of the mums, whose child I'd admitted from A&E, came onto the ward and was very agitated and I said 'Have you been down there long?' and she said she'd been down there since 10:00am and it was now 7:00pm. I asked if she had other children at home and she said she had four others and I said 'I expect you're worried about them. I offered her the chance to go and phone up to check they were all right and she said no, it was alright. So I said I'd get it done as quickly as possible so she could go home. Having four children at home, it must have been a nightmare for her and them not knowing where she was. They were all school age children, 5, 6, 7 or 8 years old and so when they came home from school, their Mummy wasn't there or they got picked up by someone else so they were probably worried about their Mum. She had the number of the hospital and we'd got her number so that we could contact her. But it's important that you appreciate that parents have other lives apart from that child, like work commitments, etc., and other family members. I don't know why, but I really noticed, and it's just like saying 'It's OK to go home. We're here to

care for your children. Because we leave you to it when you're here doesn't mean that we're not here for you, it's because you're there and you're the one your child knows'.
(Marie 12: year 3 term 3)

Marie's recognition of her role in providing strategies that could reassure her patient's mother, indicates an awareness beyond the technical and immediate demands of her task. She appears sensitive to the implications of the mother's anxiety, and in using a range of understandings brought them together to provide an outlet for her. In a different situation Nicola's acceptance of her emotionally disturbed patients and her willingness to work alongside them as part of their therapy illustrates her commitment and preparedness to learn through her own pain.

References

Aldridge, M. (1994) Unlimited liability? Emotional labour in nursing and social work. *Journal of Advanced Nursing* 20: 722–8.

Baldacchino, D., Draper, P. (2001) Spiritual coping strategies: a review of the nursing research literature. *Journal of Advanced Nursing* 34 (6): 822–32.

Carper, B.A. (1978) Fundamental patterns of knowing. *Advances in Nursing Science* 1: 13–23.

Fitzpatrick, J.M., While, A.E., Roberts, J.D. (1993) The relationship between nursing and higher education. *Journal of Advanced Nursing* 18: 1488–97.

Godkin, J. (2001) Healing presence. *Journal of Holistic Nursing* 19 (1): 5–21.

Hochschild, A. (1983) *The Managed Heart*. University of California Press, Berkeley.

Holland, K., Hogg, C. (2001) *Cultural Awareness in Nursing and Health Care*. Arnold, London.

Jourard, S.M. (1971) The 'manners' of helpers and healers: The bedside manners of nurses. In: *The Transparent Self*. (ed. S.M. Jourard), pp. 179–207. Van Norstrand Reinhold, New York.

Menzies, I. (1966) *The functioning of social systems as a defence against anxiety.* (A report on the nursing service of a general hospital.) Centre for Applied Social Research, The Tavistock Institute of Social Relations, London.

Muetzel, P. (1988) Therapeutic nursing. In: *Primary Nursing: Nursing in the Oxford and the Burford Nursing Development Units*. (ed. A. Pearson) pp. 89–116, Croom Helm, London.

Williams, A. (2001) A literature review on the concept of intimacy in nursing. *Journal of Advanced Nursing* 33 (5): 660–7.

Chapter 5
Feeling Like a Nurse

In Chapter 4 we explored how students in this research used their images of nurses and nursing to conceptualise their future role and their relationships with patients. Their images and conceptions also influenced the way they learned and worked as nursing students. Throughout their programme, students accumulated a considerable amount and variety of formal and informal knowledge. As we saw from their accounts (Helen's particularly), an intrinsic aspect of this learning was accumulating supplementary images of how nurses function and relate to patients. Students undertaking the programme had varying amounts of earlier experiences in caring activities or being cared for and consequently, had already acquired a variety of personal and professional skills and knowledge.

Jack's earlier experiences of training for two parts of the Professional Register, whilst Grace had worked as a healthcare assistant as well as undertaking six months' pupil nurse training. Their experiences had equipped them with many technical and professional relating skills. Marie had been a patient and had cared for her young nephews and nieces as well as her grandmother. As a result she had developed a concept of what a child's life in hospital would be like as well as understanding how to relate to children. By contrast, Ruth had both parents working as nurses and had cared for disabled people on holidays and so had grown up immersed in nursing talk. Through most of her university vacations, she worked as a care assistant either in a nursing home or a hospital ward. Nicola had similar experiences and family connections with healthcare professionals. She had acquired the image of mental health nursing as an ability to express feelings and to discuss experiences in a supportive environment. Helen had spent the most amount of time working as a care assistant and had also worked in an orphanage for a year.

All the students had invested a considerable amount of their free time preparing for their career choice and spending their lives on care-giving activities. Once immersed in the programme their clinical hours were used to develop their identity as nurses and to reformulate their role until they could demonstrate the skills and attributes of their chosen community of practitioners. In one sense students' personal images of how they wanted to be as nurses provided a structure or grammar for their actions and they anticipated the course would provide a means of expressing their images or provide a form of vocabulary. By encountering numerous different clinical placements, it was as if they were exposed to a range of languages expressing the ways in which nurses practised. In the process students were subjected to a variety of associated challenges which lessened as they became more able to pass themselves off as being like their qualified colleagues. The most challenging aspect of their development was how to adjust to these different social environments and whether they could or wanted to identify with their resident healthcare professionals. Students' learning was fraught with anxiety, self-questioning and doubt. They wanted to become nurses but spent most of their programme not feeling at all like a nurse. In this chapter we will explore how students responded to these periods of doubt, disorientation, confusion and their gradual progress towards a state of equilibrium. Their illuminative artwork provides graphic images of what this process was like and we will consider the kinds of knowledge and understanding students acquired whilst learning to make such adjustments and to develop as nurses. In particular we shall look at:

- how they believed they learned to be like a nurse
- whether and how their practice was influenced.

5.1 The nature of socialisation

Learning to be like other members of a community requires several kinds of knowledge. Social aspects of life are influenced by existing customs and practices that are intended to maintain homogeneity and create a shared identity. Newcomers are faced with a choice of conforming or being cast as an outsider and rejected. With students passing through several different communities this presents a considerable challenge. Their progress through their career depends on being accepted by their clinical colleagues. After all their programme is 50% practice and these people will be determining their progress when they write their assessment reports at the end of their clinical placement. Students often have very little time to make the necessary adjustments to fit in. Moving from one clinical specialty, such as working with people who are elderly and mentally frail imposes different norms than working with young substance abusers. The same kinds of schisms occur in other branches of nursing. A further dichotomy facing students when they started their course was the difference between school or employment, and university. They had no previous experience of university life. Making the adjustment from being a respected and valued member of their previous community, whether it was a sixth-form, a firm or a clinical setting presented further challenges, as Ruth in particular highlights. Further differences compounded their bewilderment such as the difference in expectations of a professional course and a subject-specific course, and of having a 50% practical component in their programme. This often meant attending distant placements early in the morning or until late evening. All these differences limited students' ability to join in with the regular and normal student activities. As Figure 5.1 illustrates, students were overwhelmed by the adjustments they needed to make in the first year of their course.

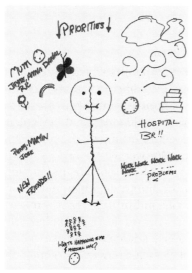

5.1a Marie, year 2 term 1 'Tensions'.

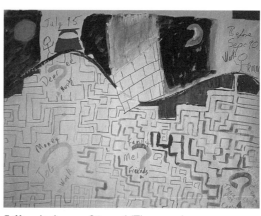

5.1b Jack, year 2 term 1 'The maze'.

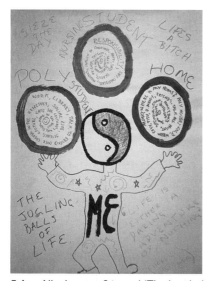

5.1c Nicola, year 2 term 1 'The juggler'.

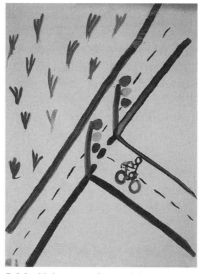

5.1d Helen, year 3 term 3 'Junction choices'.

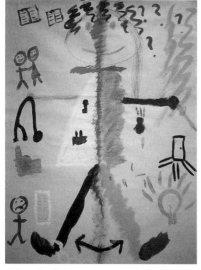

5.1e Ruth, year 2 term 1 'Split demands'.

Figure 5.1 Disconfirmation.

Socialisation is more than the outward acquisition of cultural trappings. It is concerned with identity and evolving self-image as a member of the community which reflects changes in the life cycle. Learning to become a member of a community includes adopting behaviours, language, dress and modes of thought that are characteristics of that community. The purpose is to ensure all the members maintain the status quo and they operate as a cohesive group. For example wearing shabby clothes is expected of university students but not of nursing students when in contact with patients. Nursing students face difficulties when moving between one clinical setting and another. Learning the different forms of language used, what the numerous terms and abbreviations mean and being able to use them fluently and accurately provides evidence of integration and membership. Through regular and frequent contact with colleagues or old-timers in the community of practice, newcomers begin a process of transformation. Helen reported finding one particular mentor helpful, when he explained the meaning of different terms used in patients' case notes. For Ruth it was learning not to use everyday forms of address that were not culturally acceptable in her new environment.

> I'd like to think it's just my general way of dealing with people. I accept that I often call people 'love' and 'dear'. You shouldn't use patronising terms, but then I don't see it as patronising. In the East End of London, where I come from, you get called that all the time.
> (Ruth 6: year 2 term 2)

Being told that she should not call patients 'love' or 'dear', on the basis that it could be interpreted as patronising, was a puzzling experience. It was something that Ruth was prepared to accept as part of getting used to the new cultural expectations of the profession and thus to become an invisible member of the nursing team. The visible trappings of being a nursing student did not help adjustment to the role either.

> Wearing a uniform, it tells people who you are and in what capacity. I've got those old fashioned hang-ups that nurses wear one. . . . You're never really part of the team. I felt I got on with people OK. I don't think being called 'nurse' made me feel part of the team. Just the other staff's attitude towards me and my attitude to them.
> (Ruth 11: year 2 term 3)

As Ruth's narrative indicates, one key issue is the quality of students' relationships with clinical staff and whether they hold the same values and norms expected of newly qualified nurses and healthcare professionals. The same norms and values students were expected to learn from them. However, if there was a difference then a student's failure to conform to the community's norms can have deleterious consequences as Jack reported from his first training experience (see Chapter 3, Jack: Narrative 3, page 77). As Jack and the other students discovered, it was important to become familiar with the cultural norms of each placement. Rather like the tourist going to Rome, adopting local customs enhances relationships. Learning to identify these social norms can be a challenging experience, especially in the early days of their course. Melia (Melia 1987), in her ethnographic study of pre-registration nursing students, found that they spent a considerable time in each new placement trying to identify the ward sister's preferences as well as those of the rest of the staff. A situation not always dissimilar to the students in this study as Jack recounted when comparing his earlier experiences with his degree course (see Chapter 3, Jack: Narrative 9, page 80). Adjusting to the nursing degree programme also required considerable effort.

> Working through these mazes and trying to understand things and get a better knowledge base. I see myself in this maze, it's a new course and I'm unfamiliar with this way of studying again. With the RMN (course) you knew where the target was when they gave you learning objectives and you knew whether you were aiming off centre or whether you were OK. With this (course) you have to think about a lot more and be more geared up and self motivated and confident.
> (Jack 3: year 2 term 1)

Students' worries about adjusting to the programme and to the idea of being a nursing student are part of a settling-in process. By contrast Helen's sense of uncertainty about her career choice developed as she progressed through the programme. They seem to have been fuelled by her reluctance to conform to images offered by her clinical colleagues. She stated how much she hated the flirtatious behaviour of one set of colleagues and was overwhelmed by the single-minded dedication of another. Carr and Kemmis (Carr 1986) identify six essential features of critical social experience that lead to human beings feeling oppressed, but through which they can also find liberation. Four of these are concerned with social experiences. The first feature they describe, concrete social experience, relates to Jack's early experiences of learning to be a general nurse where he felt isolated because he believed in putting patients first, and his qualified colleagues did not appreciate this approach. Secondly, personification of participants – for all the participants being accepted and able to work in some way as a team member was important. Thirdly, analysis of experience is concerned with how students interpreted their experiences and related them to their existing knowledge and beliefs. Both Jack and Helen's dilemmas about whether to leave nursing were influenced by their interpretation of seemingly conflicting images of how different nurses related to patients and their own beliefs. Fourthly, contextual operating mechanisms, or the way in which policies and practice influence students' ability to feel part of a community. Marie's experiences of the telephone affected her sense of being an outsider, unable to participate in the setting as did Ruth's feelings of being like a 'puppy dog'. Grace's financial and social difficulties also influenced the extent to which she could meet the assignment targets and so limited her ability to participate as a nursing student within the academic community.

Role acquisition – learning to become a nurse

> They didn't allocate you to patients. I felt part of the nursing assistant team, but not part of the trained nurse team, that team was a bit too elite anyway.
> (Petra 3: year 3 term 3)

In any culture newcomers may choose to accept or reject the socialisation influences of their new environment. In rejecting such influences they remain outside the cultural norms of the community. Initially the students saw themselves as university students, and then on entry into clinical practice settings initially saw themselves as something akin to healthcare assistants. Gradually they came to see themselves as nursing students. Their experiences of role acquisition were not smooth and throughout the course several seemed to be only tentatively committed to nursing. This was most evident in Natalie and Helen's narratives, but it was also true of the others. By taking a degree in nursing all students felt they were enhancing their future prospects and if they became too unhappy they had a better opportunity to transfer to a different degree rather than leave the university altogether. Three of the research participants did make the decision to leave the programme. Later, two returned to nursing after a break of a year or more and the third (Natalie) left nursing altogether. Their case studies indicate the struggle students endured to settle into the programme. Ruth, Nicola and Marie shared a similar pattern of socialisation, albeit at different rates of progress through each stage. But this was experienced differently by Helen, Grace and Jack for reasons that may be attributed to their conceptions of nursing on entry.

Over the programme, it became clear that students underwent several stages in their response to normative socialisation influences. Their adjustment to becoming nurses seemed to accelerate after longer periods in a clinical setting. In the early part of their programme students moved through several placements. This was to meet professional and European Directives requiring them to have taster experiences of the four branches of nursing (mental health, learning disability, care of children and adult nursing) as well as experiences of midwifery; home care, and care of older people. In their two-year common foundation programme students were exposed to short placements and rapid movement between placements. In reality students could afford to ignore attempts at socialisation as many practitioners were overwhelmed by the constant influx of students and were more concerned to provide supervision and experience. The timing of these placements so early in their programme meant students were anxious to do well and preoccupied with fitting in so experienced considerable discomfort if they felt unsupported. Their willingness to be influenced by some nursing colleagues depended upon their own images of nursing and how much they saw their mentors or other staff (old timers) practice in the same manner. Despite coming into nursing with such a range of different experiences and expectations of the programme, students' accounts of their transition towards becoming nurses, and their artwork demonstrate themes and stages that were common, although not necessarily taking place at the same time in their programme. Drawing on the work of Taylor (Taylor 1987) these phases have been labelled:

- disconfirmation
- confusion
- impression management
- equilibrium.

5.2 Disconfirmation

As Figure 5.1 illustrates students experienced considerable confusion and concern about the course, their role, their ability to manage the different aspects of their life, home and friends, university student life and nursing life. Taylor (1987) describes this phase as a period of 'intensive disorientation and confusion, accompanied by a crisis of confidence and withdrawal from people associated with the cause'.

Students seemed uncertain about their commitment to nursing and it was at this stage that the decision to leave nursing altogether was made by Natalie, one of the original participants. In their first year, the focus group discussions elicited strong views on what they would be doing as nurses. In many respects these views were realistic and accurately appraised the emotional pain they could experience. Perhaps as a result of media coverage, and like students in a study of traditionally prepared student nurses in Scotland by Kiger (Kiger 1993) students did not account for the extent of responsibility they would have: they anticipated that a doctor would initiate many activities. Neither did students recognise that some nursing activities could be personally stressful to implement or participate in. Activities such as invading personal, physical barriers by giving injections or enemata, caring for dying patients or people in pain, students found very difficult to cope with and for some students this was an important concern. Studies of Scottish students taking traditional programmes and participating in Project 2000 courses demonstrated very high levels of stress amongst over 25% of all students, the stress increasing during their final year and following qualification (Baldwin, Dodd et al. 1998). Students' practical sessions in a skills laboratory helped to increase their understanding and technical ability. They were also aware that involvement with university life would change once they became more actively involved with patient care. Their social life would have to take on a more serious hue.

> *Helen*: September we're going to have to work 9–5. It's going to be really hard and everyone else is going to be just like we are this year, and we've been this year and it's going to be different for us, we might get a bit segregated.
>
>   *Nicola*: I think you have to take on the responsibility that you can't go out the night before and get completely wasted, hungover. I don't mean everyone goes out and gets drunk. You have to be responsible for your actions, like a pilot before flying an aeroplane. Take responsibility for whatever and not overtire yourself basically ... I would think you've got to be prepared to be, humble, humble is the wrong word, but be able to accept help graciously.
> (Interview 0/4: year 1 term 2).

Their conversations indicate a realistic appreciation of their future, when they would have to undertake clinical activities and thus be more closely involved with the realities of healthcare practice. They also recognised that they would need help and guidance, an experience they may not have been familiar with since childhood. Their second year was extremely fragmented with students only having one placement that lasted the whole of one term. The other two terms had two or three different clinical experiences, including working in the community alongside one or two different practitioners. Perhaps not surprisingly, these experiences proved the touchstone for two more students and tested the remaining students' commitment over the year. Students had to adjust quickly to each very different social environment and achieve particular targets, or learning outcomes within a short time. Establishing good relations with different mentors every four weeks was challenging. Another challenge was learning how to demonstrate their progress using unfamiliar assessment tools. Their success relied partly on using their newfound knowledge and language appropriately and demonstrating a critical and reflective approach to their practice. Reflective practice was generally interpreted as analysis of personal feelings and so they felt even more vulnerable and exposed when they got low marks. What they needed to learn was how to identify suitable incidents taken from their practice experiences and scrutinise them critically. These learning contracts (as they were known) became a source of frustration and alienation. But they also demonstrated students' progress towards making sense of their clinical placements and to learn how to use their formal knowledge in their everyday practice.

Students' feelings of confusion and the stress of their dichotomous position were expressed by their images and subsequent narratives (see Figure 5.1). In these first pictures, Marie and Ruth drew split figures, whilst Nicola drew a juggler. Jack, who already had lengthy experiences of nursing, both in general and mental health hospitals, used a maze to demonstrate his feelings of bewilderment. In contrast to how her colleagues were feeling at the start of their programme, Helen had a different story and her images appeared harmonious, with a balance between social and nursing activities. She had included her nursing uniform 'reminding me that I am supposed to be a nurse' (See Figure 3.1a, Helen: 'Helen in the middle'; and Figure 5.4e). She does not seem to have any doubts about her intention, probably because she described how settled and stimulated by her experiences she felt, which can be attributed to her placement over ten weeks in a supportive environment. Helen's enthusiasm for nursing and her commitment gradually waned over the subsequent terms until she was faced with making a decision. It was not until she encountered the rigours of a surgical ward at the end of her second year in the common foundation programme that she was confronted with making a choice between nursing or student life. Although she described the placement with enthusiasm, she was also shocked by her experience and was forced to reconsider her choice of career. By the end of her third year she painted herself at a road junction (see Figure 5.1d).

> I was thinking about it being the end of an era in a way because it's the end of my third year and all my friends are going to go. Everyone who isn't nursing is finishing. So it's quite sad, but I'm quite happy with the way it is, but wishing in a way that I can get out onto the green grass, but I've got no choice. I know I've got another year of study and that's it. As far as the work goes, yes [I am tempted to leave]. As far as my confidence in my nursing goes, yes. (Helen 8: year 3 term 3)

Unlike the others, Helen did not seem to have a placement subsequently where she expressed enthusiasm or satisfaction or a sense of integration with the clinical team. Neither did she feel satisfied with the level of work in which she was engaged and consequently she felt less energised to study. Perhaps the others were more fortunate in that they eventually came into contact with mentors with whom they felt comfortable and could identify. It is possibly that their resolution to 'make a go of it' was sufficient to generate their mentors' enthusiasm. By contrast Helen's subsequent branch placements offered images of how nurses behaved that she found disorientating and she again began to articulate her uncertainty about her career choice. This was reflected in her conversation at the end of term 1 in her fourth year:

> [The prospect of being qualified next year is] fairly terrifying. And I don't know whether it's what I want to do either. I don't know whether that's because I haven't got any confidence or if it's the placement I was on . . . It's probably what I said before – just lack of confidence and also because I haven't got a place I really want to work . . . I'd like to have more responsibility, but I need to be pushed to have it. And I'd like to be more confident with patients, in talking to them. I don't know whether I will get that because it's my fourth year and it should have come by now. That's why I think maybe I shouldn't do nursing. I don't think I'm confident enough at communicating as much as I should be.
> (Helen 10: year 4 term 1)

Helen's expressions of deep concern seem to be associated with anxieties about her level of competence and that it could be too late to catch up with her contemporaries. Perhaps more importantly, she seemed to feel a strong sense of alienation from the images of nurses presented by her qualified colleagues (see Chapter 4, page 130). Their mannerisms seemed to repulse her and she longed for a balance between the intense, professional commitment of the surgical nurses and the contrived demeanour of the medical nurses that she perceived. Her concerns during this final year of her programme reflected the same kinds of doubts and uncertainties that her coparticipants expressed at the start of theirs. Among the research participants that completed their programme Helen was unique in her concerns. However she may have been expressing the same kinds of doubts of others in the wider community of nursing students. Certainly after reading her story other students have identified with Helen's experiences. She may have been particularly unfortunate in her placements or with her mentors. Alternatively she may not have discovered how best to work with them. The other students described feelings of alienation and isolation although they were often more fortunate with their mentors. By the end of their second year, all the other female students were feeling less uncertain about their commitment to nursing and Jack, although firmly committed to nursing was frustrated by his experiences of the academic work. Grace was struggling with her financial and family problems and had made the decision to drop out of the course for a year. She was still determined to qualify. Marie was focused on getting her degree and when asked, both Ruth and Nicola asserted that there was no way they would give up nursing. It is possible that any feelings of confusion and anger were transition points towards their becoming nurses. Ruth's own picture of riding the choppy seas of rain and sunshine in her boat (see Figure 3.6c), seemed to summarise their feelings.

> I actually think I'm where that ship is at the moment, which is coming out of a low going into a high, probably because it's end of term, coming up to quite a good time. That's why the sun is radiating on tops of the waves. That represents being quite happy and content and ease with myself. This term and at this stage of the course, hopefully I'm accepting the course for what it is and I feel I've settled down and had two quite good placements . . . hopefully with the nursing course I've gone through the total confusion and the blackness earlier this year and now will come out and enjoy it a bit more . . . Well I think for the course, it hasn't necessarily been bad but it's me learning to accept it. I think the first year was very much a jolt to the system and wasn't what I expected from the nursing course, maybe into this year as well. I wondered what the point of all the stuff was . . . I don't feel particularly competent (as a nurse) . . . Yet funnily enough I do spend a lot of my time talking about nursing.
> (Ruth 11: year 2 term 3)

5.3 Confusion

Progressing from their common foundation programme to their branch programme at the beginning of their third year was a significant milestone. Students were faced with the reality of their decision to become a particular type of nurse, whether it be a children's nurse (Marie), mental health nurse (Nicola), or an adult nurse as the other four had decided. Their second year in the common foundation programme had provided taster placements. For both Marie and Nicola their experiences had been disastrous with poor mentorship support and inevitable foreboding about their career decision. Over the intervening summer vacation most of the students worked in local hospitals or nursing homes and had the opportunity to practise some of their new skills and to gain self-confidence. They also became more confident in using the language of clinical settings and this was reflected both in the way they talked and in their approach to the programme when they came to be interviewed during the autumn term of their third year.

Throughout their third year, students were exposed to different facets of their chosen speciality. Their programmes were structured differently. Marie spent the first two terms in the community, learning about healthy children and community support for disabled children and their families. She regarded these experiences as isolating and frustrating and as a result led her to doubt whether she had made the right career choice. Disillusioned by her experiences of working in the community, her paintings were concerned with her own family and the pressures of studying to achieve good marks for her degree. She acknowledged that her concern was with the degree rather than a nursing qualification (see Figure 5.2a).

> In the corner at the bottom left hand side there's a mountain with me at the bottom in black at week nought and me at the top in purple at week 11. Because there was a massive mountain of work to do and at week nought I couldn't see the end, but at week 11 I'd finished.

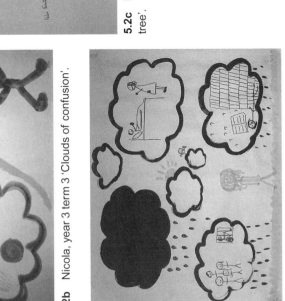

5.2c Helen, year 3 term 2 'The palm tree'.

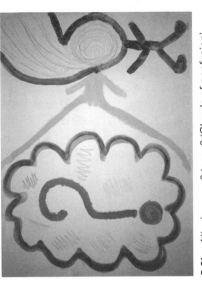

5.2b Nicola, year 3 term 3 'Clouds of confusion'.

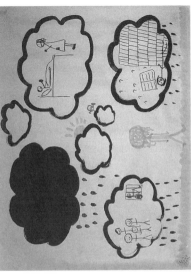

5.2e Ruth, year 3 term 2 'Shifting sands'.

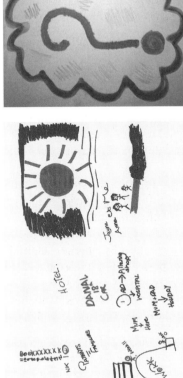

5.2a Marie, year 3 term 2 'Black mountains and sunshine'.

5.2d Jack, year 2 term 2 'Mountain roads and the rainbow'.

Figure 5.2 Confusion.

Above that there's a few books. It's just loads more to do I guess. There just seemed so much work at the beginning of term. Whether I've passed it is a different matter, but I've finished it . . . It was too short a holiday, but I don't mind coming back to [here] because I know home isn't far away. That's the sea and the sand for when we go to Tunisia. That's my excitement at the moment . . . I've done three and a half years and I'm not about to back out now. I might as well finish it. Whether I stick to it at the end of it is a different matter. Maybe I will, maybe I won't. I haven't got a clue. I've had enough. I really have. Because if all it's going to be is assessing your feelings to assess how good you are at your job I feel it's not worth it because it hurts too much when someone says 'Why did you feel like this?' But I just feel it's too personal . . . I find it very hard expressing on paper how I'm feeling about something.
(Marie 10: year 3 term 2)

Their images at the end of the second term illustrate feelings of uncertainty and some confusion. Both Nicola and Ruth worked in a number of settings where they felt uncertain about their role and their ability to practice according to their expectations, rather as Marie also identified. Ruth created an image that illustrated her uncertainty and confusion when she drew herself standing on shifting sands, surrounded by stormy clouds (see Figure 5.2e). At a similar point in her programme Nicola created a similar image describing dark clouds and arrows of uncertainty (see Chapter 3.3, Narrative, page 73; Figure 5.2b). In contrast Helen appeared to be regressing from her original happiness and equilibrium and her feelings of ambivalence and doubt began to emerge. She identified her inner conflict between wanting to be a nurse, and not knowing what else she could do. Her life had been geared up to such a career since she was 14 years old. Her image of a palm tree represents this conflict (see Figure 5.2c).

The base of the trunk, it's all about nursing. When I was a bit dodgy about whether I wanted to do nursing. The green bit is when I was improving on the ward and having lots of practical experience. Then the leaves are starting a fresh, or with new enthusiasm for nursing. Me wanting to be a student, not giving enough time to the wards and (not) taking it seriously enough. I feel I was needed and I didn't feel like an auxiliary. My mentor was saying 'Do you want to be a nurse?' What else could I do? It was quite a frightening thought if I didn't want to do nursing.
(Helen 6: year 3 term 2, adult branch)

Jack seemed to have overcome this hurdle to a certain extent after drawing his image of the rainbow and roads to two different mountains (see Figure 5.2d). Possibly he did not have to make the same adjustments to working in practice as a result of his past training experiences.

Two people are on the crossroads, both have question marks by the side of them. It suddenly dawned on me that we are almost half way through the course, half way there almost. I didn't feel like a student, I felt half way along the journey. I've spent ten weeks in one place and I've got to know the learning contract . . . I'm sitting there wondering whether to continue up to the sunshine or do I start to question the course? . . . I wouldn't quit because I've given up too much to come on this course and it would be pointless for me to quit. The only way I wouldn't complete would be if I got thrown off. [The rainbow] is getting my degree in general.
(Jack 5: year 2 term 2)

Jack's worries about the course were associated with the academic elements that he was finding difficult. Later on in his second year he was diagnosed as having dyslexia and this transformed his levels of self-confidence and subsequently his academic performance. For the other students who did not have Jack's nursing experience, feeling alone in trying to understand what they should be doing in practice was disturbing, perplexing and disorientating, leading them to question themselves and their future.

5.4 Impression management

Once students had overcome their feelings of confusion and uncertainty, Jack, Marie, Nicola and Ruth seemed to become more settled into their programme. Their confidence and understanding began to increase. Influential to their progress was good mentorship and feeling part of a clinical team and valued by its members as having something to contribute. This reflected their facility to adjust to different settings, their increased knowledge and ability to give essential care safely.

> You feel as though you can do as much as you want if you're part of the team, within limits set down. I've benefited from it. I don't feel stupid going up to someone asking something. I'd just say something like [pause] 'What's a bed pan for?' 'Where are they kept?' Whereas may be if I hadn't felt accepted I might feel stupid or very incompetent and inferior. I probably wouldn't have bothered doing anything. My learning would have been restricted.
> (Marie 13: year 4 term 1)

Ruth's clinical experiences improved and she described her mentors as supportive and stimulating, largely because they responded to her needs effectively and her confidence developed accordingly. She illustrated her development by picturing herself walking between two green fields, the past and future placements, but for the duration of her summer vacation, she was going to leave the course behind (see Figure 3.6e).

> I think I felt confident, although I don't think I've been stretched at all in my practice. That hasn't worried me, which a year ago it might have done. I actually feel quite happy generally in my ability to talk with people and communicate. My practical ability is there, . . . so perhaps I've grown in confidence there. I've not felt intimidated by the academic side so much, particularly the library and all the referencing. I feel the library was there for me to use rather than for me to drown in it with all the information.
> (Ruth 17: year 3 term 3)

Students were becoming more able to identify with other members of the clinical team and to undertake similar work. They recognised they had a lot more to learn, but they also had a better idea of what they needed and wanted to learn and so could operate more like adults, rather than like clingy children as before.

Marie's initial stage of disconfirmation had been more pronounced and longer than the others' experience and its resolution was also more intense. In the third term of her third year, Marie was allocated to a ward with an excellent mentor,

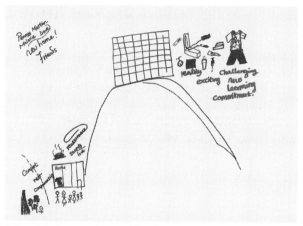

5.3a Marie, year 4 term 1 'At slope end'.

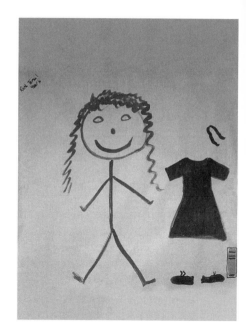

5.3d Ruth, year 4 term 1 'Pin-on nurse'.

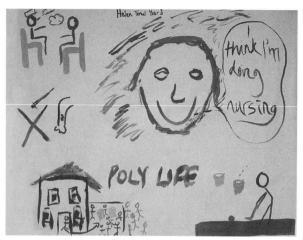

5.3b Helen, year 3 term 1 'I think I'm doing nursing'.

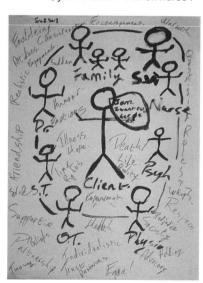

5.3e Jack, year 3 term 2 'Talking heads'.

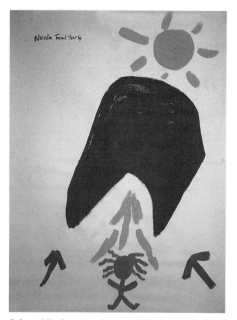

5.3c Nicola, year 4 term 1 'Sunny end of the tunnel'.

Figure 5.3 Impression management.

and they were able to develop a relationship based on trust and respect. As a result Marie felt more able to express her anxieties and her mentor was willing to take Marie with her and guide her through the different procedures and patient problems. This helped her to adjust quickly to the ward and to feel part of the team, and as a result Marie's confidence soared. At the end of her placement she illustrated her transformation with a picture of her head buzzing with confidence and for the first time as a nurse with her future RSCN qualification given pride of place (see Figure 5.3a). This burst of enthusiasm was confirmed by her narrative (Narrative 19 in Chapter 3, pages 61–2).

Jack made the same sort of rapid transition under similar conditions. In his second placement during his third year, he enjoyed recognition and status as a member of the rehabilitation team. From that period on, his confidence grew and like Marie, he became increasingly committed to a role in adult nursing, incorporating his mental health nursing skills. The transition point was illustrated by his picture of the patient surrounded by support staff and the concepts he associated with good care (see Figure 5.3e).

> It's a picture of stick men with the client in the middle and various professionals and the family round the outside . . . [and about] the placement [at the rehabilitation unit] basically and how I felt what was going on there and how I helped, hopefully, while I was there and what I got from it . . . I think it was *my* experience as well. A lot of the module was questioning our own beliefs and what we expect . . . People were willing to show you around. Maybe it was because they had the time. There was a blurring of roles almost. Although everyone had a clear identified role . . . I was involved in those [ward rounds] and in review meetings . . . It felt like I was doing something, rather like being an advocate for the patient . . . It was great. I was quite happy to chair it [review meetings] if they'd wanted. Power!
> (Jack 9: year 3 term 2)

For all these students, their sense of membership of a clinical community was central to their development of identity and enhanced their ability to learn. The process was unaffected by their supernumerary status but more importantly, was affected by the way staff responded to it. These students seemed to have achieved a watershed in their decision to nurse and were trying to act like their images. Following the summer vacation and by end of her first fourth year term, Ruth had made a big transition and illustrated her state of being with a picture of a nurse's outfit waiting to be stepped into (see Figure 5.3c Ruth).

> I think I am becoming comfortable with the idea of me as a nurse and so that's why I'm smiling and I think I am getting used and accepting the idea that it's OK for a big part of nursing to be me as an individual. Rather than trying to be someone else when I need to step into my shoes and tie my hair up and it will still be me in the dress rather than someone different. So rather than me changing to become a nurse and no longer Ruth, I was trying to show that that's me and you just superimpose the dress on it and it's still one and the same person. Maybe in the past [I] would have to become something different and adopt a different personality . . . I have to realise that as a nurse working on my own I will adopt certain styles and maybe that's the style I choose to adopt. I could choose to be someone else, put on the nurse's front, but I think I choose to be me who happens to wear a nurse's

uniform. That also comes back to deciding to be on the patient's side. I'm not on the side of the hospital staff, if that makes sense.
(Ruth 20: year 4 term 1)

As with the others on reaching this stage, Ruth continued to maintain her images of nursing and her identity as a separate person. But she also acknowledged that she could express her personality in a variety of ways, including as a nurse. For these four students their transition seemed to have been consolidated by working in hospitals over the vacation periods as they seemed to speak with increased confidence following their summer break in particular. Similarly Helen's initial feelings of confidence and ability to work as a nurse were related to spending ten weeks on a rehabilitation ward for people following major trauma. She felt well supported and found the experience enjoyable (not least because she had time to engage in student life too). Her illuminative artwork depict this sense clearly as she describes (see Figure 5.3b).

> Two chairs, I put a hat on [one] and that's supposed to be as a good nurse. I was told I was a good little counsellor. I really enjoyed the placement. It was the head injuries ward, but there wasn't much nursing involved. I really wanted to do some injections, I haven't done one yet and I'm a third year.
> (Helen 6: year 3 term 1).

Helen's transition path seems to mirror that of four of her research colleagues. It reflects her fluctuating confidence and realisation that she is not keeping up with developing the skills she believed she ought to have at the same point in their programme. Other students were able to maintain a stage personae whilst working with patients.

> I give my mentor the impression that I'm confident the whole time. But I'm not a lot of the time. [I'm] quite nervous. The whole thing is an act, I take a deep breath. Probably the whole thing of getting changed into the uniform, by the time you then walk out onto the stage you are half way there.
> (Ruth 12: year 3 term 1)

Using Irving Goffman's (Goffman 1964) description of dramaturgical action and impression management, students were faced with a huge dilemma. They desperately wanted to be like other nurses in the clinical community but also needed to be recognised as nursing students so they could gain the kinds knowledge and experience they needed. In her case study Helen descibed her worry about giving the wrong impression when she nearly fainted at the sight of blood in the accident and emergency department (Chapter 3, Helen: Narrative 6, page 36). By trying to adjust her behaviour to conform to how she thought she should behave Helen was trying to become an invisible member of her new community of practitioners. In other settings she was concerned that she may lose her humanity and sensitivity. In trying to balance her images of how to behave as a nurse and those images she saw portrayed by other nurses, Helen was seeking reassurance that she could still make a nurse. She was not alone in trying to conform to beliefs about how to be seen as a good nurse. Other students worked hard to give the impression of wanting to learn, such as Marie (Chapter 3, Marie: Narrative 6, page 53). Marie hoped that her actions would communicate her interest in nursing and then she realised that she did not need to make a special effort to convince people important to her that she was fulfilling a particular role. However a key element in helping students to fulfil their role was the social atmosphere and the support of their mentors as students' narratives earlier indicate.

The four students who painted pictures in their last year, created images of further transition and consolidation. Two students Nicola and Jack both used images of entering their final tunnel to illustrate how it felt to be a nursing student whilst they were preparing to submit their dissertations. They were also facing the final six months of their programme (see Figure 5.3c and Figure 3.4d, with Narrative 27, pages 88–90). For Marie it was having got to the top of a steep slope with the slide down towards the final six months of her course (see Figure 5.3a).

5.5 Equilibrium

At the start of her programme, Helen's very first piece of illuminative art (see Figure 5.4e) showed her surrounded by people, social friends and work colleagues. It illustrates her satisfaction at being well-supported whilst enjoying the educational and professional stimulation of her mentor. In her interview she expresses great satisfaction and enjoyment in nursing. She feels her choice of course and career have been confirmed. This mirrors the feelings of her research colleagues at the opposite end of their programme when they felt able to express similar sentiments: the expression of satisfaction and achievement of their goals. For them it is the beginning of the end of the first stage in their evolution as nurses. They appear to have developed a strong and satisfying identification with their chosen profession and a strong commitment to nursing coupled with enormous pleasure in what they were achieving.

The four who painted their final fourth year images expressed their awareness that they would soon be qualified and be expected to function according to a different role. This spurred them on to work hard in practice even though having submitted their dissertations they felt they had met their academic challenge. As Helen identified, it was a terrifying prospect, but one which for both her and the others, was clearly an incentive.

This next stage was a resolution of their worries and the exhilarating sense of achievement of successfully completing the course with registration in sight. Their satisfaction was not wholly concerned with their academic achievements but more importantly their sense of being able to operate in the same manner as their qualified colleagues. They had finally developed a clear identity as nurses. Ruth's image of the rainbow falling into a cup of tea seems to represent her transformation and views of her future (see Figure 5.4d).

> I see being a nurse more than a nursing student as part of everyday life, it's what I've wanted, probably for many years. Certainly it's what I've trained for . . . So I'm trying to get away

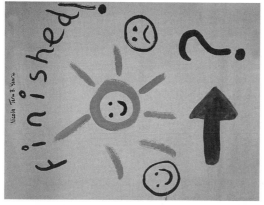

5.4c   Nicola, year 4 term 3 'The end of one road'.

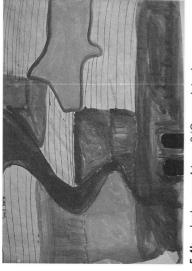

5.4b   Jack, year 4 term 3 'On peak top'.

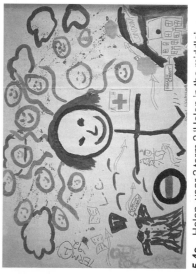

5.4e   Helen, year 2 term 2 'Helen in the middle'.

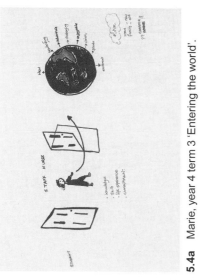

5.4a   Marie, year 4 term 3 'Entering the world'.

5.4d   Ruth, year 4 term 3 'All in one'.

Figure 5.4   Equilibrium.

from the idea that nursing is a dress you put on and go off to work in and it's a dress you take off when you get home. I still call myself a nurse and maybe it sits more comfortably (than when I saw myself split). I'm not consciously going round thinking I'm a nurse it's just one of the groups I fit into . . . It's become more one and the same person.
(Ruth 22: year 4 term 3)

For Jack it was his fulfilment of an ambition started more than ten years earlier, and his satisfaction in knowing that he had proved his old general nursing school wrong. For Jack unlike the others, this programme provided him with additional professional skills and more importantly an enhanced self-image (see Figure 5.4b).

I was aware that I had to do one [painting] when I was coming down and I had two visions in my head. One was of the earlier painting I did with two mountains and the maze in between and the other one was a feeling of coming through a tunnel to the end and the relief of coming through and achieving something . . . I remember there was a mountain at this side and a mountain at that side of the paper and I had to get from one side to the other . . . It's like this is the edge of the mountain and I'm looking straight down. These are my two feet and this is the cliff edge, greeny colour. I'm looking straight down a valley with the river and fields and I've coloured the fields in yellow because it's summer. And green and brown to make it distinctive. I have this feeling of just achieving what I wanted to achieve and feeling I suppose, on top of the world and a bit apprehensive and nervous about where and what I'm going to do next.
(Jack 16: year 4 term 3)

For Nicola coming to the end of her programme carried a realisation that her life-style would be changing dramatically and that she would be taking on new responsibilities (see Figure 5.4c). Marie expressed her recognition of being at another transition point by drawing herself in the middle of a corridor between two open doors. One closing behind her as she waited for her results to be published, freeing her to enter the next stage of her career, waiting on the other side of the second door in her picture (see Figure 5.4a, and Chapter 3, Narrative 22, page 62). Helen, also completed the course but without resolving her uncertainties and went to work in an intensive care unit where she felt more comfortable being identified with these nurses. Unlike the others she chose not to update her picture made at the end of her third year. Her last lingering image is of her on her bicycle waiting at the road junction unsure which way to turn.

5.6 Feeling and acting like a nurse

When students entered their nursing degree course they expressed a clear view of how they wanted to be as nurses and these sustained them throughout. Feeling like a nurse was a confusing and sometimes painful experience. Over the subsequent four years they gradually learned to construct personal images of how to act like nurses that were acceptable to their professional colleagues. Students' original mental images of being a nurse and how to act like a nurse provided a lens by which they perceived their nursing colleagues. In trying to manage a suitably professional impression students struggled to feel and act authentically. Sometimes they found performing according to a prescribed nursing role conflicted with their personal beliefs and they had to negotiate a different role or leave the course. This seems to explain Natalie's decision to leave nursing. She had ambitions to be both a university student and a nurse. Only when she discovered that being a nurse was different to what she imagined could she give up that aspiration. This explanation helps to understand Jack's decision to leave his initial nurse training. When he was working under pressure to meet management targets these feelings of uncertainty about his career choice resurfaced.

A second aspect of students' transition to feeling like a nurse was the extent to which they believed they behaved like nurses or at least the extent to which they could identify with other nurse practitioners. Helen's great dilemma was the internal dissonance created by a conflict between her ideal beliefs and what she perceived to be opposing and untenable models offered by two very different groups of nurses with whom she came into contact. For Marie it was feeling socially isolated and not being able to participate in nursing activities that led her to feel alienated from her clinical colleagues. Feelings of isolation were also experienced on wards (and it was mostly wards rather than home settings) where staff were unable to support students and left them to fend for themselves. Again experiences such as these caused students to review their career choice.

It seems that to become successful as a nursing student and later as a nurse, students needed to adopt one or more personalities and roles defined by several social, professional and educational communities (university student, nursing student, citizen). Students' artwork illustrates their emotional transition from disconfirmation of their initial expectations (the split person, the juggler, the maze) and of either trying to live up to their mental images or adjusting them to conform to the demands of their professional colleagues until they found some sort of equilibrium. By illustrating their feelings through paintings or drawings it was easier to detect how well students were making these transitions. Their adjustments seemed to take place in four distinct stages. The first was normally concerned with overcoming their disconfirmation and confusion and gradually settling into their programme by adjusting to a new lifestyle and learning how to juggle the different demands of studying, nursing and student life. Before they could progress through each stage they had to resolve the tensions between these different roles, and between academic work and nursing work. They also needed to recognise that they were not alone in their difficulties and that they were mostly due to external causes rather than personal insufficiencies. Their progress seemed to have been marked by feelings of confusion, anger and adjustment, perhaps not dissimilar to those of the grieving process identified by Kubler-Ross (Kubler-Ross 1970). Most important in helping them come through the process were supportive mentors who were willing and able to involve students in clinical practice and to contribute to the overall performance of the team. Opportunities to develop their practice skills with only distant supervision increased their confidence and this could be experienced during their placements or their vacations. Once students felt they really could become nurses and do all the kinds of things they saw nurses do, students then entered a phase of adjusting their self image. By the end of their programme, four of the students believed they had become nurses. They had managed to integrate their internal and external images and to feel confident in their ability to nurse in a way that they identified as 'proper' nursing. In doing so they had transformed from lay people to professionals.

References

Baldwin, P., Dodd, M., et al. (1998) *Nurses: training, work, health and welfare: a longitudinal study*. Chief Scientist Office, Department of Health, The Scottish Office, Edinburgh.

Carr, W., Kemmis, S. (1986) *Becoming Critical: Education, Knowledge and Action Research*. Falmer Press, London.

Goffman, E. (1964) On face work: an analysis of ritual elements in social interaction. In: *Interpersonal dynamics: Essays and readings on human interaction*. (eds W.G. Bennis, E.H. Schein, D.E. Berlew) pp. 226–49. The Dorsey Press, Homewood, IL.

Kiger, A.M. (1993) Accord and discord in students' images of nursing. *Journal of Nursing Education* **32** (7): 309–17.

Kubler-Ross, E. (1970) *On Death and Dying*. Tavistock Publications, London.

Melia, K.M. (1987) *Learning and Working. The Occupational Socialisation of Nurses*. Tavistock Publications, London.

Taylor, M. (1987) Self-directed learning: More than meets the observer's eye. In: *Appreciating Adults Learning*. (eds D. Boud, V. Griffin) pp. 179–96. Kogan Page, London.

Chapter 6
Learning to be a Professional

Earlier chapters have explored how these students utilised their beliefs and values about caring for patients and clients and how they adjusted to and acquired a role that enabled them to be the kinds of nurses they wanted to be. In this chapter we shall explore how they developed the professional skills they believed they needed to provide that care.

Students' stories included many references to their developing professional competence and the kinds of knowledge they needed for everyday practice as nurses: how to do the kinds of activities they found challenging, and how they learnt to do them successfully. Arriving for their interviews, students launched straight into describing their clinical practice. Often they expressed concern about the patients they cared for, or the personal and practical difficulties they experienced whilst working in their clinical placement. Sometimes they found it easy to describe how they learned to give care; at other times they found it difficult to explain how they acquired the knowledge or skills they were using. Using a metaphor taken from physiology, the process of their learning often seemed similar to the osmosis of fluids between two membranes. Knowledge and patient care became integrated into their everyday practice in a subtle, almost subliminal manner. By contrast, some learning occasions were so memorable that students were excited and inspired by their practical experiences and could easily recognise their leaps in learning. On still other occasions they went about studying some aspect of their practice that they found problematic, challenging or exciting. Not all their learning took place in the clinical environment, and instrumental to making sense of their experiences were conversations with their friends, studying in the library and completing their learning contracts. In the early stages of their programme they relied very much upon the help of their mentors to guide them and also on having time to do the same kinds of work on their own. With increasing confidence and experience they were able to identify what they needed to learn and to use a variety of resources for the help they needed.

So many people fail to recognise the complexity of professional nursing practice, partly because so many of the essential skills are also employed on a daily basis by parents and carers. The subtle difference is being able to provide the same or a higher quality of essential care to people you do not know and may have difficulty liking. To provide such care whilst also taking account of a huge range of subtle signs and symptoms, managing sophisticated equipment or dealing with emotionally distressed people makes it far more challenging, emotionally draining and complex. Being able to provide such care to groups of people, setting priorities, setting goals and then being able to manage the work-load successfully makes nursing even more demanding. However well students are prepared in the formal education setting (classroom or skills laboratory), facing the reality of an ill person and using the same knowledge and skills in busy and stressful clinical settings demands a different way of using the knowledge. It not only requires students to recognise the relevance and saliency of their formal knowledge, but also first and foremost (for these students) requires the students to know how to relate to their patients. Some situations might be amusing, sad or frightening and the students needed to know how to respond emotionally; they could not afford to respond inappropriately for fear of upsetting their clients or their colleagues. So, learning how to be professional and yet be congruent was a challenge.

Over and above these requirements was the students' concern to become viewed as valued members of the clinical team, and with this came development of their self-image as a nurse. Students' descriptions of their clinical experiences generated five specific areas of their practice that dominated their concerns. These were:

- relating to patients and their carers;
- developing technical knowledge;
- learning to bundle nursing activities together;
- developing craft knowledge;
- managing feelings and emotions (their own as well as those of patients and relatives);
- developing the essence of nursing which promotes therapeutic action;
- relating to and functioning within a clinical team.

Students' chief preoccupation was to be able to relate effectively to their patients and their carers. Their concern with this aspect of nursing dominated their pro-gramme and is the first we will consider.

6.1 Learning to relate to patients and their carers

When they started their programme each student held an image of how they would relate to patients and their carers. Despite this they had only a limited amount of actual experience in developing such relationships with strangers or ill people. It was formidable for many students to spend their first days working in a clinical setting, both challenging and distressing. As we read in Nicola's case study (Chapter 3, Nicola: Narrative 1, page 64) her first sight of mentally ill pa-tients caused her to re-examine her beliefs and motives as well as scaring her. She managed to rationalise her first reactions and to use a variety of tactics to develop her relating skills. In a similar manner, Natalie felt self-conscious when talking to children during her first placement but discovered how she could be effective:

I think once I felt relaxed on the ward, which only took a couple of days because everyone
was so friendly, once I felt relaxed in the atmosphere and surroundings and had watched
other nurses talk to the children, I could just walk up to a child and just sit down. Once I
thought the children had got to know me because there were quite a few long-term patients,
they knew my face and everything, I'd just go up and chat to them and play games with them
and stuff. I think it was just because I was relaxed with myself that I could do it. I wasn't
really tense or nervous.
(Natalie 1: year 2 term 1)

Over their programme students received extensive support to develop their interpersonal skills and were able to rehearse them in the relative safety of a classroom
environment. When they first entered practice they seemed to forget all they
had learned and used different means of developing their skills as indicated by
Natalie. Relating to people with mental problems as Nicola describes, can be
quite frightening and when Marie went to work in a mental health unit on her
first clinical placement, she was worried about how to approach patients. By
observing the experienced nurses she tuned into their successful interactions
and copied them for her own use (see Chapter 3, Marie: Narrative 9, page 55).
Marie's initial concerns about going into the unit and working with the patients
were soon allayed. As with the other students at the start of the programme,
Marie described how a good nurse was someone who could talk to patients and
get to know them and help them recover. In this narrative she is drawing on
observations that match up with her own images of how staff should relate to
patients.

This sense of consonance between personal action and ideal self-image seems
consistent with the other students' use of observed behaviours. Jack recognised
how one mentor used humour to banish feelings of self-consciousness in her
patients as they struggled with essential elements of self-care. He seems to have
been stimulated by his own discomfort at watching these patients struggle and it
motivated him to explore whether using humour could be legitimately used. The
fine balance of risk between cruelty and professional behaviour could be subtle.
Fortunately Jack felt able to challenge her approach and to understand her thinking before he decided whether to adopt the same strategy in his own practice (see
Chapter 3, Jack: Narrative 21, page 85).

Helen had a clear image of how she would like to relate to patients, but felt
inhibited by feelings of self-consciousness and inadequacy. Using a task as a
mediating tool helped her overcome feelings of discomfort. Using this kind of
approach was encouraged by students' mentors and their teachers, as was documented in Marie's learning contract:

I changed one of the patient's dressings on her self-harm wounds and I now feel I have a
'closer' relationship with that patient than I had before, as I spent time talking to her as I
was changing the dressings. I can now see that times like changing dressings give the nurses
time to talk to patients and build up a good rapport with the patients and get to know them
better. *Comment (by mentor): Well observed. Sometimes very close relationships develop in
unlikely circumstances.*
(Marie Learning Contract: objective 1: year 2 term 1)

Sometimes students had mixed feelings about which patients they could relate to. If they had extensive experience of working with the elderly (as care assistants) they would often feel less challenged by them, but feared talking to children or young adults in case they looked ridiculous or were inadvertently offensive. Helen was particularly conscious of this and as her confidence increased (and perhaps her repertoire of nursing activities), she became less daunted by talking and could commence a conversation with increased self-awareness rather than self-consciousness:

> I always think 'Oh, I don't want to talk to elderly people' but then they're quite interesting . . . on the whole [I feel less self-conscious now]. It might be because a lot of them have rooms on their own, so you can have a private conversation without the whole ward hearing. If the patient isn't easy to talk to, like the 21 year-old who wasn't that easy, but I thought I wouldn't leave straightway because he was actually talking which was apparently amazing. It's quite awkward in a way because you're in there and there's you and him and you don't want to make really trivial conversation and talk for the sake of it. You have to measure whether they want to talk or not as well. There's another patient who I found really difficult to talk to, about 50–60 (years of age), and everyone found that he wasn't communicative. So that was quite hard to know whether they want you in the room or not, and if you do go are they going to think 'She's only had two minutes to spare'. If I'd stayed longer, would he have opened up? You learn as you go along I suppose. It depends on the patient. It's quite interesting because two of my patients have been in their forties and I haven't worked a huge amount with that age group. I've got on really well with them, but that might just be them because they're easy to talk to. It's nice as well because they remember your name, which is quite amazing.
> (Helen 11: year 4 term 1)

From this narrative Helen seems to be actively experimenting and challenging herself to develop relationships with her patients. As she identifies, walking into a single room to talk to a patient could be perceived as an invasion of private space and subject to rejection. She needed to overcome the psychological as well as the physical barrier. Coping with patients labelled as 'hard to talk to' was a personal mission that she seems to have developed the confidence to achieve. Throughout her programme, Helen felt inhibited by younger patients until she worked in the rehabilitation unit where she gained new insights and developed more self-confidence.

Apart from learning how to talk to patients, students also needed to gain their cooperation in a variety of activities without feeling self-conscious. Learning how to provide care often created personal discomfort as Nicola describes:

> I think it's worse almost with someone who is younger or nearer your age than it is with someone who is elderly. I've gone bright red having to wash younger people and having intimate dealings with people, like taking bandages off or whatever. I would consider myself an unbashful person. I still get slightly embarrassed about it, but I think that's how it should be because it makes you more aware of how they might be feeling, than to have the old matron idea of 'Come on then, off with your clothes'. You need to find a happy medium.
> (Nicola 5: year 2 term 3)

Nicola's concerns about finding a suitable way to relate to patients in situations that are embarrassing bear hallmarks from media portrayals of nurses as burley matronly figures. Like Ruth she chooses to ignore such images and to find a more congruent way of relating, despite her feelings of embarrassment. This approach is more akin to that described by Carper (Carper 1978) using Buber's (Buber 1937) concept of the 'I–Thou' relationship where patients are seen as people rather than objects and to a certain extent an extension of the self. This can be a very difficult thing to achieve when students' are preoccupied with many other agendas such as technical, social and emotional as Ruth's narrative (Chapter 3, Ruth: Narrative 16, page 115) illustrates. Later on in her programme Ruth had developed sufficient self-confidence to know how to balance all these difficult decisions and activities whilst also supporting an emotionally disturbed patient:

> By the time I met David on the unit he was no longer aggressive, but much distressed by his behaviour. This time I felt confident enough to approach David. I knew that I couldn't solve his distress, but I wanted to allow him space to express his anxiety (Burnard 1988). The principle is that it is better to release feelings than bottle them up. I sat alongside David, on his bed, and said I wanted to stay with him for a short time. I wasn't trying to challenge him, but be alongside, so I adopted a non-challenging position (Cook 1970). Being at the same height made us more equal (Argyle 1983) which I felt appropriate. I was quite close to David, sitting on his bed. Writers have spoken of the personal territory patients create over their bed space (Kent & Dalgleish 1986). I was deliberately using this – entering David's intimate zone (Hall 1959) to create a sense of intimacy and security for David to express his feelings. [These are] quick and simple actions to start developing a therapeutic relationship. It strikes me that I'm avoiding the traditional nurse/patient proximity, I'm trying to make this a person-to-person contact. One that is humane. I want David to express his reaction and feelings to his current situation, since I believe this is an important part of his well-being. I want David to be a person and not just a patient. So I can take steps to help him feel this.
> (Ruth, LC: year 4 term 1)

Ruth's description of the critical incident demonstrates her willingness to question the appropriateness of her intentions whilst also illustrating how theory is being used to explore her actions. This reflective, questioning attitude to their motives was important for students and they were concerned not to make assumptions about patients' needs but to see them as individuals with their own special needs. Ruth also illustrates how her feelings of self-confidence influenced her ability to relate to David. Once students managed to overcome any natural reticence they began to feel able to relate to patients and use techniques they had learned in their formal settings. Sometimes students had to find ways of dealing with patients who were deliberately being provocative, and to respond in a therapeutic manner without feeling embarrassed. They also needed to develop skills of recognising potential danger and how to manage them whilst maintaining an outward appearance of calm professionalism. This included working in the community where there was always a risk of danger when visiting patients alone:

> We had one chap we went to, who is about 60, living on his own in a flat and he's into psy-chology and Freud and he was telling us about it and that rang bells because I reckon Freud had a lot of sexual problems. Then he started talking about how he was writing a book about prostitutes. Coming out we were saying 'Oh, I'd be a bit wary of going to him on my own' and Rose, funnily enough was saying that there were some clients they go to in twos if they're worried.
> (Ruth 16: year 3 term 3)

As students became more experienced they were encouraged by good mentors to increase their level of responsibility, and this provided new opportunities to learn about people:

> She was Iranian and didn't speak much English. I admitted her and that was another com-munication barrier. I asked what religion she was and she was Muslim, and they pray so many times a day and only eat certain foods and I asked her what she liked to eat and she said 'Anything'. So I said 'But I thought you were Muslim' but she said that in England if they were pushed that's what they would say. It's one of those things. That you always assume that people from other religions are more strict than C-of-E. People are the same all over the world really . . . So to find an agnostic Muslim was quite different really. I think especially when I've been to Saudi Arabia and see it being religiously followed. So then to meet someone saying 'We might do it, we might not' was quite strange. You should never assume anything really. It's always best to ask the patient.
> (Jack 9: year 3 term 1)

Gaining insight to patients as people also needed understanding. In particular students needed to develop concepts of patients as members of a family and a community. Their early experiences in the community helped, but more valuable were opportunities to have responsibility alongside a mentor for a patient and a whole family. This provided insights into the needs of families and relatives and how to interact with relatives, particularly when they were under stress:

> I think it's looking after the whole aspect of the child, holistically. If at the end of the day mum is stressed out, it's getting her in touch with the appropriate people to help her. You have to care for the parents as well as the child. It's not physically, but mentally caring. If they can't cope with their child's heart condition because they're stressed out or they don't know what is going on. It's mental healthcare for them and you have to make the doctors aware if there are problems. Some of them don't know how to ask questions or how to phrase it. One parent said 'I'd like to be put in touch with a social worker'. And that was straightforward really. It's little things that each day, as you get to know someone, people drop the mask a bit further and you start to see the real them. You can tell them that there are people out there who can support them. It's making them aware of the services that are available to them. They can talk to a social worker if they want to. There might be some stigma attached to social workers if they think they only deal with family problems, but if you're stressed out about your child's condition and you're saying 'I need help'. I think it's better for the child, than to hide it and keep going on and getting more stressed.
> (Marie 15: year 4 term 1)

These kinds of experiences helped students gain a broader understanding of how to relate to diverse groups of people whilst also becoming familiar with working alongside other health and social-care professionals. By the end of her community placement Marie had learned a great deal about the range of services available.

Giving bad news

Learning how to give bad news is a challenge many nurses fear and avoid. Students learned how to develop such skills by working alongside their mentor or another experienced practitioner. Seeing how they coped with difficult situations provided models of practice that they could use later. One evening when working on a specialist unit Jack and his mentor faced a dreadful dilemma and as a result, he gained experience and insight to the needs of relatives and colleagues:

> I suppose if I was in that position – if I'm asking a direct question then I would want an honest answer and that's what we decided. If he asked we weren't going to lie to him. They were fully aware how serious the situation was and you've got the worry. I can't remember why they drove all the way back [home] because they'd only been gone an hour and a bit. If you say she's seriously ill he may feel a need to jump in the car and drive all the way back and that's going to be a wasted journey. Just try and broach the subject, it's almost like giving him insight in a way. That was possibly the best example of breaking bad news I've seen over the telephone . . . there was myself, two other staff nurses, the LP and it was a case of 'What do we say?' It was a case of 'What do you think? I need help with this'. Trying to discuss it as a group worked quite well. We didn't really have time for a long, ethical discussion on the pros and cons, because he was on the other end of the phone, so it was quite hard. It's how it fits at the time I suppose. The nurse had got quite involved with the family and the doctor had spent quite a long time talking through the implications of what could happen and as I say it's almost gut reaction in how would you like to be told.
> (Jack 14: year 4 term 1)

Perhaps Jack was fortunate in being exposed to this difficult situation. He seems to have given the matter much thought and explored how he might feel in similar circumstances, having not long before experienced a sudden bereavement. Throughout the programme, students seemed to draw on their personal knowledge as a valuable means of thinking how to develop and sustain relationships and maintain an image of patients as people like them. This helped them to keep their image of patients and people and to sustain their images of caring.

6.2 Developing technical knowledge

When students first described the kinds of tasks they believed nurses perform they knew they would have to do less pleasant things such as giving injections and medications, and this created a mixture of anxiety and anticipation:

> I found my first few days really frustrating, because I was really excited about being on wards – I can get my hands into everything, and do it all. But you can't because we're not trained . . . I was sort of saying, 'Well, I want to do injections but I don't because I'm scared.' But I do want to.
> (Natalie 1: year 2 term 1)

To experienced nurses these activities may seem mundane, but to a novice like Natalie they constituted a major hurdle to overcome. Fortunately she recognised her limitations and knew when to seek help. Other activities such as bathing dependant patients were associated with caring for the elderly and many students disregarded their skill content. Mostly they saw it as a task that could be carried out by a care assistant rather than being part of the professional nurse's role. Several students had worked as carers either to relatives or in homes for the elderly. Both Nicola and Helen believed that such work was routine and that they were competent in the necessary techniques. Helen's experiences in the rehabilitation unit for older people illustrated how, with good mentorship and guided reflection, she came to review her own beliefs and underwent a complete change of perspective. Students' narratives in earlier chapters indicate that giving care formerly considered to be routine and fundamental can be sophisticated and complex when provided to people in different circumstances. For most of their programme and particularly during their first three years, students struggled to develop the necessary skills and to work as quickly as their qualified colleagues. Some of their concern were the risks of causing harm and how best to relate to patients:

> [When I gave my first injection] it was a chap of about 12 or 13 and that's even worse than giving it to a baby. I'd given injections before, but it still wasn't that nice with a boy of that age. I think I felt so vulnerable. It came home that I was only about six years older than he was. It threatened me I suppose. I was suddenly aware of how young I am really. He was in the bed and I was the one pretending to be professional about it, but it was all a bit of an act . . . I felt threatened, flustered and embarrassed. I'm not very good at hiding my embarrassment. It's just something I've got to overcome.
> (Nicola 4: year 2 term 3)

Nicola's implication that elderly patients are inconsequential was not uncommon, perhaps it was because of students' earlier experiences as care assistants or perhaps students felt more likely to be censored by younger people, whom they identified with their teachers or parents.

Sometimes students were left to muddle through as best they could, possibly because staff were too busy or because they misunderstood notions of adult learning:

> I watched my mentor do it [wash a young patient] one day and then the next she was busy and I said I thought I could manage for a little while and when I did it on my own . . . Because I was on my own and he was quite ill, with lots of tubes, I think I was careful how much I moved him. I don't think at the end, I felt I was successful and I certainly don't think I was particularly proficient at it or that I did a particularly good job . . . Just to be very gentle and careful moving him and make sure that I wasn't pulling anything out. He had a catheter and I got his shorts off and of course they were all hooked up in all the tubes and in the end I asked the Staff Nurse. I could see where it undid but wasn't sure about infection in the tubes, so I got another Staff Nurse just to take them off for me. I was very clumsy I felt, and he wasn't well so I think I was deliberately gentle. He was very skinny in the arms though. What bothered me was that half way through – and he's come in for fits – he seemed to go into a fit. Not a major one because he wasn't shaking, but his eyes would roll and that panicked me no end, so I went haring out to find someone and they came along really to

back me up, because I would have hated to think that anything happened to him. It wasn't my fault at all, but just to think that something might happen and I was so dumb that I didn't know. So that worried me a bit. It might have been easier if he'd been more *compos mentis* and he could have answered my question as to 'Is it OK if I give you a little wash?' That would have put me more at my ease. I was having to wash him when it was pretty obvious that he didn't know what was going on. I suppose there's a part of you that thinks 'He doesn't know what the hell's going on so why do it?' but more importantly he hadn't said he wanted it and I might actually be doing something he doesn't really care for. But you're always going to have those sorts of things.
(Ruth 4: year 2 term 1)

Ruth's experience is startling and her narrative identifies several important aspects of this child's care. To what extent was Ruth competent to undertake this responsibility and how aware was her supervisor of the child's safety? Fortunately Ruth recognised that she should not disconnect the various lines. She also identifies issues concerned with consent and meeting the child's needs, rather than nursing needs. At this stage in her programme it would have taken a brave student to question her supervisor for fear of being rejected. Disappointingly she missed out on a wonderful learning opportunity had she been able to participate in caring for the child alongside an experienced practitioner. Perhaps her supervisor did not recognise the opportunities that existed. On other occasions students were more fortunate:

A lot of the dressing (materials) you have heard of them, but you don't really know why they're used and what they're used for and how to do dressings. I've been doing Angela's dressing. I was observed a few times and then did it most times. It's OK knowing how to do an aseptic dressing, but knowing how to open a pack, how to open a bag, take a dirty dressing off, washing your hands, opening things, using your clean hand, putting gloves on. It's using your knowledge base. You know which is your dirty hand or clean hand, or whatever and you know how to use gloves, the actual technique. You don't touch anything else once you've put your gloves on. [I learned that by] watching Jo or Claire and then asking if I can have a go and they're there to watch me and tell me what to do properly. They can advise and guide . . . It was nice to have the confidence to do things and I suppose because I feel fairly confident I do take things on, like the dressing.
(Jack 4: year 2 term 2)

Learning how to support people with mental illness also requires a great deal of skill:

The first time I went in there I said 'Would you like a bath?' and she said 'No'. So I went and told Melisssa and she said 'If you try it in this way, then you might get a better result'. And you go away and read in the books about depression and how important it is for a depressed person to be clean and neat and tidy because you start to build up their self-esteem. So you are being slightly manipulative about getting her into the bath. Perhaps gradually she'll begin to feel a bit better about herself and other people will say 'Hey, you look really nice.' So it starts from that. [Definitely having a mentor to give you ideas] because that's the only way you learn . . . They have the ability to see a situation from quite a few angles, which is something that is quite important.
(Nicola 11: year 3 term 3)

Here Nicola deals with her concerns about the ethics of manipulating patients and draws on the literature to satisfy herself that this mentor's approach is legitimate. These students received good support from their mentors who could recognise their role in providing opportunities to learn and who were willing to share their professional knowledge. Sometimes this coaching did not work so well and students were caught in the middle of different practices:

> I did the injection with someone else and I didn't really like it. I was actually copying how my mentor does it and this lady does it differently. That got me in a complete tizzy about what we were doing. It was 'don't do that'. That was in front of the patient. 'Why are you doing it that way?' and she talked to me as if I was an idiot . . . Unfortunately at this stage I don't have that much experience. I've given four injections maybe, so I haven't really got the confidence to think 'I'm not going to do it with a swab'.
> (Ruth 12: year 3 term 1)

The discrepancy in practice was confusing and because Ruth did not feel safe with the nurse who supervised her, she was unable to benefit from the experience. Having sufficient supervised experience and practice is clearly an important issue. Many techniques become commonplace after experience but without suitable advice and guidance students can unwittingly cause pain and are in even greater fear of causing it:

> I took out quite a few [men's urinary] catheters. It was quite scary because the first time I did it I didn't know how long the tube was going to be and you don't really know what the pain is like. Being female as well and they were all men. [Deflating the balloon] that's quite easy to do though because you can tell when all the water is out. What I found the worst thing was trying to get a CSU [catheterised specimen of urine] from the catheter before I took it out. It took me hours because there wasn't enough urine in the tube. I was with a nurse who is really good and she said to bend the tube and then put the needle in and so I had to draw it back with one hand and I just couldn't do it and the patient was really anxious. I wondered what I was doing to the poor man.
> (Helen 8: year 3 term 2)

Curriculum demands made it difficult for students to attend their clinical placement every day of the week and as Jack's narrative indicates changes in patterns of hospitalisation and medical practices limit opportunities to develop skills. The shorter clinical placements of students' second and third years particularly led them to feel concerned about obtaining as much practice at clinical techniques as they would have liked. To increase their confidence, most students worked in their vacations as healthcare assistants and were exposed to a variety of practices that sometimes created a conflict with professional codes of conduct and safe practice. They also needed opportunities to work with different patients and to learn how to prioritise and manage their care giving.

Becoming skilled

Learning techniques is highly complex and requires a sophisticated range of skills and knowledge. A simple example of doing a dressing or giving an injection includes more than the physical manipulation of equipment. A practitioner needs to be vigilant and mindful of several other factors: practical issues such preventing infection, monitoring and responding appropriately to a patient's behaviour, assessing and modifying care to the area being treated, utilising evidence based knowledge, and engaging in conversation to help the patient relax and cooperate. As in mental health work where non-verbal signals may be more subtle and critical, practitioners need to be mindful of the context of their interaction, of the client's specific needs and to plan their interventions accordingly. With practice, many techniques become so refined and familiar they become tacit and practitioners no longer need to think about what they are doing. For many students being talked through the procedure and later talking themselves through it helped them to remember the stages in the correct sequence. Once they had achieved the technical aspect they could begin to think about the other elements of the procedure:

> I think because before I did it I'd seen Sarah do it so much that it was a bit like, 'Oh yea just do this now.' A bit like old hat sort of thing. So it'd be me talking myself through the stages, telling her what I was going to do. Saying well, I'm going to clean the wound, the dressing now, now I'm going to put this padding on. I've got this padding on because the wound is not weeping like it was. I've only used one. And she'd say 'Yea that's OK.' So I'd be talking myself through it, but telling Sarah what I was doing.
> (Marie 3: year 2 term 1)

Transforming practical information into taken-for-granted-knowledge or tacit knowledge (Polanyi & Prosch 1973) took place in two stages. The first stage in Polanyi's terms entailed learning the necessary but subsidiary skills. Most skills consist of several components as Jack described earlier when talking about doing a wound dressing. Once students had practised and refined their ability to carry out each subsidiary skill so that they no longer needed to concentrate on them, they could then develop the focal skill by combining all the different subsidiary skills into one nursing task; and could then combine all the different tasks into providing individualised and holistic care. Developing relevant craft knowledge or a repertoire of knowledge of different but associated case examples enables students to adapt their practice according to each patient situation-at-hand. Once students were able to relax their concentration on both the subsidiary skills and the composite focal skill, then they had the psychological space to recognise what they needed to learn. Or they could begin to make connections between what they were experiencing in their practice with their formal knowledge from school or from their reading.

Having a coach to help them through these experiences speeded up the transition from what felt like a cack-handed novice to skilled practitioner. Once operational competence was achieved students needed to practice their focal skills to refine their performance and learn to contextualise their knowledge; how to adjust skills and knowledge according to the particular needs of a patient and the situation-at-hand. This form of thinking about practice and contextualising it on an individual case basis requires considerable practice and skill. On a relatively simple level Keller (Keller & Keller 1993), describes this process of evolving cognition in his black-smithying when forging a metal object. To achieve satisfactory results, a blacksmith is constantly evaluating the strength and heat of the metal and its readiness to be shaped. Throughout the process he is drawing on all his knowledge about metals, heat and pressure and what the final design will look like. In the same manner healthcare practitioners constantly monitor a huge range of signals and symptoms from their patients whilst also evaluating how they are responding to care as it is being delivered. They too draw on a wide range of knowledge whilst deciding whether to modify or change the process. Schön (Schön 1983) calls such activities 'reflection-in-action'. Benner (Benner, Tanner et al. 1996) describe the same sort of activities when researching expert nurses in action. They used the term 'active contemplation': a state of being 'present-at-hand'.

Becoming competent in a wide range of professional skills applicable to numerous clinical settings over a three-year programme provides a very short time for students to become independent and autonomous practitioners. Most other professions have a far longer period of supervised or supported practice both during and following qualification, and many practitioners are not expected to reach the same levels of professional maturity for a considerable time after qualifying. Relatively less complex activities such as athletics and opera singing are reckoned to take a minimum of eight to ten years of rigorous training before peak performance can be reached (Ericsson, Krampe et al. 1993). These researchers and others (Dreyfus & Dreyfus 1986) argue that expertise and skilled performance can only be developed following repeated exposure and practice, supported by good feedback from knowledgeable practitioners. Meeting this educational need is more and more difficult with changes to the organisation of healthcare and with the employment of fewer registered nurses undertaking care delivery. With healthcare becoming increasingly complex, mistakes become more commonplace, owing to practitioners working under greater pressures with often limited peer support or guidance. It also raises questions about the kinds of expectations managers hold and the extent to which they are realistic or whether they are based on expediency and a shrinking workforce.

6.3 Learning to bundle nursing activities together

Without appropriate support from their mentors, students had difficulty developing and refining their psychomotor skills and this seems to have influenced their ability to take on more complex activities such as organising and providing care to small groups of patients. With increasing competence the groups of patients became more complex in their needs and required more sophisticated knowledge and care. Managing such caseloads is described as 'bundling nursing activities together'. Nursing care is prescribed as a holistic package for patients. Past criticisms of organising nursing care on a task-allocation basis included patients being frequently disturbed, aspects of care being neglected and care often being substandard. Learning to carry out a nursing care plan for one or more patients over a shift requires considerable skill and time management. Providing care to a number of patients with different care needs and levels of dependency is even more sophisticated.

> I could actually see someone from admission through to going up to surgery without constantly having to ask what to do next. I could virtually do the pre-med, but I just needed the countersign and I could fill in all the forms and I would just double check. It wasn't as though they were leading me by the hand. I was going off on my own, but obviously getting it checked. I spent the first few times with my mentor and then I'd take the easier cases on my own. That would be a case of us both saying hello to the patients and I'd come back and maybe she'd say 'What are you going to do this morning for this person?' and we'd go through it, agree it and then I'd go off. Depending on what it was, if it was a dressing she'd supervise me, but if it was assisting someone to the toilet I'd go off. Actually there was a time by week six or seven that she said I could do more. My mentor said I didn't really need to ask because I knew what's what. You get a feel for what you can and can't do, but it's still difficult as a student because if something does go wrong . . . It was nerve wracking and I wondered what I was getting nervous about. A lot of it is common sense, the daily things you would do at home. So before you tell Mr. Bloggs he can go and leap in the bath like we'd all do, then you find out that because of the surgery he's had he mustn't go near the shower for six weeks. And you suddenly realise you've just told him he can have one!
> (Ruth 13: year 3 term 2)

As with the other students, Ruth learned a great deal more than just the technical aspects of care by having opportunities to work alone. Even Jack, who had worked for eighteen months as a general/adult student nurse, and also as a registered mental nurse, had so many more much-needed opportunities to learn how to plan and manage prescribed care, and he was anxious to be allowed to do so.

Having a caseload of patients gave students opportunities to practise their skills with different patients and to identify aspects of care as problematic or requiring more information. Perhaps more importantly it gave students a sense of self-confidence and worth that was highly motivating and stimulated their learning:

> It's the first one I've really got into. In the third week I was going out by myself with my own patients and feeding back to Iris what had happened and what I thought should happen and seeing the doctors and referring to dieticians, going to see the consultants with them. It was really good and I had a good rapport with most of them. In the end they were telling me things that I fed back to Iris and she would say 'I didn't know that. They haven't told me that before'. So I thought it was really good and I really enjoyed that module. I feel that my personal development had really shown this module. I was linking in things from my psychology in my first year and the first term this year and relating in my science and exploring lots of issues. I really felt it was good.
> (Marie 11: year 3 term 3)

Being supernumerary meant that students could seek help from the patients' named nurse and work at a pace that allowed them to think about what they were doing. They were able to see patients as people rather than as work objects as Helen had once described her patients in the nursing home. Being supernumerary and having their own caseload of patients gave students time to talk to them, to understand their dilemmas, to learn about them and to develop new understandings about their medical conditions for their practice.

6.4 Developing professional craft knowledge

Experienced practitioners draw on a range of knowledge derived from a variety of sources. Much of it comes from learning in practice through watching other people, reflecting on successful or unsuccessful actions and reading patients' case notes, relevant texts and more recently using the internet. This practical everyday experience, otherwise known as fingertip or craft knowledge is best underpinned by formal theory that has been contextualised to the situation-at-hand. Practitioners use this knowhow according to the situation-at-hand and mould it accordingly. Students are exposed to a vast amount of formal knowledge during their programme. Much of it has been decontextualised from everyday practice and documented. Their curriculum was designed to help students apply this information to their practice using several different strategies such as action inquiry/problem-based learning, reflective practice, case studies and seminars. Students needed to learn how to recognise the saliency of this knowledge to their everyday encounters with patients and their carers. With practice they learned to notice the signs and symptoms of patients' conditions and to relate formal knowhow to the situation-at-hand. Over time they learned to refine their repertoire of knowledge by recognising case examples and knowing how to modify their practice to meet patients' individual needs. Formal knowledge alone is insufficient in support this kind of development, irrespective of the manner in which it is delivered. A fundamental element in supporting students' learning of professional craft knowledge is coaching from a knowledgeable and experienced practitioner. By working alongside such a practitioner whilst giving care, students can pick up tips that reflect the situation:

> Some things are so obvious and you don't think. Like doing the post-op checks for the first few weeks – you know you concentrate on the blood pressure fine, and she [mentor] said 'Did you check the wound site?' and I didn't look at that. He'd had major abdominal surgery and I suddenly thought how obvious it was. She would say 'What I do, Ruth, for post-op is the observation as per the chart, but more than just the chart. This gentleman has had a big operation on his leg, so look at his leg. His temperature might be fine for the next five minutes but he could be bleeding profusely the whole time.' That's so obvious and I didn't think of it.
> (Ruth 13: year 3 term 2)

The earlier narratives in this chapter and the students' case studies in Chapter 3 provide examples of how they picked up information incidentally whilst working with their mentor or another practitioner. Sometimes this was through preparatory sessions before taking supervised responsibility for a group of patients as described by Jack, or in debriefing sessions (for example, Marie's experiences in the community). Students used such experiences to expand their knowledge by going back to their text books to learn more about their patient's problems and so expanding their knowledge base. Being supernumerary provided the emotional, physical and social space for them to learn in a way that being part of the workforce makes impossible.

Curriculum and learning

The curriculum for this particular programme had been structured to promote integration of theory and practice. Lecturers who were also practitioners were responsible for teaching nursing so could share their expertise and knowledge of current practices and theories in the local clinical setting. Classroom learning also sensitised students to their practical knowledge:

> You get into really bad habits of talking over the patients in the nursing home. I think I've realised just from talking to people how much power nurses really have. A lot has come out of our seminars. Like the way you feed them and whether you let them help themselves. Just from a time-consuming point of view, getting them dressed in the morning. Some patients in the nursing home I'm sure could dress themselves if they were given time and a bit of help ... Having a seminar once a week helps as well. Each one was really helpful, especially having the lecturer–practitioner on my ward. She'd talk about patients and say 'Now look at how you lift such and such with the hoist' and it's so much more specific. Although it was in the room something like this, the hospital is just over there and you know the patients they're talking about and it's really relevant. A lot of times we didn't come to any conclusions. Should you feed someone if they don't want to be fed? What rights do we have? Then we'd talk about how powerful nurses could be and how you have to be careful and that we should just give them as much leeway as possible. Then we'd talk about experiences of one patient and they were interesting.
> (Helen 1: year 2 term 1)

Evidently, Helen is drawing on a variety of sources and is using critical incidents from practice to trigger her learning. As with the other students she became more sensitive to her own practice and as a result was able to compare different nursing practices and relationships. By using experiences as critical incidents students could demonstrate their level of competence and achievement required by their course learning outcomes as Petra describes here.

> [My objective is] improving my communication skills. It's very short, I just recognise the [importance of] non-verbal communication. At first I didn't think she wanted to talk to me and I found her very hard going. I realised that with mentally ill people they often don't want to talk and then I decided to try again. I tried to use some of the communication skills I'd read about in Chapman and Hore, and that I'd learned from my seminar. I used lots of eye contact and posture towards her to show that I was interested the second time I talked to her. Although she never looked directly at me she was directing her attention towards me. I think she was more comfortable with me. I felt I was establishing a beneficial relationship and also being therapeutic. In future conversations I had with her, she even smiled on one occasion.
> (Petra 3: year 2 term 3)

Petra illustrates how despite several setbacks from working with this patient she went back into her placement and used information from several sources to help her achieve a successful outcome with her patient. Students mentors had responsibility for verifying that the materials they discussed in their learning contracts represented their clinical performance.

In other situations, writing their learning contracts could be frustrating, for several intrinsic and extrinsic reasons such as lack of preparation, a heavy assessment schedule, lack of support, or poor access to the necessary literature.

> What I try and do at some stage that day, if not the next morning, is just write a summary of what I've done and try to reflect on it. Then I don't forget . . . At the end of the day you try and fit your learning contract round what you do. I'm still dubious and open minded about it. I've done quite well. I think I'm on the right track and I can't deny it does make you think. So the theory is getting a lot better. The learning contract has to be about practice and I'm sure with practise we'll all get better.
> (Ruth 4: year 2 term 1)

> This time I've made more of an effort to write down everything that happens on the shift and I've been using the spider diagram. I'll put something in and draw my points from it. There's been so much I can put in that I don't think it's going to be a big problem writing it. [the spider diagrams summarise experience on the shift] what happened and my immediate reaction. Most of it [my reading] has been for essays for developmental psychology and I did a presentation on the Mental Health Act. I've got a couple of books out on counselling and I've been reading them, but I haven't read very much directly related to my placement as of yet. I will do though. I've been looking everywhere for books on self-harm and I can't find anything. I'm going to have to look in journals I think. I'm really quite enthusiastic about it all.
> (Nicola 8: year 3 term 1)

Their learning contracts demonstrate how students were able to develop their professional knowledge despite their often intense frustration. As they indicate, such knowledge was not necessarily at their fingertips when they were working with particular patients and when they first needed it. But their learning contracts provided a means for students to develop their craft knowledge and so their ability to care for their future patients experiencing similar kinds of problems, and this helped them to anticipate patients' needs better. As we have seen, students' learning was not only motivated by their assessment but also by their encounters in practice.

6.5 Learning to manage feelings and emotions

> I know I get attached to little children too easily, and I know I've got to harden up to that, because you can't get attached to patients. I hope that I'd be able to think to myself, 'Well this child has got this and he's going to be feeling bad.' And just hopefully [I'll] be able to do my greatest help to try and get him through, all the way through it. Well lots of people have said to me, 'You've got to harden up, or else you're not going to cope'. When you've seen something really horrible, with some two-year-old child for six weeks and they finally don't

make it, they said 'You're not going to cope, you're going to be a mess'. When this time, while I've been on the wards, I'll be going home, going, 'Oh there's this gorgeous child, he's so lovely!' And everyone's saying, 'You can't do that Natalie, you've got to just see them as patients. Because if they do die or anything, then you're going to be in a mess'.
(Natalie 1: year 2 term 1)

Natalie's feelings and fears about caring for children or adults who die was a common worry for the students. Not only death but any form of human distress and discomfort could leave them feeling helpless and frustrated. Students were concerned about how to cope effectively and professionally with such situations. But they were also concerned by a range of dilemmas, ethical, legal and moral as well as the emotional issues identified above. Students' other concerns were associated with supporting grieving patients or relatives, coping with anger and abuse that is directed at them but that possibly represented years of frustration or a multitude of other emotions that lay people can walk away from. Yet these students needed to learn how to respond professionally to them. Natalie's story echoes the public view of nurses as hardened or indifferent to suffering. Helen's concern was that she might become hardened and lose her feminine attributes of compassion. Outsiders often describe nurses as drama queens because of the stories they tell their friends, perhaps to debrief from dreadful scenes that have not been debriefed at work. Throughout the programme students were struggling to come to terms with a huge range of perplexing and often distressing dilemmas to which they had little exposure before they started nursing. Whilst they had worked as care assistants they were unlikely to receive much emotional support from the staff (see, for example, Helen's story). Learning how to provide care that is empathetic to a patient's experience and sharing it without feeling pain is a demanding and perhaps unrealistic expectation of healthcare professionals. Small wonder that so many students and new staff experience mental health problems (Baldwin, Dodd et al. 1998). Being able to provide emotional support whilst also attending to the needs of several other patients requires a special approach and sophisticated professional skills. Natalie's friends realised that it was a skill she needed to acquire if she was going to protect herself. Helen was afraid that acquiring such a skill, meant losing her sensitivity, perhaps by misinterpreting her older colleagues' responses. Nevertheless, students learnt how to develop such skills by talking to friends and colleagues. Here Marie describes her feelings after learning about the unexpected death of a baby following a routine investigation. She had looked after him earlier and knew his parents:

> I was so stunned, it just knocked me back. If it had been expected may be I'd have said, why? What happened? But I was so shocked. And I had to keep it shut out of myself the whole shift because I'd be in the office and I'd start thinking about him and the way he'd been and I'd nearly burst into tears and I knew I couldn't do that on the ward. Not because on the ward I had to keep my professional whatever, but because I knew that if I burst into tears on the ward I wouldn't be able to concentrate for the rest of day. So I kept trying to shut it out at the back of my mind and when I got home I thought about it and it made me accept what had happened. Not really grief stricken . . . I had to keep saying to myself he'd gone to a

better place, his parents hadn't to go through so much pain . . . I didn't feel like talking to anyone in the flat and Penny, the only person I would have talked to wasn't there. She was on a late shift. I spoke to Martin (my boyfriend) on the phone and told him. It was nice to be able to talk to someone. It was supportive, but it wasn't as supporting as talking to Penny, because she understands what I am going through. She'd had to cope with quite a lot of death. I felt more comfortable talking to her about it. Maybe because it was face-to-face and there was eye contact and all the other non-verbal signals.
(Marie 13: year 4 term 1)

As for most people, students' first encounter with death can be emotionally traumatic and Marie sought comfort and understanding from someone who understood the situation. Clinical colleagues can provide such help but often students feel more comfortable with peers. Pam Smith's research into emotional labour in nursing (Smith 1992; Smith & Gray 2001) identified how 'feeling rules' exhibited by a charge nurse sets the emotional climate for a clinical setting. She argued that if nursing students feel nurtured and supported they are more able to provide care that nurtured and supported patients and their carers whilst helping them learn effective ways of coping without suffering burnout. With students working alongside mentors and opportunities to develop friendship and trust this kind of immediate support is more likely to be available. Marie did work in such an environment and did receive support from the staff; but both she and Helen needed a more personal kind of support. After the death of patients they knew well, both Helen and Marie describe how they tried to suppress their distress until they found a suitable moment to go through their own grieving. Hochschild (Hochschild 1983) describes this process as an essential skill of undertaking emotional labour. She argues that in service industries (such as air-hostessing) effective practitioners should learn how to deal with strong emotions as well as how to induce personal feelings such as friendliness, kindness and so on. In this way practitioners are acting out their professional role, showing interest and caring to their clients. Hochschild identified three particular elements of emotional work:

- face-to-face contact with the public
- producing an emotional state in the recipient, such as gratitude, relief, stress-relief, by the worker;
- control over the worker's emotional activities through training and supervision by the employer.

In their daily involvement with the public, nursing practitioners are constantly supporting people in distress. However support for practitioners tends to be limited with little training or effective and continuing supervision. Learning how to increase their self-awareness is a critical skill that reflective practice develops. When responding to people with mental illness this skill is crucial:

I did [feel frightened in the ward]. I don't now because I try and avoid getting myself in a situation where I am actually in danger. I'm sure I will be frightened in years to come and will probably end up being in the wrong place at the wrong time. But as yet I haven't. I suppose

someone bigger than you taking a swing at you. And I find that difficult when someone has very sexual behaviour or is sexually disinhibited. I find that very difficult. I get embarrassed and unfortunately I blush and there's no way I can hide being embarrassed. I feel out of control then . . . But if there's danger you just push the emergency button and hopefully lots of people will arrive.
(Nicola 14: year 4 term 1).

Learning how to cope with such feelings and dilemmas strengthened students' sense of being nurses and helped them to contain their feelings. In some respects as they developed they created a form of professional membrane. This is perhaps a clumsy metaphor to describe the process whereby students were able to retain their sensitivity to patients, whilst retaining their own integrity. Of being present with them in their distress and yet not becoming enmeshed by it and to suffer as a consequence. Such an ability has been described in various ways, Peplau (Peplau 1991) describes it as an attribute of maturity as a nurse. Godkin (Godkin 2001) describes this ability to empathise with patients and their carers as an important element of having a 'healing presence'. She describes this form of being present with a patient, as intuitive and subjective, having a phenomenological understanding of the patient's needs. These female students needed to learn how to develop such compassion whilst preserving their own mental health and well-being. Learning how to respond to such situations could best be achieved through support from their mentors and supervisors whilst engaged in clinical practice. Learning to respond to different events within a community is influenced by how other members of the community normally act. Nursing students wishing to enter a community of healthcare practitioners, have to relearn old habitual responses that would be regarded as normal behaviour in their home or university communities, and adjust to those of each new clinical setting. Regular contact and support from 'old-timers' or people who are established members of the community of practice (the ward or department and so on), such as their mentors and clinical colleagues helps them achieve this (Bruner 1990; Stearns 1995; Wenger 1998). Helen's eventual insight that adopting a stoical approach did not necessarily result in hard-heartedness, was perhaps important for her own progress towards learning and becoming a nurse, and could only have been acquired by regular, close contact with her mentors and other nursing colleagues.

6.6 Learning to cope with ethical dilemmas

Students were deeply troubled by some patients' experiences beyond the shock of witnessing them or the responses they encountered. They sought to take a broader perspective, using their understanding by drawing on their own beliefs, values, philosophy and religious values as well as their learning about ethics and so on. When faced with a conundrum they examined the situation rigorously to find their own solutions.

> I sometimes wondered about the quality of life and whether it's worth resuscitating people and how far medical science can save people if the quality of life after you've saved them is

going to be crap. Are you doing anyone any favours really? It's all very well having these high tech machines and being able to save people's lives, but if once it's saved . . . I know one of the guys on the ward was really pissed off and angry because people used to say 'You've done really well' if he'd walked three steps. Before he had the accident he was able to weight lift or run God knows where. He was only young too. I think that's the problem, that there isn't the money put into rehab. It's seen as an expensive luxury rather than a necessity and in a way the money is probably better spent in the rehab. than in saving their lives.
(Jack 10: year 3 term 2)

Students' encounters with patients stimulated much thought and questioning as Jack's incident above indicates. On a more everyday level:

If someone says 'I don't want to eat this today' then fine. But you're told in mental health that what they say isn't really what they want. And you end up thinking 'God, what the hell is going on?' It was very good for me as it showed me an important lesson. One lady I was with came in quite depressed and she just didn't want to eat. I was asked to help her eat. She was quite good about it because if I got the spoon up to her mouth she would take it, but she would say to me 'I don't want this. I don't know why you're wasting your time on me.' She got better and started feeding herself. When I sat chatting with her in the afternoon I said 'Do you remember you weren't eating at one stage?' and she said 'Oh, I'm so glad you did feed me. I'm feeling so much better now'. That was good to hear because my gut reaction is that if someone says they don't want to eat, then I don't think they should be made to. I believe that quite strongly. The only way I think I can justify them, is going back to the professional code of conduct and saying 'I'm a professional and it's my duty to keep them fed'. So I suppose that's where I take my guidance from.
(Ruth 6: year 2 term 2)

This approach indicates the conflict Ruth experienced with her own image of 'being there for the patients'. As a last resort, perhaps to salve her conscience, she used guidelines that had been prescribed. Also on a personal level, students expressed concern about their ability to remain congruent with their aspirations and guiding images. Helen's fear of becoming hardened and indifferent reflects one important aspect of their concern. Finding a means of coming to terms with traumatic events whilst remaining sensitive and congruent to patients' identified needs was challenging and required courage. For all the students, there was an internal struggle to come to terms with what they encountered. Sometimes this was concerned with how care was provided and other times it was because they had to witness the decisions of other healthcare practitioners:

Even though I realised that he had to be up and mobilised I felt guilty about moving a patient who was in pain. He was having painkillers and they didn't seem to be having any effect. I presume they were, but the more anxious he got . . . I discussed this with Louise and she said maybe we rushed him sometimes and we should have spent more time with him and assessed him better. But I realise that because she's busy it's difficult for her. So I reflected on that and how I felt about mobilising and I realised it was the right thing to do. When the patient's complaining of pain it's a bit heart-rending. Maybe it would be better if I just left him in bed. We like to empower our patients and get them to tell us what they want, but sometimes we have to say 'Look, you need to be up and about'. I try and say to myself 'If he stays in bed, even if he is in pain, he'll develop a pressure sore perhaps, he might develop a chest infection'. You can get wasted limbs and stiff joints not moving around, so it would be

far worse in the long run. If you explain all these things to him it would be far worse doing what he wanted. If you explain that it's important for him to be up and about despite the fact he's in pain. That's how I reassure myself that we're doing the right thing. That's empowering them isn't it? If he's in that much pain and normally a patient will go along with what you want – but if he's in that much pain and that unwell I don't think it's fair to drag them out of bed everyday. It's difficult.
(Grace 4: year 2 term 3)

I went with my lecturer–practitioner. There were so many people and nobody introduced themselves to the patient, and one of them was even talking over her when she was under anaesthetic. She had so many self-harm marks that they said 'Has she been sexually abused?' It was nothing to do with them.
(Petra 3: year 3 term 3)

He's got a couple of years and not everyone wants to know because it might alter things. But I was talking to him and his sister and he was saying 'I don't know whether I should go back to work or perhaps I should go and do something that I've always wanted to do and enjoy myself'. That was really hard because I knew something about him that he didn't and it was really strange . . . The wife didn't even know. But now he's not going to know he's ill.
(Helen 11: year 4 term 2)

Situations like these raise serious concerns for students and learning how to reconcile them with their knowledge and understanding of best practice can compromise their position.

6.7 Developing the essence of nursing and therapeutic action

In Chapter 4 we explored students' visions of how they would be as nurses. Having the time and energy to give care in a manner that was faithful to such visions was promoted by their supernumerary status. Their course philosophy embraced and required students to develop skills of reflective practice. Their assessment strategies encouraged students to develop self-awareness. In the process they became critically aware of the extent to which their ideals could be realised or were appropriate. In most instances they strived to remain faithful to them. Their essence was to provide care that was holistic and empathetic to their patient's needs. With increasing understanding and skill they became more proficient. Throughout their programme students found the process of learning to become reflective practitioners challenging and sometimes painful, necessitating students to appraise and question their experiences. Perhaps Nicola was the most vulnerable of the participants as she was the most conscious of using her selfhood when working with patients. As she identified, among other things, she was frequently discomforted by her patients' socially inappropriate behaviour. She was conscious that she needed to develop a strategy that safeguarded herself without jeopardising her therapeutic role:

But thinking about me as a nursing student and me as Nicola, a lot of them over-link. But definitely the way you talk to people is different from the way you do at home and that's

healthy and good. You have to be professional about it and do your job. I'm not trying to sound callous, but you've got to be very careful to make some boundaries and keep them separate, otherwise you just take everything home with you and that's not good. It's not good for the client either. You're not doing them any favours. But some of the skills you've learned being a nurse might be of benefit outside where you communicate with people. It might help. I'm trying to get more in touch with my feelings, like 'Hell, I found that really hard', so therefore I need to take some time out for a few minutes just to get my head round it. I've got to know that that's work and then I've got an outside of my nursing life and that nursing isn't always first and foremost. Most of the time it's top of my list, but I want to be me before anything else.
(Nicola 13: year 4 term 1)

Nicola's strong awareness of the boundaries of her role and relationship with patients is reflected to a lesser extent in the narratives of other students as they developed their role. As they became more confident in their knowledge and technical skills, their ability to provide care which was in keeping with their images of good practice began to inform their approach more fully. Students were exposed to a range of theoretical models for nursing practice, all of which advocated a holistic approach to patient care. Their narratives illustrate how students strived to achieve this. Their development seems to have been derived from a range of sources beyond the technical or managerial. They saw ways in which they could act as well as to try and implement their own beliefs about therapeutic practice. As students became more experienced, their workload changed and they were faced with a sense of regression as they struggled to implement patients' prescribed care. Jack' expresses the challenge they all experienced:

I think you're trying to give high quality care. This lady is depressed. I think I could really help her. This morning she's a lot brighter. I don't think that's anything I did because I was on yesterday morning looking after her and she was totally flat. And this morning she's totally different. Maybe it's the anti-depressants starting to work because she's been on them just under a week. But I suppose that's the thing that's lacking. You're giving her good physical care and looking after her that way, but that isn't enough, but you could spend half an hour just sitting chatting to her and I haven't got that time. She does need quite a lot and you wash her. I'm spending a lot of time trying to motivate her, so I am putting the psychological bit in there while I'm doing the physical bit. It's all aimed at her getting to do a wash and you're asking how she feels and she says 'I don't know, I'm fed up'. But it's just that still isn't enough in a way. I suppose it's because it's an acute medical ward.
(Jack 15: year 4 term 3)

The essence of nursing and of giving such care was students' ability to be 'present' with their patients and to see and respond to their needs effectively. It would be unreasonable to anticipate that they were able to deliver such care all the time but it was evident that they held it in mind and provided great personal satisfaction, despite being difficult to articulate. In Chapter 4, pages 135–6, Marie describes how through her own experience and insight she could fulfil her caring responsibilities towards parents of in-patient children in a manner that went beyond the technical and immediate demands of her task. She was sensitive to the implications of the mother's anxiety, and in using a range of insights and knowledge was able to suggest a means of resolving some of her conflicts. Students' willingness to work alongside their patients and carers, and to use themselves therapeutically, illustrates their commitment and preparedness to learn through their own pain. Such combinations of intimacy, reciprocity and partnership relate to Muetzel's (Muetzel 1988) description of therapeutic nursing and characterise the artistic dimension of nursing described by Carper (Carper 1978). Carper's four fundamental patterns of nursing knowledge: empirical, or scientific knowledge; the moral or ethical component of nursing; aesthetics or the art of nursing; and personal knowing. The earlier sections of this chapter illustrate students' struggle to utilise and develop their knowledge and understanding of the scientific aspects of nursing whilst also becoming technically competent. In being able to combine these two elements and to reformulate their knowledge to their everyday practice, they began to develop their professional craft knowledge for everyday use with patients. Throughout their programme students were constantly questioning practices that they observed and they explored them in relation to their own values and beliefs as well as in relation to their newly acquired and developing professional and legal knowledge. As they felt more confident and were able to make a greater contribution to the overall work of their clinical colleagues they were more able to relax, to take note of what was happening around them and to think more widely about the way in which they were delivering care.

For these students the more subtle attributes of caring and nursing were concerned with the manner in which care could be offered and the ethos they created through interactions with patients and their carers. Jourard (Jourard 1971) describes nursing as a special case of loving, through an ability to be open, honest and in touch with self, which promotes self-development. However because these students had insufficient case knowledge or exposure to sufficient examples and variations of the same sorts of patient problems they were not yet at a stage of being able to manipulate their understanding and refashion it to plan and provide holistic care for individual patients. They were probably better able to identify and read their patient's less subtle signals. For example, Grace was able to sense her patient's reluctance to move because of insufficient pain relief, even though her mentor had apparently overlooked the signals. They had not yet accumulated a repertoire of knowledge of what could or would not work for each patient and when to act. Such knowledge is described as characteristic of expert nurses or nurses who have a healing presence (Benner, Tanner et al. 1996; Godkin 2001). Achieving such expertise requires considerable practice and experience. These students had moved beyond the novice stage (or in Godkin's terms the stage of lay/bedside presence) and had progressed into the professional domain and developed their ability to provide a clinical presence.

6.8 Developing interprofessional relationships

Students' entry to their clinical placements was a key factor influencing their success and this will be discussed in greater detail in the next chapter. As they progressed through their programme they engaged in more collaborative relationships with different members of the health and social care team. As they acquired their skills and knowledge and undertook more sophisticated and more complex nursing activities for patients, so their contacts broadened. In the process they developed a greater understanding of the different roles of other healthcare professionals and were better able to liase with them when planning care. This had a significant impact on their identity and their self-confidence.

Throughout their programme an important influence on their access to clinical placements was the university timetable and freedom from lectures and tutorials, as well as the accessibility of their mentors. Even following careful planning shifts were changed and students encountered difficulties:

> I have to do weekends because you have to get in 20 shifts and it's hard to get them in at the best of times. The Sister said 'You pick your days don't you. There's nobody here at the weekends.' That wasn't very nice. Not even a 'Hello, nice to see you' and I just thought 'Roll on 3.00pm.' But you get that at work. In that situation I'd just maybe laugh, certainly wouldn't make a deal out of it. I find it's quite intimidating. I wouldn't make an issue of it, probably go bright red and feel a complete idiot and sit quietly in the corner and wait for handover and keep out of her way.
> (Ruth 12: year 3 term 1)

Ruth's experience was common and illustrates the difficulty clinical staff had in understanding the curriculum students were following. More often than not students overcame their embarrassment, but not without a great deal of personal discomfort, especially if they were mature students, used to being treated with respect. To increase their acceptance by clinical staff, students regularly engaged in minor activities that could be seen as helpful and would in some way reciprocate the staff for the time they felt they were taking up:

> I was there for ten weeks and I didn't mind doing whatever needed to be done. There was an auxiliary off sick and at dinnertime I would help the auxiliary, get everything ready, make cups of tea, do the washing up if it needed doing. I'd do anything that needed to be done. It was as though I was part of the team. If I didn't feel comfortable with something, I said so. They were all there if I needed any help. It was as if all the team were my mentors. If I wanted any help from them you could go to any of them for literature, etc. and that was really good. I felt part of the team and it was a good feeling. I felt I'd achieved a lot more than just getting on with the patients. It increased my confidence as well, which was really nice.
> (Marie 5: year 2 term 3)

Occasionally because of ward closures or change in clinical use students were moved to a different setting during their placement. Students were often disturbed by such moves, losing the confidence brought about by incidental but important things such as knowing where to find equipment and being familiar with the different staff. These could be important in an emergency. Jack had this experience but fortunately in this instance his mentor was also moved.

> I didn't particularly know what was going on. The machines that go beep and it feels quite disabling. I think it was disabling also to be moved half way through [the last placement]. In a way it was quite good because I had the same mentor, but things were different. You

couldn't get continuity because half way through you suddenly got changed and suddenly had to get used to a new ward again. Where do they keep things? Just as you feel comfortable you get moved and then the term finishes.
(Jack 10: year 3 term 2)

With increasing use of healthcare assistants or nursing auxiliaries to replace the student workforce, supernumerary students inevitably worked alongside them:

Certainly the associate [registered] nurse had very similar standards [to my mentor]. A couple of the older nursing auxiliaries weren't the same, but there were two new auxiliaries and they were really willing to learn and they came to listen to my mentor when I was with her and I thought we learnt a lot together. Two of them came two weeks after me, which made it even better because they didn't think 'Who's this coming and invading us?' Because I'd been there a bit before them. We got on really well and that really helped. Obviously their standards are not the same as my mentor's at the moment, but they're willing. One is in the same situation as me, having worked in a nursing home and she was talking to me saying how true it was that they treated them differently in a home. We realised it wasn't really nursing as a trained nurse should act.
(Helen 2: year 2 term 1)

As students gained in self-confidence they felt more able to contribute to the overall function of the unit and this exposed them to more members of the clinical team:

I will do these things, take on responsibilities, help share the ward work and be useful to them to try and get in on their team because I just think it affects the nursing care. It certainly affects how I get on with people, the ward staff as individuals and as people. Maybe at the end of the day it doesn't affect client outcome, but I think it does. If you have a happy committed workforce and a work team that values you as a member I'm sure you get more out of your placement than if you're not. [When I've been able to make a contribution] I've felt more comfortable definitely and if I feel that, I feel more confident and I think I can help patients more. Particularly, say in your relationship with the doctors, if I have a patient I'm not sure about and I don't feel confident with the ward staff it's twice as hard to go and say to the Sister 'I think I need a doctor here'. I hope I will call them, but I'll think twice about it. Whereas if I'm confident with the team and they're confident with me and I know the doctors I don't have the hesitation about phoning them up and saying 'Look, it's Ruth, the student, and I'm worried about this person'.
(Ruth 20: year 4 term 1)

Ruth seems to summarise the concerns all students had as they became more familiar with nursing work. Their relationship with members of the clinical team had a strong influence on their confidence and development. Throughout their programme students came in contact with different members of the healthcare team, ancillary workers, doctors and other practitioners. During their placement at the rehabilitation unit, Helen and Jack, developed a diffused identity about their own role and how it related to their other colleagues which was a unique experience. Jack was stimulated and refreshed by the experience, feeling that he was valued by the team and able to make a contribution on behalf of his patients.

Even in the ward rounds when people come in I'd chip in if I didn't agree with what was being said. People would respect what you said and take it on board. You felt you were being listened to, be it just as a student or a nurse. It was interesting because on the ward rounds the consultant would say, 'Right I want to hear from the nurse, the physio, OT etc. and then the medics would be last, if at all'. Rather than at the [main hospital] where the medics come first. That was the way it was done. Very much 'Where are we going?' Definitely more of a partnership than anything else and the rights of the client, what they wanted. If they didn't want something you might explore why they didn't want it and try and encourage them that it was in their best interests, but if they were adamant. . . .
(Jack 10: year 3 term 2)

Working in a democratically managed environment helped students to settle in quickly and to learn and also to make a contribution to the overall success of the setting.

6.9 Developing professional knowledge

Students' professional growth was complex and development of each area identified here was interrelated rather than wholly sequential or linear. These students' principal concern was to fulfil their vision of how nurses relate to patients and their friends and their family and how to conduct themselves in a therapeutic manner. Faced with a reality of practice, they struggled with feelings of self-consciousness and embarrassment when dealing with unfamiliar and difficult situations. Helping them to gain self-confidence and begin to match their vision with their practice, was their increased professional competence in technical knowledge and ability to bring together a range of complex activities when caring for a single patient and later for several patients. By the end of the first half of their branch programme they were sufficiently confident to organise and manage their own work, knowing how to bundle their activities of nursing together. This was particularly noticeable with Marie and Nicola who had been members of a small group of students following their particular branch programme. As a result there were relatively fewer students going through the same clinical areas and so received much better mentorship support than adult branch students. Another influential factor was the structure of their programme. This allowed for longer, more intense periods of practice time. Once students felt technically skilled, they all began to recognise the relevance of their observations in practice to the theory they had acquired. This helped them to increase their craft knowledge and with it their self-confidence in relating to patients and to enjoy more equal relationships with colleagues in their placement settings.

Another area of importance in their development included the extent to which they could manage feelings and emotions, and this helped them to perform in therapeutic ways. These factors represent areas with which students were frequently, consistently and specifically concerned throughout their programme. It was also evident that students' development was influenced by their emotional state and the degree of confidence achieved in each placement area of practice.

Some of the influential factors affecting students' development were existential and others, perhaps from the perspective of this study the most important, were largely beyond the grasp of educators and curriculum planners and remained primarily and irrevocably within the remit of clinical practitioners. Subsidiary factors that influenced their development included their supernumerary status, and opportunities to discuss their experiences with peers, with practitioners and also with their teachers. Each group of factors offered different and unique media for learning. It is these that will be discussed next.

References

Baldwin, P., Dodd, M. et al. (1998) *Nurses: Training, work, health and welfare: A longitudinal study*. Chief Scientist Office, Department of Health, The Scottish Office, Edinburgh.
Benner, P., Tanner, C.A. et al., Eds. (1996) *Expertise in Nursing Practice: Caring, Clinical Judgement and Ethics*. Springer Publishing, Cambridge MA.
Bruner, J. (1990) *Acts of Meaning*. Harvard University Press, Cambridge, MA.
Buber, M. (1937) *I and Thou*. T & T Clark, Edinburgh.
Carper, B.A. (1978) Fundamental patterns of knowing. *Advances in Nursing Science* 1: 13–23.
Dreyfus, H.I., Dreyfus, S.E. (1986) *Mind over machine. The power of human intuition and expertise in the era of the computer*. Basil Blackwell, Oxford.
Ericsson, K.A., Krampe, R. Th., et al. (1993) The role of deliberate practice in the acquisition of expert performance. *Psychological Review* 100 (3): 363–406.
Godkin, J. (2001) Healing presence. *Journal of Holistic Nursing* 19 (1): 5–21.
Hochschild, A.R. (1983) *The Managed Heart: Commercialization of human feeling*. University of California Press, Berkley.
Jourard, S.M. (1971) The 'manners' of helpers and healers: The bedside manners of nurses. In: *The Transparent Self*. (ed. S.M. Jourard) pp. 179–207. Van Nostrand Reinhold, New York.
Keller, C., Keller, J.D. (1993) Thinking and acting with iron. In: *Understanding Practice: Perspectives on activity and context*. (eds S. Chaiklin, J. Lave) pp. 125–78. University Press, Cambridge.
Muetzel, P. (1988) Therapeutic nursing. In: *Primary Nursing: Nursing in the Oxford and the Burford Nursing Development Units*. (ed. A. Pearson) pp. 89–116. Croom Helm, London.
Peplau, H.E. (1991) *Interpersonal relations in nursing: A conceptual framework of reference for psychodynamic nursing*. Springer-Verlag, New York/Berlin.
Polanyi, M., Prosch, H. (1973) *Meaning*. Chicago University Press, Chicago.
Schön, D. (1983) *The Reflective Practitioner: How professionals think in action*. Arena Ashgate Publishing, Aldershot.
Smith, P. (1992) *The Emotional Labour of Nursing*. Macmillan, Basingstoke.
Smith, P., Gray, B. (2001) Reassessing the concept of emotional labour in student nurse education: role of link lecturers and mentors in a time of change. *Nurse Education Today* 21: 230–7.
Stearns, P. (1995) Emotion. In: *Discursive Psychology in Practice*. (eds R. Harré, P. Stearns) pp. 37–54. Sage, London.
Wenger, E. (1998) *Communities of Practice: Learning, meaning and identity*. Cambridge University Press, Cambridge.

Chapter 7
Supporting Professional Development

So far we have explored students' perceptions of how they wanted to be as nurses, the progress they made and the kinds of knowledge they believed they needed in order to become nurses. Chapters 3 to 6 have presented detailed views of six individual students' professional development and case-study perspectives on all eight participants in the research. These illustrated experiences, joys and difficulties that are different from normal experiences of everyday life. Preparing newcomers to a healthcare profession is challenging, and no matter how graphically the reality of everyday practice is described, people still need to find their own truths through experience. These earlier chapters illustrate how much personality and other existential factors can motivate students to pursue their vision of ideal practice. In this chapter we shall look at the key extrinsic factors that students found most influential in supporting their professional development.

Inevitably the most significant influence on their development was the nature and quality of students' acceptance by clinical nursing staff and their relationship with clinical colleagues who supported them in their practice, particularly their mentors. Students' mentors were clearly the key to their progress irrespective of which stage in their programme they had reached. There are several key mentoring functions that describe the extent of their role and will be discussed here. Inevitably other practitioners with whom students came into contact also influenced their development to a greater or lesser extent and this was affected by their mentor relationship. In addition to good mentorship there were several other factors influential to students' progress, such as their supernumerary status, and what they termed as 'flying solo' or working independently under the distant supervision of their mentor, and learning by story-telling and associated reflective activities, such as the assessment strategy, where they learned through action inquiry and solving problems based on their clinical practice. These will be explored in this chapter.

7.1 Breaking through

When students first commenced their clinical placements, they were excited and enthusiastic at encountering the real world of nursing. Their first-year placements were concerned with understanding health and healthy living in the community. To widen their understanding students either visited identified families accompanied by a family health visitor, or on their own, and they also engaged in community activities. They made several taster clinical visits to observe the kinds of nursing that they would be learning when they progressed to their anticipated branch of nursing. Students believed their second-year branch placements were more significant, primarily because they believed they were doing 'authentic nursing work'.

Despite introductory discussions and opportunities to meet lecturer–practitioners before commencing a clinical placement, students reported feelings of confusion and bewilderment at their unfamiliar experiences. They often described a sense of alienation that was related to how accepted they felt by the clinical team. Such feelings are not surprising when students were being exposed to communities based on a different culture of values, language, modes of dress and social structure. Feeling alienated is a painful experience and can often lead to newcomers leaving unless they are able to readjust and learn to adopt the practices of their new community. To be successful in their chosen career, students needed to fashion a new approach to viewing themselves and their relationships with other people so that they could pass off as members of their adopted community. Changing their clinical placements once, twice, and in their second year three times in one ten-week term was challenging and disruptive and not surprisingly caused considerable confusion and discomfort. Changing mentors could be equally disruptive. Whilst students were adjusting to their clinical placements, they were also trying to establish themselves within two new peer groups, within two additional communities, that of their programme group and that of their peers within the university at large. Certainly for the first three years of their programme, all the participants believed they needed to earn their place within the clinical team, to legitimise the amount of time staff gave to support them. They seemed to believe this was a necessary strategy to repay staff for their efforts of tolerating and teaching them.

> But when you're actually getting your hands into the muck so to speak, and getting doing things, you feel as though you're of more use. Otherwise you feel you're wasting your time and theirs, the ward's time and you shouldn't really. What's the point of you being there? It's simple things like answering the phone in the office. Say you're doing something, like last night, the phone was ringing quite a lot, and the phone calls, a couple of times were wrong numbers. It's so frustrating because you feel as though they're like, 'You were sitting right next to the phone, why didn't you answer it?' I'm not saying that is what they're thinking but that's how you feel because you're not being of any use. Even though it's just answering the phone. Say it was someone phoning up to see how someone's operation went or something, but I didn't know the answer. That is part of my learning, recognising that I need to ask questions. Going to you or whoever and saying, 'It's so and so, and they've had an operation', or whatever, and then I'd also learn from you saying 'Well, this happened' or 'That happened' and then I could say to you afterwards, 'Well, why did this happen or that happen?' It's part of the learning process, to recognise your own limits.
> (Marie 6: year 2 term 2)

This particular and exemplary incident described by Marie characterises the fear many students faced when feeling excluded or unable to 'buy' the attention they needed or to reciprocate the support they were given. Marie's frustration was concerned with a number of factors:

- feeling isolated by her mentor and other members of the staff;
- wanting to be included by contributing to the work of the clinical team;
- feeling unwanted, de-skilled and useless because she is not allowed to undertake even a simple task;
- feeling guilty and then angry by her experience of being rejected;
- feeling despair and disillusionment with having such a bad experience at her first opportunity to learn about children's nursing (her chosen career path).

As with most of the other students, Marie believed acceptance as a member of clinical placement teams depended upon her usefulness to the ward staff. Students tried to find small tasks that did not distract their mentor or other staff but were essential such as answering patients' call bells, the telephone or doing simple nursing or ancillary tasks. Marie's incident characterises her sense of isolation from her mentor and the ward team. For her in that situation the telephone became an important symbol of the barrier between her and the staff. She was told that she should not answer the ward telephone even when she was sitting next to it or when it was clearly inconvenient for other members of staff to do so. Conscious of the effect of the impression she was giving, she felt their denial maligned the impression she was giving to the clinical community. On this particular ward Marie came to feel that her role as helper both to her mentor and to the ward staff was forbidden with the result that she felt that she had no legitimate claim to membership of the ward team. Marie's placement mentor (Lilly) described how she saw her role:

> I find it very difficult. To me, my role is to show people what's on the ward, what's on offer. Talk about their experiences, discuss what their aim is, and facilitate the other resources that we've got, and show them the other people on the ward, get the resources, teaching resources as well as books, and experience. We work very much as a team here. I don't know, I find being a mentor quite difficult, I suppose especially as I'm unclear about what it really is about. It depends very much on the person. The best thing is to do, if they're just happy enough to go and do things on their own.
> (Lilly, [Marie's mentor] 6b: year 2 term 2)

Marie's mentor had not realised the significance of her relationship with a student or how much help they needed to adjust to a new clinical area and to find their role. She did not seem to have an image of working alongside her student, sharing her nursing work, her decisions and her knowledge. Instead she saw herself rather like a signpost, directing students to other people or resources. Later on when Marie reviewed her three clinical placements over the term she was still upset by this particular experience:

> It was just so like 'You're invading our [space]'. I just felt so out of place. 'You shouldn't be here, what were you doing there?' I found it really, I mean normally I find it really easy to talk to people and that, and I just found it so hard, so awkward. I think if I'd have had a different response from the beginning, or maybe if my mentor had said 'Well, I've spoken to

so and so', or if I'd felt part of the team, maybe I would have been more like, ready to go along and say 'Oh I'm here as a student. I need to know X, Y or Z'. Then I think, I just felt so totally alienated from the whole thing that [pause] it didn't really make me want to work. I just felt 'Well, if you can't be bothered, I can't be bothered.'
(Marie 7: year 2 term 2)

It is clear that such experiences can have a negative influence on students' ability to learn. Narratives from other students indicate how commonplace such experiences were, and how much they affected students' professional development unless they were able to rescue the situation. Many students might just not have returned, but with increasing pressure to demonstrate clinical hours students are caught in a no-win situation, unless they can talk to someone who is willing to negotiate on their behalf. Probably the most challenging experience for any newcomer is to develop their identity and their role within their new community. By changing placements over their programme these students were entering and needing to become members of at least twelve different communities. More recent changes to nurse education have reduced this number of placements to just a handful. Even so, students need extra special care and support as any changes are difficult, even for practitioners who already possess the necessary professional skills. For people who are learning new skills, the task becomes almost insurmountable unless they receive some form of social support or sponsorship. When students receive sponsorship to their clinical placement community by a named and experienced member of the community (a mentor) then they are more likely to develop a sense of self worth, confidence, commitment and enthusiasm.

Sponsorship to a community

Several researchers investigating how people settle into the workplace, have identified the importance of good social support, particularly when people are new both to the community and to the work (Van Maanen 1976; Lave & Wenger 1991; Wenger 1998). A human characteristic is wanting to become an integrated member of their society (however fleeting), and to work on its behalf and thus (re)gain their identity through so doing. Thus newcomers cease to feel exposed and vulnerable and enjoy the protection and support of their colleagues. In her case study Ruth uses the metaphor of behaving like a 'puppy dog' running behind her mentor illustrating her dependence and loss of identity. She also described her need to be recognised as rather like 'nudging her way into the community with her elbows'. Many newcomers to nursing, especially if they have enjoyed some status in their previous role, and have been encouraged to strive for personal success and distinction, find adjusting to their new status as nursing students to be potentially even more stressful.

Being accepted by a new community imposes the necessity to conform to its normative style. Part of this includes looking like their new peers (like a nurse or a university student) and acquiring the language, the jargon and terms that only insiders use. Helen reported finding her mentor helpful, telling her what the terms meant in patients' casenotes. Likewise Ruth had her language corrected being told that calling patients 'love' or 'dear', could be interpreted as patronising. Despite feeling puzzled, she was prepared to accept it as part of getting used to the new cultural expectations of the profession and thus to become a (invisible) member of the nursing team. Learning to adopt different ways of behaving is perhaps even more difficult especially if it is to be effective at a deeper psychological level. Adjusting to the role of being a nursing student is not confined to appearances alone as many students find and as has been described in Chapter 5. Helen's learning contract for her first placement includes a reflection on this:

> I have had much experience with the elderly. However, my attitude has noticeably changed since my first few weeks working on the ward. One tendency was to treat all patients the same, and especially those with similar illnesses; however, having worked on the wards I have realised that each person should be treated as an individual as for example some elderly people have more self-respect than others. A simple example I found was that the majority of patients are called by their Christian names. It seems the accepted format. However, I met a new patient a few days ago and she introduced herself as Mrs Graham, as opposed to Anna, her Christian name. It made me realise that it is quite important to ask the patient what they like to be called when they first come to the hospital and not just assume that they like being called by their Christian name. Another patient may find it very formal and impersonal to be called Mrs, and this can be just as distressing for the patient. We must be aware of empowering the patient.
> (Helen: LC, year 2 term 1)

When students worked closely with their mentors and were able to contribute, their satisfaction and their learning soared:

> I just don't think I realised the huge difference between last term and this term. I knew it was going to be harder. Doing a full eight-hour or more shift. I was learning so much, at the same time because we were so busy I felt I was needed. I didn't feel like an auxiliary. My mentor was so busy. I wanted to help her as much as possible. I felt I was learning a lot but wasn't reflecting enough with my mentor.
> (Helen 7: year 3 term 1)

These concepts of 'breaking through' and 'sponsorship' help to explain the students' somewhat ambiguous situation, neither integrated members of the clinical community, nor of the community of university students. As a result they found themselves in a kind of limbo on their own. Their choice was to either develop their own nursing student identity, as did the three younger students or remain on the periphery like Natalie and for different reasons the three older students. Few students met in their placement settings and friends from their peer group could not provide supplementary support when they were in practice, and so they needed an alternative support system. Nicholson's (Nicholson 1987) research demonstrated how change and adjustment is a cumulative process influenced by the extent to which workers are encouraged to implement their learning. His finding reflect these students' expressed concerns. They often became frustrated by what they felt were obstructive practices, which deterred their progress. However, most of them were able to compensate when they moved to a different setting. Perhaps Helen was less fortunate and this may explain her enduring loss of confidence through most of her branch programme.

7.2 Mentorship

Providing sponsorship to incoming students were experienced practitioners. These mentors had responsibility for inducting students to their clinical setting, planning their learning agendas and assessing their progress. Mentors, in essence, were students' key informants to the setting. The extent to which each mentor understood their role and could manage to free sufficient time to work alongside their student made a significant difference to their student's progress and no doubt to the quality of care the students gave. Being able to feel comfortable, emotionally and socially with their mentor influenced the extent to which students could admit their learning needs, and indeed their fears, as well accept comments on their performance. So the quality of student–mentor relationships influenced students' progress. In successful mentor–student partnerships students were able to learn from their mentor and then practice independently under their mentor's distant supervision. Such opportunities provided inspiration, confidence and motivated students to study harder to learn more about the clinical speciality and the patients they were caring for. Good mentorship depended upon students' willingness to learn and to take some initiative for their own learning. Elements that made up good mentoring included four specific characteristics: *befriending, planning, confederacy* and *coaching*.

Befriending in mentorship

> I thought Michelle was someone I could actually say what I thought [to], whereas others I could talk superficially to but I couldn't open my heart. It helped because it was quite a technical placement, so we were doing things [together] – the drugs, techniques and she would go through it all. 'This is the drug chart, this is what it means'. We might look up a drug because neither knew what it did. It struck me as much more of a learning situation. I really felt there I was not a burden on her, I was working with her, I was helping her.
> (Ruth 11: year 2 term 3)

Students' narratives and the discussion in Chapter 6 illustrate how important their assigned mentor was to their progress throughout each placement. Like Ruth above, Helen's first placement with an experienced and supportive practitioner freed her both emotionally and socially. As a result she was able to acknowledge the limitations of her earlier beliefs about caring for older people. Her account is so striking and complete that it provides an exemplar of all the students' accounts of good mentoring. Relationships like this are more in tune with a learning climate where emotional deterrents to learning, such as fear and shame are replaced with encouragement and openness. Students are handled sensitively and affirmation is considered paramount. Mentoring relationships of this nature were fundamental to students' eventual survival and success. Being greeted by a willing sponsor when new to a clinical setting helped students adjust quickly. It also gave them an identity and a place within the team. As a result other staff members also related to them and students felt able to seek help from them if their mentor was busy. Befriending in mentorship involves more than the relationship, it confers a social status and is made up of several attributes.

Attributes of befriending in mentorship

- *Democratic relationship:* mentor and student are able to relate to each other on an adult–adult basis rather than as parent–child. This models the kinds of relationships students are expected to develop with their patients. With mutual levels of trust students feel more relaxed and open about their learning needs. It also allows mentors to delegate suitable activities knowing they can rely upon the student. As a result everyone benefits from the student's presence.
- *A secure base:* with a partnership based upon mutual trust, students are more able to feel sufficiently confident to take on responsibilities relevant to their educational needs and to widen their circle of contacts within the setting. This frees them to work independently, to learn from others, to acknowledge their limitations or their fears. All of which enhance patient care and the work of the team.
- *Sponsorship:* providing social and professional support, so students can get engaged in a whole range of activities that might otherwise be missed. Following effective sponsorship student's personal and professional development increases as other members of the community of practice are willing to involve them in their own work as well.

Democratic relationship and a secure base

By creating and sustaining a mentor–student relationship based on mutual caring and trust, students were encouraged to develop the same kinds of relationships with their patients. The professional relationships developed by the ideal nurse and the ideal mentor have close similarities with the ideal therapist in counselling relationships. Research into effective adult therapeutic relationships substantiates the importance of an empathetic and supportive practitioner (Howe 1993). Only by developing trust can clients express deeply-felt fears and anxieties, to challenge their assumptions and to learn. A mentoring partnership with such characteristics is very similar to those described by Bowlby (Bowlby 1988) in his theory of attachment as central to creating a 'secure base'.

A secure base provides a foundation for relationships from which clients can progress. This seems congruent with mentoring processes that students found most helpful and educational, as Marie's narrative illustrates:

> I think it's important that you need to know that we're not expected to know everything, ... and you're thinking 'Am I really stupid because I don't know that?' I think it's important that people don't make you feel stupid for asking questions because if they do you're not going to ask questions and you're then going to become unsafe.
> (Marie 17: year 4 term 3)

In placements where students felt attached to their mentor through a secure and supportive relationship, they became confident to participate in clinical practice and to learn from other members of the clinical team. The social and emotional security provided by such caring relationships enabled them to express their worries, fears and learning needs. As a result they were in a position to receive help and to mature both professionally and personally.

Sponsorship

> I feel part of the things that go on. The really nice thing when you come on and they allocate patients they all put 'Luke and Petra'. I just felt part of what's done really.
> (Petra 3: year 3 term 3)

Once reassured by their mentor's willingness to sponsor them into the new clinical setting, students could participate effectively within the clinical team and were acknowledged as legitimate members of the community of practitioners.

Without effective sponsorship and befriending, students had difficulty engaging with other members of a clinical team unless someone became a substitute. Irrespective of the stage in their programme, students missed out on relevant clinical activities, not knowing what was safe or appropriate for them to do. If they tried to use their initiative, it often meant they undertook activities below their capability and so had difficulty meeting their learning outcomes for the placement. Without sponsorship they became socially and professionally invisible to the rest of the clinical staff. By contrast they felt highly visible and like a spare piece of a jigsaw puzzle, shunted around the board unable to fit in and thus sidelined. They became overwhelmingly self-consciousness, and remaining in the setting was often unbearable. Returning for subsequent shifts created high levels of anxiety and as a result they lost any ability to function effectively. Such experiences correspond with findings of Fuhrer (Fuhrer 1993) in his studies of newcomers. Even more painful for students in such alienating situations was to know that their development was being stunted. Most students were able to compensate for these unfortunate placement experiences later on. However unless they could do so fairly quickly they would accumulate something akin to a debt of competency, stunting their professional development and condemning them to cycles of increasing incompetence and alienation, such as described by Nicholson (1987). Ultimately there would be a point where it was impossible to recover fully, with inevitable consequences for their development as nurses. Helen identified her anxiety at being a third-year nurse and unable to fulfil the sort of responsibilities she imagined her peers would be able to achieve. In her fourth year she was comforted by the knowledge that other newly qualified nurses also felt uncertain and insecure in their knowledge.

Effective befriending influences students' levels of self-consciousness, enabling them to gain confidence and self-awareness. Rather than be preoccupied with their internal lives, their fears, anger, disillusionment and so on they were free to see beyond their immediate personal concerns. Through this process, students became more self-aware of their relationships with clients, their contribution to the overall workload and also to see what was happening in the clinical setting and to learn.

Planning in mentorship

> At the beginning we worked together and when she [student] felt comfortable on her own, we'd sit at the beginning of the shift and discuss what she wanted to do and what plans she'd got if any, and see where she wanted to go. In the end she saw someone through until they'd discharged him. Every time she was on [duty] the same [patient] was assigned to my student and she saw what he was up to. She'd watched someone else admit and she felt confident in doing this admission. So I let her do it. When she admitted him, she felt he wasn't really appropriate [patient] to be admitted. She said 'He seems OK at the moment'. I said 'Go and see what the doctor says'. She came out with a totally different picture. [The doctor] was asking him how he managed at home and whether he heard voices and what they were telling him. [The student] was just gob-smacked because it was like something she hadn't thought about really. We discussed this and that the doctor was asking questions with a different emphasis and background and was probably more experienced in asking questions and what to look for. [The student] would say 'Oh yes I wouldn't have thought to ask that'. At the end of every shift, or once or twice after every second shift, I would make a special effort to sit down with her and go through her concerns and see where she was up to, what she was doing and what she planned to do, her caseload as it were.
>
> (Jack 15: year 4 term 3)

Jack's account describes how he provided mentor support to his own student whilst working on a mental health unit and taking a mentor preparation course. Drawing on his own experiences of being mentored he realised the importance of assessing his student's capability before leaving her to work under distant supervision. By planning his student's agenda for learning they were able to identify what she needed to learn and what kinds of patients could help achieve her targets.

Jack describes how his student's views changed after seeing her patient in a different light. It is also likely that she learned a lot more about the patient's needs and how to use questions to find out as much as possible about patients as well as about how other healthcare professionals work. Having experiences such as these extend students' understanding and capability. But it is not possible without adequate assessment of their practice and current knowledge and then identifying and agreeing an agenda of practice for their placement. To achieve this students and their mentors need to engage in some form of planning.

Properties of planning in mentorship

- providing a menu of experiences available in the clinical area;
- assessing a student's capability;
- helping students identify areas of curriculum interest;
- identifying skills that a student needed to develop or develop further;
- agreeing an agenda for learning to meet students' overall educational aims for the placement as well as short-term learning outcomes;

- planning suitable legitimate (and possibly peripheral rather than central) activities and patients and perhaps members of the clinical team for students to work with;
- helping students organise learning opportunities or to organise visits (to clinics or other departments etc.).

Students entering different clinical placements bring a variety of experiences that are unique to their particular personal curriculum. They follow the essential aspects of their programme but unless students all take the same placement at the same time they will have been exposed to variations of patients, mentors and clinical situations making each students' experience of their curriculum idiosyncratic. Student's clinical placements are normally planned to provide specific learning experiences according their stage in the programme and their learning needs. Making an assessment of students' capability when they arrive in the clinical community provides a baseline for future assessments as well as providing data for decision-making. When such activities are carried out effectively they can help students to integrate their formal learning with their clinical experiences. Achieving this requires mentors who have considerable understanding of the students' curriculum as well as understanding of their own work. Mentors need considerable expertise, guidance and support to recognise aspects of personal practice that are relevant to students' learning, to reconceptualise it sufficiently to talk about it and to teach students how to learn from practice. Careful assessment of each student's performance and discussion about their learning needs enables effective planning for their placement. With supported practice and ongoing assessment of their progress these plans can be reviewed and a new agenda for their learning can be developed. Planning is a cyclical process of evaluation of observed practice, discussion, agreeing an agenda for practice, practice and collaborative teaching followed by debriefing and record-keeping. The more frequently mentor and student engage in this cycle of activities the more successful the student is likely to be (see Figure 7.1).

Planning is a discrete and important part of the mentoring relationship in that it acknowledges the individual needs of each student so that they are not depersonalised but recognised as travelling by a unique route through the programme. Again this activity emulates the ideal relationship with patients that the profession aims to promote (Redfern 1996). Building on students' earlier unique experiences and planning a programme of learning that is most relevant to their needs is central to such an activity and promotes successful induction (Spouse 1990). The examples of Ruth and her mentor, and Jack working with his mental health nursing student illustrate how this relationship can work successfully. Australian research by Hart and Rotem (Hart & Rotem 1994) indicates that many mentors have difficulty appreciating the importance of this role, for example, Marie's mentor Lilly, described earlier in this chapter.

With increasing self-confidence in their own skills and familiarity with the curriculum, students became more able to prepare for their placements. Even so, they continued to need support from their mentors' expert local knowledge to

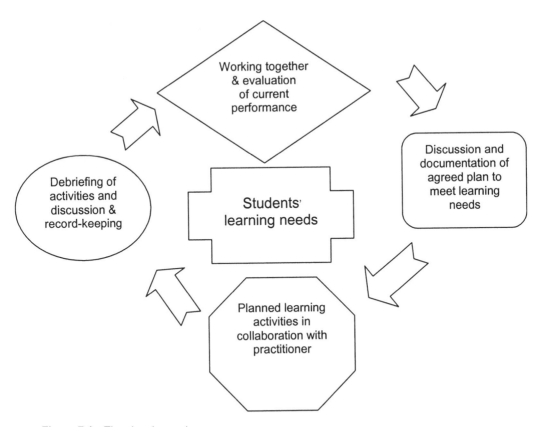

Figure 7.1 The planning cycle.

implement their learning plan. They also needed guidance as to who they could work alongside to develop their professional craft knowledge.

Confederation in mentorship

Working in confederation is concerned with student and mentor working together in tandem whilst giving care. Confederate activities are normally planned to meet the student's learning needs. Mentor and student work in partnership whilst delivering care. The mentor is the key actor in this setting and the student is delegated a peripheral role but also contributes to the overall care being provided. The important aspect of this confederate activity is providing planned experiences of practice that meet the student's learning needs and that also provide access to the mentor's craft knowledge.

> Veronica's been really good this term, because we'll do something together and she'll turn round and say 'What do you think of that?' I'll tell her [how] I thought it went and we'll have a bit of discussion about it. She does quite a bit of CBT (cognitive behavioural therapy), that's her speciality. So I sat in on her several times when she's been doing that with

a patient and she's been quite good, talking me through what she's doing whilst she does it. So I suppose I am learning all the time, but it doesn't seem like learning. It's just like I've opened my pores up to being receptive to everything that's there. People are just feeding me really with all this knowledge and information.
(Nicola 15: year 4 term 3)

The kind of learning that Nicola describes here would not be possible without working in confederation with her mentor. Confederation does not have to take place only with the student's mentor but with any other healthcare practitioner who is willing to share their professional knowledge with the student. Confederation has five specific properties:

Properties of confederation in mentorship

- a trusting relationship exists between student and practitioner;
- the student works in a partnership whilst giving care;
- the focus on the activity is practitioner-initiated and led, in that this person plans and delivers the care and the student assists;
- the practitioner thinks aloud (as appropriate) whilst conducting the care-giving, sharing their craft knowledge about meeting the patient's care needs and the manner in which they are being met. This normally takes place with the mentor articulating thoughts, instincts and knowledge about any observations, processes and procedures, and conclusions for future action;
- the student is delegated to and undertakes legitimate aspects of patient care which contribute to the workload, commensurate with their level of capability (actual or potential), whilst working alongside a practitioner.

Through these confederate activities students learn in a social context, and as Nicola identified above, can absorb knowledge and understanding almost by virtue of being present. Watching how their mentors relate to patients, how equipment is manipulated, how care is delivered, provides students with powerful images of practice. Having a legitimate role empowers them to feel valued. From a practitioner's perspective, confederation provides a mentor with valuable information about their student's confidence, communication skills, professional knowledge and so on. Confederation permits a mutual exchange of information about practice, meeting the patient's needs as well as the student's.

Their knowledge is a lot greater than mine so I always feel that what they say is a lot more substantiated because of what I've read and the limited experience I've had. So it's nice to hear how they would deal with situations that I've not encountered. Like the lady with the terminal care and how they're dealing with that.
(Ruth 16: year 3 term 3)

Ruth identifies how such experiences are valued and motivate students to explore situations further and generate questions.

Using this approach to supporting learning in practice mimics the natural way all humans learn. From childhood humans participate in social activities and absorb a huge range of information. Children watch their parents interacting with other adults and learn how to recognise those who are friends or foes, how to use language, adopt mannerisms and a range of other more subtle skills. By watching others in action they learn about childcare if there are other siblings, they learn about nutrition, how to prepare and eat food, how to care for their environment and so on. Adults also learn in a social context, modifying and developing their behaviour from the signals they pick up through social interaction. Anyone who has watched a cookery or gardening programme on television will have used this approach to learning, albeit from a distance. Learning in this manner is described as cognitive apprenticeship and theories underpinning it are derived from the Russian psychologist Lev Vygotsky's work (Vygotsky 1978). These will be discussed at the end of this chapter in Section 7.3. Nicola's story at the beginning of this section describes her experiences of learning to use new psychiatric nursing skills even towards the end of her programme and illustrates the importance of cognitive apprenticeship, irrespective of seniority. Inevitably there are always new skills or new knowledge to be learned throughout life.

Coaching in mentorship

With increasing confidence students were able to spend more time working independently consolidating their knowledge and clinical skills. As they made progress and undertook more complex activities they continued to need direct support from their mentor or another practitioner but in a different way.

> I took this man's stitches out and it was really difficult, it went inside. It was a continuous one. I know how to take stitches out, just the ordinary ones. She went through it in a lot of detail. Why you need to cut it close to the skin so that I'm not dragging it through, the dirty part. So if I cut close to the skin then I'm pulling through a minimal part, and how to do it to get it out easily and why we did it that way. [It was] brilliant. I mean I felt a bit guilty talking over the patient's head, but he didn't mind either. At least he understood that I was a student and that's why we did it like that.
> (Grace 5: year 2 term 3)

Grace describes one type of situation where she needed help with a technical procedure. At other times she may have needed a different type of support, perhaps helping a patient who was confused or aggressive, supporting a person receiving bad news and so on. Clinical support from mentors through their coaching activities differs from confederation as students are in the lead role and their mentor is supporting them.

Properties of coaching in mentorship

- coaching supports learning of additional and complementary skills or understanding, either during care delivery or afterwards;
- during care delivery the student leads and is supported by a more experienced and knowledgeable practitioner;
- coaching takes place within a supportive and secure environment based on mutual respect and trust;

- coaching includes specific guidance, information or reflective questioning associated with clinical practice and is intended to support perspective development or transformation;
- evaluation of performance is discrete and developmental.

Students found it invaluable to have their mentor or a trusted practitioner, coach them and talk them through procedures. On other occasions being able to plan or debrief from care-giving helped them to think through their actions and to explore alternative approaches. In clinical situations, such as the one described by Grace earlier in this section, patients are witnesses to the event and so students are more self-conscious of making mistakes, or being rude to their patient. Schön's (Schön 1987) three modes of coaching, 'collaborative', 'follow-me', and 'hall of mirrors' are described as taking place in the relative privacy of the equivalent to a skills laboratory. In clinical settings with clients or sick patients present such coaching activities can be difficult to undertake, and students' learning may be inhibited by overwhelming feelings of self-consciousness. Part of Schön's strategy was to help students learn what good practice felt like, to achieve an affective understanding of skill. This is why the mental health student, Nicola's, experiences of coaching were concerned with helping her to recognise and acknowledge her own feelings and to work with them, so that she could come to understand those of her clients and how to best help them. Through easy access to her mentor Nicola could share her difficulties and talk them through and supplement her ideas with her reading and discussions with her peers. As a result she came to develop a stronger self-image and thus a clearer sense of boundary between herself and her clients. Clinical techniques can also be learned in this way, especially in the safety of a clinical skills laboratory. But learning how to use the same skills with a patient needs careful coaching until students can feel confident in their skill and are safe to practice alone.

Another aspect of coaching is the dialogue between student and practitioner during planning and debriefing sessions. This is a particularly valuable way for mentors to assess how much their student understands and what extra help they may need. By encouraging a student to talk through their intentions or their rationale for action, both can recognise where more help is needed. Realising what they did know was also encouraging.

> She was more of a good friend, but that didn't affect her criticising my work. We went through my contract and she would say 'In here we can do this'. Or 'I'd phrase it like this'. Then again she was positive about it and said things were good reflections, she wasn't totally positive or negative.
> (Marie 4: year 2 term 2)

> She helped me by saying 'What would your plan of action be for that person?' and I'm beginning to think 'What would I do if I were her? What are the key issues I want to address?' which is quite good.
> (Nicola 11: year 3 term 3)

> [She'd ask] 'What's happening here, Jack?' And it was just to draw out what I'd done in science and relate physical symptoms to the patient's experience. We had a teaching session

where she focused on the patient's experience of chest pain and what we do and how it affects them and giving them this makes them feel like this etc. I suppose I am bringing out my knowledge and 'Yes I do know this'. Of course we had done the heart in anatomy and physiology last year and it was drawing on my knowledge and experience and making me think a lot and bringing them to the fore, which was good.
(Jack 14: year 4 term 1)

These three examples of coaching illustrate how students learned to relate their formal knowledge and to their practice.

7.3 Explaining good mentorship

Knowing how to support students using the four stages, befriending, planning, confederation and coaching described earlier is not easy, especially when clinical practitioners are preoccupied with providing patient care. Many mentors did not recognise or did not have the knowledge and skills to provide this kind of mentoring support. There were, however, many who did, either knowingly or not. The kinds of theories that support this approach to learning, known as cognitive apprenticeship, are described as sociocultural theories of learning. These theories are derived from Vygotsky's work (Vygotsky & Luria 1970; Vygotsky 1978), and are used to explain development of cognitive processes through social interaction and speech. These theories are based on the assumption that human beings are constantly seeking meaning from their experiences and their knowing can take several forms. In this context professional craft knowledge and formal (or decontextualised, generalised) knowledge are two important and recognisable forms of knowing. Both are derived from practice and are dependent upon good theory to support them. Theory and practice are inextricably linked and mutually dependent. Without theory it is hard to talk about practice and without practice, theory has no meaning (Moll 1990).

Talking heads – the social aspects of learning through talk

Thinking of language and theory in this way demonstrates how inextricably they are bound together. Using language as a mediator between formal and everyday knowledge helps clarify the relationship between students as newcomers and their adjustment to nursing. Without having a vocabulary of nursing and medical language they found it impossible to discuss what they were encountering or to give language and meaning to what they were experiencing. When first working alongside experienced practitioners, the gap between a student's knowledge and the supervisor's knowledge was considerable, and trying to fill it with unfamiliar practices, or with information or with theory left students confused and overwhelmed. As they accumulated more clinical expertise, knowledge and information they could begin to relate it to their experiences and understand what they were witnessing. As we have seen students learned best when they were supported by a mentor able to make links or to provide opportunities for links to be made, between a student's existing knowledge and the culture and practices of the clinical placement, or perhaps more fundamentally to professional practice. Students also learned through other forms of social interaction such as talking with their patients and carers, other members of the clinical community as well as with friends. Through their conversations they picked up snippets of information that could be saved for future use. Working and studying in a community of healthcare practitioners, they were exposed to a range of different practices and attitudes as well as to visions of people experiencing a range of diseases and discomforts. Sometimes they recognised the significance of what they saw and heard, and other times they did not. Recognising situations as being relevant relies on having prior knowledge. When students learned about depression or breathlessness they were more likely to see examples of people suffering from the disorder. When their mentor drew their attention to people experiencing these conditions they are more likely to remember and to learn from the experience. These forms of social interaction and social exchanges of knowledge relate to Vygotsky's (Vygotsky & Luria 1970) argument that learning is a social activity and takes place in two stages: the social or interpersonal (otherwise known as intermental – between two heads); and the intramental (inside one's own head).

Interpersonal speech and intermental learning

We have read several examples of interpersonal speech and intermental learning in the preceding pages. When we discussed the interpersonal activities of confederation, students described how effective it was to have their mentor thinking aloud whilst working. It helped students feel involved and excited about what they were doing and learning. In the other stage, coaching, students again described their satisfaction at being able to learn from this form of social interaction during placements. Sometimes the nature of their mentor's coaching made students think deeply and draw on knowledge they perhaps had not yet used; sometimes it made them use knowledge in different ways. By having to talk through what they knew, they came to recognise or be helped to identify some of the loopholes or errors of their thinking. Talking and writing about their practice (for their assignments) helped students internalise their knowledge and use it in relation to practical situations. Using this approach is made better with some sort of framework to structure thinking so increasing chances for success and covering the essential points. In situations like this students are using the intramental stage of learning where knowledge becomes internalised. Reflective practice when students debrief following a clinical event, or when they write up their reflective journals or their learning contract assignments also encourages students to take this intramental approach to learning.

Intramental learning

Intramental speech Vygotsky argued, promotes *higher mental functions* of problem-framing and solving. These are skills that are invaluable in clinical situations where students need to compare different cases or draw on formal knowledge to understand what they are experiencing, or their patients are experiencing. Another way in which humans use intramental speech is as an internal organiser of behaviour and the more sophisticated the activity the more egocentric the speech (Vygotsky & Luria 1978). Marie's narratives in Chapter 6 (*6.2 Developing technical knowledge,* page 168) and here demonstrate this process well:

> When I do things at home, I talk myself through what I'm doing anyway, like, 'Put the onions in the pan now, add this' sort of thing. So whenever I'm doing this sort of thing, I talk myself through it anyway.
> (Marie 3: year 2 term 1)

Having an initial external voice such as their mentor explaining and highlighting significant aspects of the operation helped students become familiar with new procedures or to learn unfamiliar terminology. Marie's activity of thinking aloud whilst she practised unfamiliar procedures allowed her to internalise her actions and begin to assimilate some of the associated language and concepts.

Linking theory and practice – a two-stage theory

Most people know more than they can actually say. This is usually because material they have learnt has not yet been sufficiently internalised to become useful or available to be manipulated. People are often able to carry out a procedure better than they can describe, or justify its relevance. Most of us have tried to explain how to find a house or road with poor success, but can easily take someone there. Using knowledge and talking about it require different skills and understanding. Vygotsky (1978) argued that people learn socially and mentally and sometimes one form of knowledge is in advance of the other, which needs guidance and support to be used. So for example, the knowledge students learn in formal settings such as through reading, learning in tutorials or discussions and so on has to be contextualised and have its salience demonstrated by a colleague or perhaps a patient. This knowledge-in-waiting (Spouse 1998) needs to be teased out and used in relevant clinical situations. Both confederate and coaching activities provide ideal opportunities for students to make connections between what they are seeing and hearing with what they have learned earlier. The reverse is also true. When students are exposed to practice situations they can with guidance learn about the underpinning knowledge either through debriefing sessions, tutorials or reading independently as several students describe. This two-stage process of learning relies upon students' intellectual development and whether they are ready to move to the next stage.

Two-stage learning – the zone of proximal development

Helping to transform learning from the knowledge-in-waiting stage to knowledge-in-use, needs assistance from a more experienced person – hence the social aspect of learning. Vygotsky (1978) conceptualised this process by describing what he called a 'Zone of proximal development' (ZPD, see

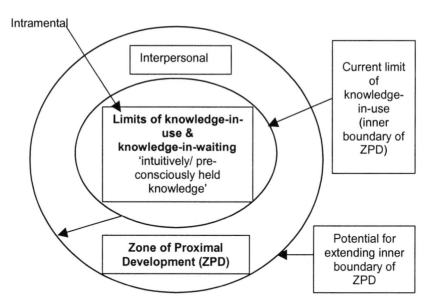

Figure 7.2 Inner and outer boundaries of a Zone of Proximal development (modified from Spouse 1998).

Figure 7.2). Within the inner zone students carry existing knowledge-in-use such as their lay images of how nurses should relate to patients, and any technical and theoretical knowledge they are already bringing into practical use but have used in only a few settings. Also within their inner boundary is their knowledge-in-waiting, which is still decontextualised – such as knowledge of nutrition, psychology, pathology, nursing theory and so on. Confederation and coaching activities of more experienced colleagues, or through discussion in peer groups provides what is called scaffolding and helps students bring their knowledge-in-waiting through their ZPD and transform it into knowledge-in-use.

Scaffolding learning through a zone of proximal development

Scaffolding practical or theoretical knowledge provides a way in which learners can work intramentally to transform knowledge-in-waiting into knowledge-in-use. Scaffolding is provided in various forms such as framing questions that require knowledge application, learning by working alongside an expert practitioner (confederation) being coached, formal teaching, reflecting on practice, writing assignments. Wood, Bruner and Ross (Wood, Bruner et al. 1976), coined the term '*scaffolding*' to describe this process of providing experiences or challenges that move learners' knowledge-in-waiting to knowledge-in-use (from within the inner boundary to the outer boundary of their ZPD). The concept of scaffolding has since been developed in a number of ways but the case studies and our discussion throughout this book illustrate how important good mentorship is to supporting learning in this way. Thinking aloud when undertaking care delivery either by the student (such as with Marie) or by a mentor is a further example of scaffolding learning.

Scaffolding practice

When students were delegated nursing activities that were easily within their capabilities their learning often remained undeveloped. Quite frequently students were left to get on with doing observations or talking to patients without purpose or any guidance about what they could achieve. By contrast, when they were delegated activities that they were assessed to be safe to undertake but which stretched their ability, and challenged them to think differently and motivated them to study further, their learning increased rapidly. Being supervised whilst undertaking such activities helped them reach their existing level of potential and to transfer knowledge-in-waiting to knowledge-in-use thus preparing them for a further cycle of learning and a new ZPD.

Monitoring students' readiness to learn is quite sophisticated and does not rely only on their willingness but also on their knowledge base. Mentors need to know what students have been learning in their course (students' knowledge-in-waiting) so complementary clinical educational activities can be planned and tailored to their educational needs. When mentors assess their students they will identify their level of development potential and plan an agenda for learning accordingly. Sometimes this means modifying language, activities and so on to accommodate any deficit. A novice who is, say inexperienced in a clinical specialty, needs some form of induction whilst working with a mentor so they can learn the language as well as the specialist nursing practices. When novices are unable to interpret instructions correctly or fulfil implicit directions, then either the nature of verbal guidance (language used) or the task needs to be reviewed. For example it may be that mediating language used to describe the required activities is beyond the student's comprehension and so different, perhaps lay terms need to be used. Alternatively, the task may be new and too complex and so a lesser, legitimate, but more peripheral activity needs to be offered. In both situations the expert assesses and reassesses their student's level of understanding or potential to learn and refines the nature of instruction offered. By identifying students' knowledge-in-use and knowledge-in-waiting in this way the mentor uses the idea of two-stage learning and the zone of proximal development as a diagnostic or analytic tool (Hedegaard 1996).

7.4 Learning by flying solo – being supernumerary to the workforce

> It's just now, over the past couple of weeks, that my mentor gave me my own client or two to look after, which is quite nice. Although I was still responsible for her and she would say 'How are things going Jack, and what are you going to do next?'
> (Jack 3: year 2 term 1)

Developing professional skills and receiving sponsorship does not mean students either need or want to practice alongside their mentor all the time. An essential part of undertaking clinical activities that are legitimate (perhaps also peripheral) is for students to work on their own under their mentor's more distant supervision.

Properties of flying solo

- Based on assessment of their practice the mentor identifies a caseload that is commensurate with the student's level of development but is not too heavy to cause exhaustion or disillusionment;
- the caseload includes several opportunities to practice a variety of skills embedded within holistic care needs of one or more patients;
- the caseload provides opportunities for interprofessional collaboration and learning;
- selected patients give their consent to having a student as carer;
- the mentor or other members of staff are available to discuss the care planning, implementation and evaluation;
- the caseload is sufficiently challenging for students to utilise their knowledge-in-waiting and to extend their zone of proximal development by motivating them to read and question unfamiliar or taken-for-granted practices.

Working independently, or as Jack called it, flying solo, provides opportunities to care for a group of patients with dependency levels that are both within their capability but which also stimulate further learning, both of practical skills but also case knowledge and associated theory. As a result of such experiences, students develop managerial skills, learning how to bundle different nursing activities together, even at a very early stage of their programme, providing the nursing work matches their assessed capability and their learning needs. Alongside these experiences are opportunities for students to work with other healthcare professionals and to learn from them and with them. Having a specially selected caseload of patients who offer students relevant learning opportunities can stimulate their learning further.

> My patient-study man has had a stroke and the occupational therapist comes in every morning and watches him get dressed. It takes a long time and his wife comes in as well because they're about to move into a flat. It's like a lot of the independence has been taken away from the patients in the nursing home by pampering them and it's not always the right thing. In hospital it's orientated towards giving them back their independence and putting them back into the community.
> (Helen 1: year 2 term 1)

At this early stage in her programme Helen is able to learn how to work alongside other healthcare professionals and to understand their role within a patient's healthcare pathway. As students progressed through their course, and with increasing responsibility for patient care so their contacts with other healthcare professionals changed. By engaging in collaborative team working students were able to gain their own professional identity whilst also acknowledging and understanding that of other professional colleagues.

These quotes illustrate the excitement and feelings of being part of a clinical team that good delegation brings. This form of scaffolded learning activity has to be carefully planned on the basis of assessment of students' practice and identification of their learning needs. When preparing to give care, students benefit from preliminary discussions with their mentor to explore how they are going to manage the care planned, work out their priorities and plan how they are to meet targets set for the shift. As safety and quality measures, mentors have to ensure patients are consenting to their arrangements. They also need to check their student is managing and is sufficiently competent to undertake the assigned work. Debriefing patients and student at the end of shift provides time to evaluate what has been undertaken. It also provides time for reflection on what has been achieved and learned. Using these opportunities to review a student's professional knowledge means student and supervisor can identify new developmental needs and select ways of providing appropriate experiences.

Advantages of working independently

Working independently, students need to have clear boundaries of responsibilities and know where they can gain help. Ruth's narrative of bathing a patient in the hoist lift (see Chapter 3, Ruth: Narrative 17, page 116) illustrates the potential for problem-solving that working independently offers, but it also illustrates the potential difficulties students may encounter without suitable preparation and support. Through repetitive practice students can begin to see patterns in their experiences and to develop their own professional craft knowledge. Marie's experiences in the community of working with a small number of families gave her a sense of responsibility that both thrilled and motivated her to study hard. As with the other students in the same situation, she found her theoretical material began to have relevance and application. Being in a safe position to make mistakes and being able to discuss them with a respected member of the team also helps students learn and develop. Having opportunities such as these are important motivators for students to become active agents in their own learning, providing they (and their patients) are able to enjoy physical and psychological safety whilst students experiment with practices that are new to them.

By increasing students' encounters with practice, students are confronted with situations that can challenge their assumptions and cause dissonance and thus learning. Nicola's experience with the woman who deliberately harmed herself (Chapter 3, Nicola: Narrative 12, page 68), raised questions about her therapeutic relationship and increased her understanding. Ruth's concerns about removing her male patient's urinary catheter (Chapter 3, Ruth: Narrative 20, page 117) caused her to reflect on her professional role and relationship with him. Helen gained an opportunity to question ethical issues arising as a result of being party to knowledge about one of her patients. Without exposure to experiences like these students would not have recognised their own capability or began to question their own practice.

Scaffolded experiences like these provide intellectual and practical stimulation. They are examples of effective negotiations following assessment and correct diagnosis of each student's potential for development. As a result students can consolidate their knowledge (within the boundaries of their existing ZPD) and extend their knowledge-in-use to develop a new field of learning from their practice. Working and developing in this manner helps students organise their work, develop their theoretical knowledge and learn how to meet and prioritise patients' nursing needs. They also develop an increased understanding of their role as nurses. Benner (Benner 1982) argues that it is only through systematic examination of their repeated exposure to case experiences of a similar nature that advanced beginners can develop professional knowledge. By contrast, the mindless burden of repetitive practice where both patients and students are reduced to work objects is very different from these kinds of scaffolded practice experiences. Working independently enables students to get to know their patients more closely than when their mentor is present and as a result they gain greater insights to experiences of illness and healthcare. For example Helen's experiences with the physically disabled clients gave her insights that she may not have achieved otherwise (see Chapter 3, Helen: Narrative 13, page 39). Being able to learn to practice independently is far more educationally stimulating and satisfying – providing expert support is available to discuss their activities. With such support students develop self-confidence and become excited about their learning.

7.5 Learning through story-telling

The idea that learning is a social activity is not confined to learning and working in clinical settings. Throughout the study, students described their immense satisfaction with and the benefits of sharing stories about their practice. The students each had someone they felt they could talk to about their work. Grace, Helen, Nicola and Marie each had a best buddy and a strong peer group, with whom they shared experiences and debated issues that were keenly important. The two older students developed networks of their own; in Ruth's case her mother, who was a nurse; and Jack talked things through with a friend who was a paramedic.

> I think you need to be able to say you've had a bad day. It's nice to go away and talk to someone who has nothing to do with it. They may ask really obvious questions that you haven't thought of like 'Why are you doing it then?' or you know what the good points are. (Jack 3: year 2 term 1)

These contacts helped students make sense of their clinical practice, through describing and discussing their experiences. In the process they gained additional insights from the telling and from the responses their audience provided. Sometimes they shared experiences with non-nursing flatmates and as a result gained insights from a lay perspective. This was not always beneficial as sometimes their non-nursing peers misunderstood and misinterpreted students' accounts as overly dramatic or socially unacceptable, because they were beyond their own life experiences. Helen for example used her non-nursing peers, who were sympathetic when she needed emotional support, but it was clear that the nature of her work set her apart from them and her peers sometimes found it difficult to understand her attitude.

Properties of story-telling – content

- provokes strong emotions such as distress, enjoyment, guilt or failure;
- seems confusing or inexplicable;
- questions their identity;
- may be useful for their assignments or others' learning.

Because of the large group size and their wide distribution over several trusts, students' modular curriculum provided limited opportunities to develop a peer group that could support them throughout their programme. Those students who lived in residential accommodation were able to develop supportive peer networks, often generated from chance contacts with neighbours who were also nurses. In the third year of their programme an important component of the course was a module of learning concerned with interpersonal skills. Students met in small seminar groups on a weekly basis over two or three terms and brought issues from their practice. This provided an immensely valuable aid to their sense-making and was facilitated and supported by experienced teachers.

> Mostly ethical points or dilemmas that we'd come across in our work and things that had upset us or whatever. It was quite personal stuff in the Interpersonal skills group . . . Sometimes we carry on with the Interpersonal skills down at the pub afterwards. You can't talk nursing all the time though, I think you need a break from it. You just see how everyone else is getting on and see how they're coping in different fields. You can discuss the funny and sad points. Most of the time it's quite useful to get different view points on things and see how everyone else is tackling it.
> (Nicola 9: year 3 term 1)

Nicola's experience of her peer group illustrates its value in a variety of sense-making activities. They found it helpful to share experiences that they found uncomfortable or incomprehensible and that they could compare their own feelings with those of their peers. Through story-telling, students could construct and rehearse their thinking. Story-telling gave students opportunities to disengage or stand aside from their experiences so they could take a more objective view. Their stories provided opportunities to learn from each other:

> My mentor actually gives me facts and information that are useful for my skill. Whereas when I'm talking to friends, some of the discussions we've had I might remember it more easily because it was an interesting talk.
> (Helen 1: year 2 term 1)

Story-telling or sharing experiences (critical incidents), seemed to be important to learning because the stories carried a reality which was heated by their immediacy and engaging qualities. This was, for them, more influential and touching than a good piece of fiction or drama. Students could actively engage in their story at any point by clarifying and enlarging aspects of interest or rehearsing parts that were particularly pertinent. For the narrator they offered opportunities to review their role and define new ways of being, much as in the psychotherapeutic relationship or in action-learning group work. For the listeners, story-telling might reflect their own experiences or provide information they could use in the future. Experiences such as these are common in everyday life. We tell our children parables and fairy stories to help them learn about the world. We tell stories about important events that have touched our lives to help us make sense of them. American psychologist Jerome Bruner (Bruner 1990) argues that it is only through story-telling that human activity can be understood. As with fairy stories, parables or other forms of literature whether biographies, fiction or non-fiction, stories contain elements that teach us about ourselves and our lives in a manner that is more accessible and memorable than lectures or text books. By exploring their experiences through exchanging stories with their peers, students could develop concepts of themselves in different roles according to who they were talking to. As a result they could get several perspectives and several different stories of practice that provided a broader sense of nursing and even insights into practice that they had yet to experience. Students' interactions with their peers, especially where they enjoyed equality meant they could debate and defend their perspectives and thus develop new perspectives and frameworks for thinking and acting. By resolving any feelings of dissonance, they could reframe their self-image and their experiences into more acceptable ways of thinking and feeling and thus further develop their professional understanding.

Peer support as emotional support

Having an integrated self-image seems an important aspect of the transition to becoming a nurse when students are confronted by their inability to function as they see others. This may explain Jack's frustration at not being able to maintain his image as an autonomous professional; Helen's concern not to faint when she saw a 'bobbly finger'; and Ruth's concern not to be told what she ought to do to get an A, by her colleague. All appear to be symptoms of needing reassurance that they are operating at an acceptable level. Part of the function of story-telling in a peer group is to test out a sense of progress by exchanging insights, knowledge and experiences as if at a metaphorical tennis match of competence. Missing out on a lob of experience or a backhand slice of knowledge, signals a deficiency that needs to be rectified if the student is not to fall too far behind. Being able to talk about their practical experiences influences students' perspective of self within their community of students, and perhaps influences their decision whether to continue. In a sense, their social status as students causes them to realign their self-concept according to unfamiliar models. It is not until they can develop sufficient confidence in their ability to use the language and to understand their practice in the same way as their peers can they become comfortable. Talking about personal experiences in the safety of a friendly peer group also helps students develop self-confidence, helps them develop their critical thinking and learn how to develop arguments. Peer support seems to be an essential component of learning to nurse, not only for the opportunity to share understanding and to learn from each other, but also to ease the process of becoming nurses.

7.6 Learning through assessment of theory and practice

> I've been writing notes as I go along, but I think my learning contract won't reflect the amount of knowledge I've learned this module because I can't get it in. It's not a diary as such, more a page with the patient's name and lots of issues coming off it. When I've read up on a certain disorder I'll write notes on there. If I'd looked after a child with diabetes I'd read up on it.
> (Marie 15: year 4 term 1)

Marie's quote illustrates some of the activities described by Vygotsky's two-stage theory of learning, the social and the mental. Here she is describing how situations in her practice have triggered further learning, thus helping her extend her (ZPD). It also helps to explain the benefits of using reflective practice to demonstrate learning and understanding as students' use of stories illustrate. Their story-telling helped them prepare for their assignments as much as for their practice, by providing opportunities to rehearse their knowledge (interpersonal learning), develop skills of critical thinking and thus extend their ZPD. Students' end of placement documentary evidence of their clinical experiences provided a further form of intermental activity. The curriculum use of learning contracts (LC) is based on work by Malcolm Knowles (Knowles 1975). In this programme students were encouraged to become action-inquirers (Winter 1989; McNiff 1993) and include not only a statement planning their experience but also demonstrate what they had achieved.

> You have to think of a learning opportunity that fits the competency or sometimes you can get a learning opportunity that expands the competencies. But you then have to think 'Right, think of an example' and then it brings up the competencies. Then you look at it the other way and you've got to find out all this literature in the library. You could spend hours doing that and basing it on whatever and maybe then argue 'Does that help the person in the long term?'
> (Jack 5: year 2 term 3)

For each of their practice placements students had to identify critical incidents that related to specific course learning outcomes. Learning outcomes for each placement were negotiated and agreed with their practice mentor. These were related to the outcomes for entry to their branch programme or the competencies for entry to the professional register, laid out by the professional statutory body. Using relevant critical incidents taken from their own clinical practice, students conducted investigations of the literature and wrote a detailed analysis of each incident demonstrating achievement of the relevant learning outcome. Critical incident analysis was a form of problem-based learning generated by students' own practice. As a strategy to integrate practice with theory it was successful. Monitoring students' progress and verifying documentation of practice was the mentors' role.

Despite careful induction and preparation, practitioners still held different conceptions about their role and how to interpret the guidelines. Perhaps this was inevitable when trying to introduce a radical tool across a wide range of placements and mentors. Another difficulty was the limited library resources as several narratives illustrate. Jack experienced more difficulties than the other research participants because of the late diagnosis of his dyslexia. The learning contracts occupied a great deal of students' energy and dominated their placements. They frequently expressed frustration at having to write about a learning outcome or a competency rather than an incident that they found meaningful. Despite these difficulties, extracts from students' learning contracts illustrate how they used their clinical experiences to develop their professional and personal knowledge.

Students' learning contracts provided a two-fold medium for scaffolding their learning. They encouraged students to become actively involved in their own learning right from the start of each placement. Using learning contracts in this way, students also needed help from their mentors and so helped mentors develop their own knowledge.

7.7 Students' professional development – the influential factors

Throughout this chapter the voices of the participants have continued to describe and account for their experiences. The most important external factors promoting their development have been the nature and quality of social interactions between clinical staff and other nursing students. Of secondary importance were curriculum issues such as students' supernumerary status and the assessment strategy.

Of prime importance was the quality and nature of the *mentorship* they received. Few mentors had received similar support in their training programmes and faced with an unfamiliar assessment strategy, many struggled to develop their own role. Some were extremely successful, as students' accounts give testimony; others either misunderstood their role, or misunderstood the nature of adult education and supernumerary status; and others were just too preoccupied with their own clinical responsibilities to be helpful. The research highlighted four important elements of the mentorship role. When mentors provided good support through sponsorship and befriending they gave students legitimacy within their clinical setting and so opportunities to learn. When such structured support was missing students floundered, unable to gain necessary access to practice or to professional craft knowledge. Their learning was further increased when they spent time working alongside their mentor in a confederate relation-ship, watching and learning from the care delivery. Once they became settled and safe to practice on their own, coaching sessions with their mentor or another experienced and knowledgeable practitioner stimulated and challenged their thinking and increased their development.

Students' supernumerary status freed them from the worker role to explore their relationships with patients and colleagues as well as the literature. As a result they were excited and stimulated by their experiences and worked hard to develop their understanding. Frequently in their efforts to reach levels of achieve-ment with which they could be satisfied they spent far more hours than required by the course programme in their placement areas. Their enthusiasm was partic-ularly noticeable when they were given manageable caseloads of their own which challenged their existing knowledge and stimulated further practical and theo-retical learning.

All the way through their programme, students strived to make sense of their experiences and even though they used their mentors for some aspects, and gained from the literature or through their assessments in others, their chief resource was the support from peers. Their story-telling of good and bad experi-ences, provided new personal insights for future practice, reduced their sense of isolation from university colleagues and strengthened their commitment to nursing.

References

Benner, P. (1982) From novice to expert. *American Journal of Nursing* **82** (3): 402–7.

Bowlby, J. (1988) *A Secure Base: Clinical application of attachment theory*. Routledge, London.

Bruner, J. (1990) *Acts of Meaning*. Harvard University Press, Cambridge, Massachusetts.

Fuhrer, U. (1993) Behaviour setting analysis of situated learning. In: *Understanding Practice: Perspectives on activity and context*. (eds S. Chaiklin, J. Lave) pp. 171–211. Cambridge, Cambridge University Press, Cambridge.

Hart, G. & Rotem, A. (1994) The best and worst: Students' experiences of clinical education. *The Australian Journal of Advanced Nursing* **11** (3): 26–33.

Hedegaard, M. (1996) The zone of proximal development as a basis for instruction. In: *An Introduction to Vygotsky*. (ed. H. Daniels) pp. 171–95. Routledge, London.

Howe, D. (1993) *On Being a Client: Understanding the process of counselling and psy-chotherapy*. Sage Publications, London.

Knowles, M. (1975) *Self-directed Learning: A guide for learners and teachers*. The Adult Education Company, Cambridge, New York.

Lave, J. & Wenger, E. (1991) *Situated learning: Legitimate peripheral participation*. Cambridge University Press, Cambridge.

McNiff, J. (1993) *Teaching as Learning: An action research approach*. Routledge, London.

Moll, L.C. (1990) Introduction. In: *Vygotsky and Education: Instructional implications of sociohistorical psychology*. (ed. L.C. Moll) pp. 1–3. Cambridge University Press, Cambridge.

Nicholson, N. (1987) Work Role Transitions: Progress and outcomes. In: *Psychology at Work*. (ed. P. Warr) pp. 160–77. Penguin Books, Harmondsworth.

Redfern, S. (1996) Individualised patient care: Its meaning and practice in a general setting. *Nursing Times Research* **1** (1): 22–33.

Schön, D. (1987) *Educating the Reflective Practitioner: Towards a new design for teaching and learning in the professions.* Jossey Bass Publishers Inc, San Francisco.

Spouse, J. (1990) *An Ethos of Learning.* Scutari Press, London.

Spouse, J. (1998) Scaffolding student learning. *Nurse Education Today* **18**: 259–66.

Van Maanen, J. (1976) Breaking in: Socialization at work. In: *Handbook of Work, Organization and Society.* (ed. R. Dubin) pp. 67–130. Rand McNally College Publication Co, Chicago.

Vygotsky, L.S. (1978) *Mind in Society: The development of higher psychological processes.* (eds M. Cole et al.) Harvard University Press, Cambridge, Mass.

Vygotsky, L.S. & Luria, A. (1970) Tool and symbol in child development. In: *The Vygotsky Reader.* (eds R. Van der Veer & J. Valsiner) pp. 99–174. Basil Blackwell Ltd, Oxford.

Wenger, E. (1998) *Communities of Practice: Learning, meaning and identity.* Cambridge University Press, Cambridge.

Winter, R. (1989) *Learning from Experience: Principles and practice in action research.* Routledge, London.

Wood, D., Bruner, J. et al. (1976) The role of tutoring in problem solving. *Journal of Child Psychology* **17**: 89–100.

Chapter 8

Enhancing Nurses' Professional Learning

If research findings are to be used as evidence for policy development they also have implications for the design, organisation and funding of nurse education. The case studies presented in Chapter 3 illustrate six very different individual experiences of learning to become a nurse. Perhaps with other or less eloquent participants these narratives may have been different. Evidence of their transferability has come from many nursing students studying in countries such as Canada, Eire, Switzerland, the United Kingdom and the United States. These students have each found at least one case study that described their own personal journey through their particular nursing programme. The value of such case studies lies in their representativeness and so far they seem to offer existing students encouragement and a sense that they are not alone in their struggle. Researching and creating the case studies was part of a process of trying to understand how nursing students develop their professional knowledge. Better understanding may be achieved from models of the kinds of knowledge they felt they needed and how they developed their professional knowledge; and of how clinical education may be enhanced to support students in their quest to become professional practitioners. Possibly as a result of beliefs about the so-called theory–practice gap, simple remedies have been sought to resolve policy failures, with teachers being used as scapegoats. Alternatively the problem has been identified as a deficit in the quality of the learning environment, or the ability of entrants. It is probable that all these factors contribute, but the process of how students learn to become nurses has remained largely ignored. Perhaps the questions need to be more carefully formulated and research presented here indicates how multifaceted are the nature and content of professional development. The four broad questions used to frame the research design reported here have provided some understanding about how nursing students develop their professional knowledge. These were:

- what conceptions of nursing do students hold on entry to nursing and how do these frame their professional development?
- what kinds of knowledge and understanding do students acquire whilst learning to nurse and how do they believe they learn to become nurses?
- what are the major factors that facilitate their learning to nurse? What is the nature and extent of supervisory, peer, personal and activity factors?
- how can the professional development of nurses be better understood and what are the implications for the design, organisation and funding of nurse education?

Findings from this research indicate that students' entry conceptions of nursing have two particular and significant influences on their progress. Firstly they appear to affect their decision about whether nursing is the right career choice for them and whether they decide to remain or leave their course. Secondly their conceptions provide a form of template for how they want to be as nurses and how they want to relate to their patients and carers. These images appear to be very powerful and influential in maintaining their commitment and also conform to contemporary attitudes to patient care and professional relationships. As a result they should be explored and fostered as far as possible.

The second research question concerned investigating the kinds of knowledge and understanding students acquired whilst learning to nurse and how they believed they learned to become nurses. Students described seven particular forms of knowledge that was essential to their professional development. These were concerned with:

- relating to patients and their relatives;
- developing technical knowledge;
- bundling activities of nursing together;
- developing craft knowledge;
- managing feelings and emotions (their own as well as those of patients and relatives);
- providing therapeutic care;
- relating to and functioning within a clinical team.

Factors that influenced their professional development and knowledge acquisition were most importantly related to the quality of sponsorship they received from knowledgeable mentors. This was based on effective befriending that permitted assessment and planning of future clinical educational activities, such as working in confederation with their mentor and then subsequently through coaching whilst undertaking legitimate clinical activities that were part of the overall workload of patient care. Three other important factors that facilitated professional development were: opportunities to fly solo and work in a supernumerary and independent capacity whilst under the distant supervision of their mentor; engaging in story-telling with peers about their clinical experiences and learning from each other; documenting their action–inquiry and problem-based learning in clinical practice.

Having discussed findings arising from these three research questions this chapter addresses the final research question: How can the professional development of nurses be better understood and what are the implications for the design, organisation and funding of nurse education?

8.1 Conceptualising nurse education

From our discussion in Chapter 1, it is evident that there has always been tension between the employers and professionalisers within health service factions. Traditional nurse training schemes were based on the belief that learning by doing alone was sufficient to prepare women [sic] to undertake tasks that were natural to them. Several governments and professional organisations commissioned investigations to understand why women were unhappy with nursing as a career and why they left. The same kinds of findings kept being rediscovered, principally that nursing cannot be learned by doing alone and that students need to become valued and educated members of a learning community of practitioners.

Assessing practice

The preoccupation of nurse educators and researchers with theory–practice issues highlights some problems associated with overreliance on procedural matters and assessment of skills. In trying to define good and bad performance and to measure outcomes of learning, both the professional statutory body and the department of health in its various guises, have identified guidelines for elementary standards of performance in the form of outcomes and competencies. Reductionist strategies taken from industry that influence distribution of workload and deconstruction of activities into tasks and skills have also influenced attitudes to competence and to assessments. Standards of this nature may be useful for specifying quality assurance guidelines or minimum levels of performance. When they are used to define boundaries of practice they can become restrictive and limit professionals' ability to respond to developments resulting in fossilisation (Sutton & Arbon 1994). Certainly by deconstructing common nursing tasks, their complexity becomes more evident. For instance, Dunn's analysis of giving medication via an intramuscular injection arrived at 34 subprocesses, or subsidiary skills, needed to achieve the focal activity (Dunn 1970). Whilst skill development forms an important aspect of learning to nurse, in focusing exclusively on skills the human aspects of nursing become hidden and the relationship to nursing activities of other considerations such as context and salience is denied. As the students' case studies and Chapter 6 indicate, whilst they were preoccupied with developing technical competence, they were even more concerned to develop practice that was therapeutic and patient/service-user centred.

In continuing to be concerned with competency and its consequent implications of training for a specified skill, several agencies have developed broader definitions of competency which include a range of attributes such as knowledge, skills, attitudes (Sainsbury 2000; UKCC 2000). These provide a basis for curriculum development and to monitor access to professional Registration as well as prescribing standards of performance. By focusing on achievement of specified outcomes in competency-based assessments there is an assumption that standards of expected performance quality can be described and that judgements will be consistent. Unless specifications are couched in generic terms they may represent outmoded ideals of practice. Assessment of competencies are frequently planned and conducted with a belief that practice settings are a flat playing field untroubled by everyday events and turmoils. In reality nothing could be further from the truth as illustrated by Phillips et al. (Phillips, Schostak et al. 2001). So choice of assessment strategy, the assessor and timing of assessment become critical to the validity and reliability of evaluating performance and certifying readiness for progression or fitness for practice and purpose prior to professional registration. More realistic assessment of practice has to be designed and practised in a manner that takes account of a student's response to unpredictable contexts of practice, as well as fluctuating levels of expertise when faced with unstable situations.

Students' descriptions of writing their learning contracts indicated their frustration with being confined to specified competencies which did not reflect their experiences and when their practice was much more diverse and fluid. Despite their grumbles, as well as difficulties caused by large numbers of mentors providing (different) guidance on how their learning contracts should be written students learning contracts demonstrated significant learning. These provided evidence of their ability to engage in action–inquiry, problem-solving, reflective practice and their overall professional development. They were an effective and influential means to developing students' professional knowledge and understanding. In the early stages of their programme it was evident that competency statements provided useful guidance to what students and mentors should consider and plan. As both became more adept at identifying areas of interest and relevance, the competencies were increasingly believed to be restrictive, inhibiting students' ability to discuss problematic and educational incidents. Using suitable assessment tools to ensure satisfactory standards are being achieved and maintained throughout the profession presents difficulties, as research commissioned by the ENB demonstrated (Phillips, Schostak et al. 2001). Their research showed that assessment tools are often implemented with little knowledge of how professionals develop their practice knowledge. Their research also demonstrated how few practitioners understand or have time for their role as assessors or understand the educational potential of assessment for student learning. In some instances it is hard to know to what extent assessments are accurate predictors of professional performance. The advantage of accumulating evidence of suitable performance rather than relying on incidental assessment results helps to resolve some of these problems. By relying on misleading and simplistic mechanistic assessments of outcome performance the process of learning to nurse is oversimplified denying the importance of planned and supported clinical experiences by experienced clinical practitioners after effective presentation of theoretical and practical material in formal settings. Research shows what a complex undertaking it is to become a professional nurse.

Doing and writing about practice

A further concern of students was related to a potential disparity between those who were good at writing about practice and those who were better at doing it. Their irritations reflect a complexity of monitoring performance that is more sophisticated than skill achievement or academic skills alone. It may be that by the very nature of their practical and interpersonal inclinations, nurses are much better at using non-textual modes of expression and that formal, academic assessment strategies fail to provide a suitable vehicle for students' cognitive achievements to be acknowledged. This is not to belittle scholarship but to raise questions about overreliance on written evidence alone. It seems tragic that Jack only became aware of the cause of his academic difficulties when his dyslexia was diagnosed half-way through his programme. This discovery was fortuitous and came about due to the caring approach taken by a highly skilled lecturer–practitioner who was a children's nurse. Her sensitivity and collaborative approach to student support caused her to seek a deeper meaning to Jack' academic difficulties and thus to identify the necessary support. It would be interesting to know the extent to which other students suffer the same difficulties but are less fortunate in understanding the cause or getting the necessary help that is available and who as a result experience similar forms of unnecessary discrimination. By acknowledging and identifying the existence of literacy and numeracy problems in large numbers of students entering higher education, both students and teachers can address such needs and alleviate enormous personal distress as well as saving on resources.

8.2 Researching nurses' professional learning

In trying to understand how nurses develop their professional knowledge several questions come to mind such as how much does students' classroom learning influence their development in practice? At what stage in the curriculum should different topics be introduced and are there any key aspects that should be considered first. Another question is the influence of contact with different client groups and whether timing of such contacts should be planned differently. We have no knowledge of how the sequencing of placement experiences influences professional development or whether students' clinical experiences could be completely reconceptualised. With increasing recruitment to nursing of adults with more life experience to what extent does their age and previous experience influence their professional development? Could it be more beneficial for younger students to be given different placements at different stages in their development from those to which older students are placed and how would this influence their adjustment to the many stressful aspects of nursing? Another concern is the effect on peer-group relationships when there is a mixture of students with different amounts of prior nursing experience. It could be that the influence of experienced healthcare practitioners on students who have little previous experience of nursing is not always helpful. To what extent does the choice of client groups and timing of placements affect students' learning? Is it better to learn and work with some client groups than others? And what are the benefits or otherwise for the service users and the clinical staff? Traditionally, older people have been the target of inexperienced students. Similarly the policy of early taster placements helping students reevaluate their career choice means they are often working with more vulnerable people when they are least experienced, and as we have discovered, sometimes with insufficient support. By changing the student–worker relationship by making all students supernumerary, and with effective mentor support, risk to patients should be minimal. The benefits to students being supernumerary are enormous and seem to foster a healthier attitude and commitment to patient care. But so far there is little information about the function of the mentor and the consequences for staffing clinical units and skill mix. We need to identify and map the advantages and disadvantages for staff who mentor students, especially in times when shortages of registered nurses mean there are fewer available to provide educational support in clinical settings. We also need to consider the implications for nursing students' professional development of using healthcare assistants as the major care deliverers.

Personal aspects of professional development

Students' images of ideal practice seemed to encourage and sustain them, even through moments when they were close to giving it all up. Why did some students leave the course and to what extent could it be attributed to a lack of vision, or visions which conflicted with their clinical experiences or those promulgated by their teachers? To what extent are personal images appropriate and realistic for meeting service users' healthcare needs and influential in developing effective healthcare practitioners? On the other hand, to what extent is it possible for the profession to promote a realistic and attractive image of nursing? To what extent is prior experience of nursing (as care assistants or informal helpers) instrumental in promoting success as nurses or desensitising them to the unique and personal needs of their patients? The most enduring analytical impression gained from the students' conversations about their lay perspectives of *being* nurses was the sense that they were responding to a sense of vocation. Their feelings of frustration were bound with feelings of despair that their visions could not be realised. These were concerned with providing everyday essential nursing care to patients in an humanistic and therapeutic manner that promoted healing. Their first ambition did not include ward management or supervision of unqualified workers.

Affective aspects of nursing appeared to be more important than the instrumental aspects. Whilst students were deeply concerned to develop the necessary technical skills, their paramount concerns were more to do with relating to patients and their carers. Students' images seemed to help them recognise when they were functioning effectively. Their ability to be nurses as well as doing nursing was important. *Doing nursing* was influenced by the extent to which they could undertake the same range of nursing practices they observed in their mentor or other members of a team. Feeling able to contribute to the aims of the whole team and their workload was important to students' morale. Feeling like a nurse and *being a nurse* were more subtle than doing nursing, and seemed to involve personal identification or immersion in the whole process. Possibly by satisfying subliminal, kinaesthetic and affective experiences, students were willing to make greater investments of self (Goleman 1996). When there was congruence between everyday practice and their ideal practice students seemed to merge their identity as everyday folk and their identity as nurses. Most students wanted to and seemed able to develop a closeness with their patients which required personal involvement, commitment and a use of self which is unusual in most everyday encounters. In using their ability for therapeutic purposes, participants came to *feel like* nurses or to understand at a deep or psychic level what it was like to be a nurse. As they accumulated an experiential wealth of such sensations it seemed that their ability to feel congruence with their role also developed.

Working and learning in practice

The nature of the students' curriculum was innovative and their progress was idiosyncratic, in some instances more so than others. The nature and amount of clinical experience was ostensibly the same but interpreted in different ways. Some of the students supplemented their hours by doing more clinical work than required by the curriculum and also by working in their vacations. Not having to worry about their assignments when they worked in the vacations was constructive in helping them concentrate on practising their skills rather than having to find suitable literature to explore their practice. However as in other research, students expressed shock and concern at the inappropriate supervision they were given and the nature and quality of nursing care that was being delivered (May, Veitch et al. 1997). Their successful development relied heavily on effective mentorship support. This was particularly important whilst students were developing self-confidence and encountering unfamiliar experiences especially during their early placements in the programme and at the beginning of all their placements.

Students who leave nursing

Those research participants who left the programme prematurely offer some interesting perspectives on students who stay and those who leave. Unlike Jack, Petra and Grace left owing to personal family worries that preoccupied their energies and distracted them from studying. They were effective in practice but failed academically. Like Jack, both later returned to nursing, with Grace qualifying two years after her research peers. Petra returned later to a different programme in another institution. When embarking on longitudinal research it is difficult to anticipate which students will survive a programme. Capturing the students' images of nursing from the point of their entry has been unique to this study and having more data of the same nature would provide a better understanding of factors influencing decisions to leave.

8.3 Curriculum issues

Changes in healthcare provision

Of striking interest throughout students' narratives was the amount of time they spent involved in providing traditional, essential care to patients. Common perceptions of nursing have tended to diminish the art and science of nursing associated with meeting intimate personal health and sickness needs of service users. With increasing use of technology, advances in healthcare and changes in utilisation of health services as well as changes in demographics of age and culture world-wide, nurses have to work in a responsive and flexible manner. The experiences of these students indicate that they are well prepared for working in the twenty-first century. But they were more privileged than many of their contemporaries. Recognition of the influence of social context on healthcare is becoming better established and the support of kith and kin is now recognised as essential. Patients are now designated as experts in their health needs and are in a position to make a greater contribution to determining their healthcare needs as well as to service provision. Furthermore, because of escalating costs of healthcare or sickness care, greater emphasis is being made on public health and prevention of disease. Consequently nurses are engaged in a more sophisticated and complex relationship with their patient's social environment.

High throughput of patients means professional relationships need to be established quickly and are only transitory. In some clinical units staff work 12-hour shifts to provide continuity of care, making clinical work intensive and emotionally as well as physically exhausting. Working at such an intense level requires great skill and knowledge and this has been recognised in the burgeoning number of post-registration, specialist nursing education programmes, but less so in the kinds of day-to-day peer and emotional support nurses need to survive successfully.

Having neophytes visiting or working in such busy clinical units or in delicate situations such as home settings create additional burdens on clinical and educational staff to ensure that students are safe and have suitable opportunities to learn rather than be neglected. This makes the sequencing of students' placements even more critical, especially with single entry points to courses for large groups of students and a limited number of placements. Overcrowding placements with a range of different students with many different educational needs diminishes both the quality and the range of experiences to which they can be exposed.

Students in this study sometimes sacrificed their academic time to ensure they could attend when others were absent. Clinical staff also suffer from such pressures. Research into the implications of these changes in healthcare provision and in staffing levels for optimum numbers of students allocated to clinical areas will help to clarify these issues. Finding alternative clinical experiences that reflect the broad base of healthcare provision have exercised education providers as well as service providers and needs further research to identify the benefits and costs (in educational, human and material terms) of such placements. Attachment to families or small communities may provide a more valuable (possibly supplementary) means of ensuring practitioners are suitably prepared for their future role offering insights into overall health needs and care in home settings as well as hospitals.

Future developments in nurse education

Recent investigations of the UKCC Post-Commission Development Group (UKCC 2001) were partly concerned with changing current structures for initial training and the five branch programmes. Amongst their six options they modelled a generic initial programme with clinical branch specialisation at post-registration level. This is in line with other European and many English-speaking countries. By creating a generic initial programme students have potentially more time to develop their professional knowledge and understanding whilst further protecting the public. Such practitioners would be grounded in community and hospital practice across the spectrum of age groups, thus multiskilling nurses and enabling them to support family units more flexibly than current educational provision allows. It also fosters a more economic use of the workforce, a constant and increasing concern for governments. With current emphasis on collaborative interprofessional learning, a common initial preparation course for all healthcare practitioners and different stepping on and off points leading to professional qualification, provides a model that offers greater flexibility and cost-effectiveness. The data from all eight students demonstrated that apart from Marie (the children's nurse) and Jack who was preparing for a second registerable qualification, students were not necessarily committed to a specific branch of nursing on entry. Nicola's dilemma was as much to do with whether she wanted to be a nurse or an occupational therapist. Having joined the nursing programme she took some time to be sure of her commitment to mental health nursing. Perhaps with more time and greater freedom she and the others may have felt more confident about their final career choice.

Preparation for practice

The nature of students' preparation for practice is also crucial. The discussion on measuring levels of competency indicates a preoccupation with technique rather than with overall nursing ability. Whilst technical aspects of care were an important concern for students, skill development was incidental to their wish to give holistic care and it distracted them only until they could operate effectively in practice areas. Their mentors often assumed students possessed a level of skill that was unrealistic and possibly they did not recognise their own role in teaching skills. Many mentors were good at helping students apply skills to their area of clinical practice and this perhaps differentiates current practice from that studied by Gomez and Gomez (Gomez & Gomez 1987) when they argued that skill transfer from laboratory to practice did not take place. Schön's examples of coaching implied his learners were already competent in basic techniques and that their coaches were helping them to develop artistry in their use (Schön 1987). Polanyi's (Polanyi & Prosch 1973) constructivist approach to the development of tacit knowledge indicates that students need to master technical skills and procedures before entering practice and then to develop focal skills associated with actual care provision. With mentorship support, they are more able to concentrate on bundling the technical and other activities of nursing together. This is reflected in current provision of laboratory skill preparation using simulations and virtual reality. However even if students arrive in clinical placements well-rehearsed in relevant skills, being able to relate and use their skills with specific client groups will continue to require expert support and guidance from clinical practitioners. This is necessary to help students contextualise their skills and, as importantly, to benefit from their mentor's craft knowledge. It cannot be substituted. Research also needs to be undertaken to investigate the optimal preparation for students to develop tacit knowledge of skills, their professional craft knowledge and their readiness to practise holistic care.

Supernumerary status of students

Students' supernumerary status protected them from the burden of unrealistic workloads which have characterised past programmes including the Diploma course preregistration (Project 2000) students. In conditions of nurse shortages and replacement with agency staffing, students have been frequently the only members of a clinical team familiar with patients. As a result their professional development suffered both in practice and in time or energy available for study (May, Veitch et al. 1997; White, Riley et al. 1993). These supernumerary students found their delegated caseloads, when carefully planned, provided appropriate development and were stimulating and satisfying. They used their spare time to read about their patients' medical and nursing needs. Their familiarity with an action–research approach to professional practice, generated by course assessment strategies, encouraged them to broaden their understanding of patient circumstances. With changes following recommendations of the UKCC Commission on Nursing and Midwifery Education (UKCC 1999) students now have fewer, longer placements and with their supernumerary status they can, with their patients' consent, follow them through their healthcare pathway (to their homes or to other areas of healthcare). Students' development becomes effectively patient-centred and holistic, bringing them into contact with a whole range of professionals and resources in social and healthcare services. By encouraging students to take an action–inquirer/reflective-practice approach to their learning and clinical experiences, they develop and draw on skills of problem-based learning and thus the skills of lifelong learning.

8.4 Conceptualising mentorship in nurse education

Spending their clinical experiences as supernumerary to the workforce meant the quality of mentor support students received was significant to their progress.

When they were sponsored and supported by knowledgeable and confident practitioners they could settle into the clinical environment and learn more effectively. Their relationship with other members of the team was also more mature and productive. Several mentors were hampered by insufficient understanding of how to interpret concepts of self-directed learning and adult education that the curriculum used and were unfamiliar with their role as key informant to the clinical practices for students. This is not an unexpected finding and reflects a widespread uncertainty arising from the implementation of new programmes (Maggs 1994; Phillips et al. 2001; White, Riley et al. 1993).

Influence of workload and clinical skill mix

An important factor that seemed to influence mentors' readiness to support students was their workload. Clinical staff rarely received a reduction in their caseload when supporting their students and as a result struggled to find time to plan their experiences or to discuss their work. In several instances mentors found it difficult to accommodate students in their daily activities and abandoned them. Having an understanding of an ideal caseload and of the influence of mentorship responsibilities on practitioners may help resolve this issue. It would also be useful to understand whether better education and preparation of mentors can help them manage their workload and their mentoring responsibilities differently. Where this study took place there were few care assistants employed to supplement nursing activities. As a result all nursing care was carried out by registered nurses and this provided many good opportunities for students to observe and participate in high quality practice.

During their vacation periods students worked as healthcare assistants and frequently encountered staffing situations where qualified staff were in a minority. Care was provided entirely by healthcare assistants. Often these students were responsible for administration and management of care that the hard-pressed clinical managers delegated without assessing their capability and thus the safety of their patients. Earlier research has indicated that students and qualified nurses working under such conditions are more likely to leave nursing within six months of completing their programme (Reid 1985). The short-term financial gain of employing unqualified staff perhaps hides a long-term cost that merits investigation. Opportunities for effective supervision or even education of nursing students may also be affected, if it is even possible at all. Early indications suggest that students have difficulty accessing clinical experience where healthcare assistants provide most of the nursing care in surgical wards (Wakefield 2000).

Benefits to mentors

Despite workload constraints some mentors were extremely skilled at creating time and turning situations into everyone's advantage, with students enjoying opportunities to share their mentors' workload through engagement in legitimate activities. Mentors benefited from such contacts and their own learning was enhanced. In several cases mentors found it helpful to have students stimulating them to review their practice. On the rare occasion when a mentor had been in practice for less time than a fourth year student owing to different lengths of their preparation programmes, they worked together to resolve clinical problems. This was not necessarily educationally beneficial to students on the degree course, but it meant that they could learn from each other's experiences on a collegiate level that they may not have achieved by working alone in the clinical team. Whilst this may not be ideal or commendable, it allows cross-pollination of experiences and ideas through scaffolded activities.

Knowledge of practice and assessment

Many mentors whilst extremely competent and experienced were not necessarily used to having to account for their actions. Students often found it hard to obtain such knowledge without feeling that they were being rude or challenging. As a result they felt inhibited from asking questions. Some mentors had a facility for talking about their patients and explaining their actions and clearly enjoyed encouraging students to question or discuss their experiences. Their approach was a mixture of challenge and support. They used challenging activities in their coaching role by asking students to think through their actions or testing their knowledge. This helped students to recognise the relevance of their formal classroom knowledge to their clinical situation and to use it in different but similar situations. By working together, either through collaborative care-giving or through preparing students to undertake legitimate clinical activities, effective mentors were able to support students in their decision making and planning as well as promoting their understanding of what they had encountered and achieved. In supportive relationships students were willing to accept and internalise comments on their work and progress. Assessment and collaborative activities of this nature by mentors was inevitably more effective than assessment activities by a less familiar practitioner.

Mentor education

Many mentors either could not articulate their practice or did not have sufficient language to rationalise and discuss their actions and so help students develop their own craft knowledge. Sometimes this was not a problem if students felt at ease within their environment and could approach other members of staff. However, access to other clinical practitioners or even access to planned care-giving depended upon sponsorship from their mentors. Without it students had difficulty recognising or benefiting from learning opportunities. Frequently neither mentors nor students appeared aware of the complexity of the nursing situations they encountered. Possibly they did not know how to explore the potential difficulties or the potential range of explanations for what they encountered in practice. Students' concern with taking up too much time by asking questions, or mentors' concern with giving detailed explanations may have influenced this. It may also be that few practitioners were familiar with questioning what they did on a daily basis and that they also required help in learning how to conceptualise their practice. Those mentors whom students described as particularly good or outstanding were often in senior positions and had considerable experience. In many respects, they seemed to bear the characteristics of proficient or expert practitioners described in nursing by Benner (Benner, Tanner et al. 1996) and by Titchen (Titchen 1998) with her concept of critical companionship. Researching how mentors and practitioners achieved such effectiveness would contribute to our understanding of education in clinical settings.

Facilitating mentor development

Most mentors in the study had attended a two-day course designed to prepare them for their role. These courses included discussion of the curriculum as it related to their area of clinical practice. In addition, most mentors had undertaken a programme designed to develop skills of teaching and assessing. The majority had completed the ENB 998/997 short course, others had taken the City and Guilds Certificate in teaching (number 730). The dominant paradigms of learning that appear in most nursing education texts are concerned with behaviourist approaches to learning, competency and assessment (Spouse 2000). Very few of these texts address nurse education in clinical practice with more than a few pages and most of the discussions and recommendations are more relevant to classroom interactions and recall of formal, decontextualised information. Reports by many practitioners indicate that these materials are of little benefit when dealing with students in clinical settings. Neither courses or texts are concerned with the unpredictable and demanding environment of clinical practice. This research demonstrates that mentorship is an interpersonal relationship of primarily confederate and later coaching activities and practitioners need help to learn how to achieve this. Staff also need help to articulate and develop their craft knowledge so that they can communicate it effectively. By using reflective practice and action inquiry to investigate and learn about their own practice practitioners are in a better position to provide mentor support. Recent initiatives by the English National Board for Nursing Midwifery and Health Visiting in collaboration with the Open University (OU 2001) have transformed this situation with publication of a set of learning materials designed to support mentor preparation and based on research by Phillips et al. (2000). The materials can be used as part of a longer programme of preparation or as a means towards developing evidence of meeting the advisory standards for mentors and mentorship (UKCC 2000a, 2000b). The model of supervision offered as a result of this research and indeed reflected in the English National Board learning materials for mentors demonstrates that a collaborative approach will bring benefits to both student and qualified practitioner alike. With increasing emphasis on quality in healthcare through clinical governance, investment in the continuing education of existing practitioners has become an acceptable and mandatory requirement of all healthcare practitioners and healthcare providers.

8.5 Research and the future professional development of nurses

This study has raised a number of questions concerned with the professional development of nurses. Research projects commissioned by various professional organisations throughout the UK have influenced the development of current programmes and their delivery by educational institutions. By transferring nurse education out of the service-delivery cycle of deprivation, other influential factors have become more apparent that are less clearly understood. This study demonstrates some of the key factors that are influential to nurses' development, and highlights the continuing and inevitable dependence upon provision of the same facilities that promote high standards of care. It is perhaps unsurprising that so many questions are raised considering the nature of the profession. With the growing emphasis on professional practice and evidence-based practice, it must be of concern that students in this study had difficulty gaining access to practitioners' craft knowledge and in many instances were dependent upon their assessment strategy and access to library facilities to develop their own professional knowledge. The consequence of this, with increasing pressure for such scarce resources and declining expenditure in higher education, is not encouraging for the future. This gives rise to the need for intensive study of practitioners who offer good mentorship support, to explore the factors which characterise their performance and the extent to which they are commensurate with their performance as practitioners. Evaluation of how mentors influence student performance and thus patient care is also relevant.

Other findings arising from this study are concerned with curriculum issues. In particular the effectiveness of large-scale education of preregistration nurses at degree (and diploma) level and the impact on service delivery and educational support is now becoming better recognised. The importance and benefits of supernumerary status for students and the value of their engagement in reflective practice (or action–inquiry) have been recognised by the Commission on Nursing and Midwifery Education (UKCC 1999). Evaluation of new approaches to professional education once the programmes have been established long enough to overcome preliminary difficulties could provide answers to many of the questions posed. In addition exploration of the continuing development of new nurses and their first years of practice will provide a better understanding of the long-term influence such education has on practice.

Another area for future research is to explore the relevance of existing educational programmes for students' future role. There has always been a discrepancy between the required practice of students during and following their development to registration. With widespread adoption of the principles of professional nursing, current nurse education programmes are highly relevant and effective, providing newly qualified practitioners are given the appropriate recognition and support that has been prescribed by the professional statutory body and that newly qualified practitioners do not fall victim to staffing inadequacies. However a different mode of preparation may be needed if the majority of care is going to be given by appropriately prepared and regulated healthcare assistants under the supervision of nurses. Good nurse supervision and education will remain essential if advances in the management of disease are not going to be squandered through poor staffing and nursing care.

A fourth area for future research is to explore the different modes of knowledge development and knowledge acquisition in which students engage, and how their learning may best be supported. Little research has been conducted in this area. Our understanding is both minimal and based on inappropriate models. The complexity of developing and using a range of different types of knowledge, competencies, attitudes and personal knowledge has only begun to be identified and described. Practitioners' achievement of identity as nurses, evolving from their role as student and from nursing student to nurse and the influence of personal vision are little understood, and this may contribute to explain anomalies in recruitment and retention of staff.

Several other considerations for future research that this study has highlighted include: the profound importance of story-telling narratives in peer relationships and how these may be fostered to encourage professional understanding. The educational nature of confederate and coaching activities undertaken between student and mentor and its influence on students' understanding of practice. The nature of discourse between student and mentor and the extent to which it needs to be fostered through structural aspects of the programme. Some institutions have compensated for insufficient educational input to clinical settings by making joint appointments between school and service. These are not without their difficulties for similar, though contextually different, reasons (Lathlean 1997). The lecturer–practitioner role was well established in institutions used for this nurse preparation programme and it was assumed that they would figure strongly in students' accounts of their professional development. It came as a surprise that this was not at all the case and lecturer–practitioners were only mentioned in connection with classroom teaching or validation of students' learning contracts. This suggests that in their educational capacity, they have taken over the role of the nurse–tutor in monitoring students' progress and have thus increased the schism between school and practice and have isolated nurse teachers even further. The difficulties experienced by lecturer–practitioners documented by Lathlean (Lathlean 1997), suggest that the role is overly complex and perhaps its clinical aspect could be more justifiably undertaken by well educated and prepared clinical managers intent upon staff development and professional practice and who are supported by nurse educators. More recently a new practice-based post has been established that also links education and practice, the practice educator and the less expensive version the practice facilitator. These are essentially clinical practitioners with responsibility for supporting clinical staff and students and they frequently cover very much larger areas than lecturer–practitioners but usually without the managerial or educational responsibilities. Initial reports indicate that these posts are successful in trouble-shooting activities as well as having a monitoring and advisory capacity.

Nurse education has had to adapt to momentous changes over the past decade and this is likely to continue as demographic and technological influences become more profound. The Post-Commission Development Group (UKCC 2001) reported on recommendations arising from the earlier Commission's work (UKCC 1999). It recognised the educational difficulties caused by insufficient resources for clinical placement experiences. Rapid developments in management of sickness care alongside unprecedented changes to the demography of the population as a whole and the healthcare population are being tackled with a radical revision to how healthcare is provided. More care will be provided in people's homes and the community, and nurses will be assuming a different role in monitoring and advising people on how to maintain and improve their health as well as on their ill health. NHS Direct and walk-in clinics are nurse led. Such practitioners will need the kinds of skills developed by the students in this study. Their ability to investigate their practice and to both utilise and generate research-based evidence for their decisions enables them to arrive at best practice. Developing essential academic and clinical skills are more likely when initial preparation is at degree level. The UK government White Paper *Working Together – Learning Together* (DoH 2001) emphasises its commitment to interprofessional preregistration education and in particular development of core skills such as communication, at the earliest possible stage in the students' programme through both academic and clinical activities. The paper also urges collaboration between regulatory bodies, employers, education providers and patient representatives to ensure initial preparation programmes are dynamic and responsive to changes in healthcare as well as public expectations. Exhortations such as these require clear evidence of their merits and further research such as that commissioned by the professional statutory bodies is needed to support future decisions. Coupled with adequate financing and resources throughout the system nursing and other healthcare professions are more able to respond flexibly and effectively rather than as in the past at enormous individual cost and consequent high attrition rates. Having evidence to justify nursing practice is important but can only be effective if the profession also has the resources to undertake necessary research to understand the nature of nurse education and the nature of nurses' professional development in particular. And then it is only effective if resources are also available to implement the findings.

References

Benner, P., Tanner, C.A. et al. (eds) (1996) *Expertise in Nursing Practice: Caring, Clinical Judgement and Ethics*. Springer Publishing Company, Cambridge MA.

DoH (2001) *Working Together – Learning Together*. HMSO, Department of Health, London.

Dunn, M.A. (1970) Development of an instrument to measure nursing performance. *Nursing Research* 19 (6): 502–10.

Goleman, D. (1996) *Emotional Intelligence*. Bloomsbury Publishing, London.

Gomez, G.E., Gomez, E.A. (1987) Learning of psychomotor skills: Laboratory versus patient care setting. *Journal of Nursing Education* 26 (1): 20–4.

Lathlean, J. (1997) *Lecturer Practitioners in Action*. Butterworth-Heineman, Oxford.

Maggs, C. (1994) Mentorship in nursing and midwifery education: Issues for research. *Nurse Education Today* **14**: 22–9.

May, N., Veitch, L. et al. (1997) *Preparation for Practice: Evaluation of Nurse and Midwife education in Scotland, 1992 Programmes.* Department of Nursing and Community Health, Glasgow Caledonian University. Funded by the National Board of Nursing, Midwifery and Health Visiting for Scotland, Glasgow.

OU (2001) *Assessing practice in nursing and midwifery* (K521). K350: Assessing practice in Nursing and Midwifery. School of Health and Social Welfare, Open University for the English National Board for Nursing, Midwifery and Health Visting, Milton Keynes.

Phillips, T., Schostak, J. et al. (2001) *Practice and Assessment in Nursing and Midwifery: Doing it for real.* English National Board for Nursing, Midwifery and Health Visiting, London.

Polanyi, M., Prosch, H. (1973) *Meaning.* Chicago University Press, Chicago.

Reid, N.G. (1985) The effective training of nurses: Manpower implications. *International Journal of Nursing Studies* **22** (2): 89–98.

Sainsbury, C.F.M.H. (2000) *The Capable Practitioner – A Framework and List of the Practitioner Capabilities Required to Implement the National Service Framework for Mental Health.* Sainsbury Centre for Mental Health, London.

Schön, D. (1987) *Educating the Reflective Practitioner: Towards a new design for teaching and learning in the professions.* Jossey Bass Publishers, San Francisco.

Spouse, J. (2000) *Challenges to professional education: Learning in workplace settings. Improving student learning: Improving student learning through the disciplines.* Proceedings of the 1999, 7th International Symposium. C. Rust (editor). Oxford, Oxford Centre for staff and learning development. **7**: 364–76.

Sutton, F.A., Arbon, P.A. (1994) Australian nursing moving forward? Competencies and the nursing profession. *Nurse Education Today* **14**: 388–93.

Titchen, A. (1998) *A conceptual framework for facilitating learning in clinical practice.* Institute for Practice Development, Royal College of Nursing, Oxford. Occasional paper No. 8.

UKCC (1999) *Fitness for Practice.* The UKCC Commission for Nursing and Midwifery Education. United Kingdom Central Council for Nursing, Midwifery and Health Visiting. Chair: Sir Leonard Peach, London.

UKCC (2000a) *The Nurses, Midwives and Health Visitors (Training) Ammendment Rules Approval Order 2000.* United Kingdom Central Council for Nurses, Midwives and Health Visitors, Statutory Instrument 2000 No. 2554, London.

UKCC (2000b) *Standards for the preparation of teachers of Nursing, Midwifery and Health Visiting.* United Kingdom Central Council for Nursing, Midwifery and Health Visiting, London.

UKCC (2001) *Fitness for practice and purpose. The Report of the UKCC's Post Commission Development Group.* United Kingdom Central Council for Nursing, Midwifery and Health Visiting; Chair: Valerie Morrison: 94, London.

Wakefield, A. (2000) Tensions experienced by student nurses in a changed NHS culture. *Nurse Education Today* **20** (7): 571–8.

White, E., Riley, L. et al. (1993) *A detailed study of the relationship between teaching, support, supervision and role modelling in clinical areas within the context of Project 2000 courses.* London, Kings College London & University of Manchester. Research commissioned by the English National Board for Nursing, Midwifery and Health Visiting, London.

Index

academic skills 49, 87–88, 94, 107, 216
academic work 54, 61, 64, 71, 74, 76–77,
    79, 87–88, 92, 94, 101–107, 109, 111,
    114, 120, 122, 153, 156
access course 92, 104
achievement 155
active contemplation 169
accommodation 41, 51, 110
action inquiry 58, 171, 208–209, 214, 216,
    222, 226
actor 152
adult nursing 9, 34–49, 64, 75–91,
    107–123
adjustment 146, 151
aesthetic knowledge 180
affection 98–99
affirmation 190
agenda for learning 193
agenda for practice 193–194
agony & ecstasy 84, 96
aggression 68
alienation 53, 145, 186–188
anger 192
anxiety 52, 64, 96, 101, 138, 180, 192
art 9, 23–24, 34–35, 49–50, 71–74, 103,
    120–121, 142, 146, 148, 156
art work 48, 61–62, 146, 148
artistry 126, 133, 180, 220
assessment 40, 55, 87, 102, 116, 134, 138,
    144, 173, 178, 193–194, 205,
    209–210, 214–217, 224
assignments 101–102, 110, 122, 207,
    219
attachment 191
attitudes 42, 46–48, 64–67, 140, 189
attrition 3, 124–125, 129–130, 142, 145,
    148, 156, 219
autonomous 169

auxiliary nurse 34, 42, 91, 93, 95, 112,
    116, 133, 141, 146, 165, 167, 174,
    181–182, 189, 218, 223, 226

bad news (giving) 164, 197
befriending 127, 190–193, 210, 214
behaviour 168
beliefs 141
body language 68, 98
branch of nursing 186
branch programme 209, 221
breaking through 185–190
bundling nursing activities together 45–46,
    159, 169–171, 204, 222
burn out 175, 210, 220

capability 83, 193–194, 204, 221, 223
care assistant 34, 42, 91, 93, 95, 112, 116,
    133, 141, 146, 165, 167, 174,
    181–182, 189, 218, 223, 226
care 34, 83–84, 93, 124–136, 137, 158,
    164, 177, 179–180
career choice 34, 41, 48–50, 61–62, 64–66,
    70, 73–74, 76–78, 91–93, 107–109,
    124, 136, 137, 144–145, 148, 153,
    156, 214, 217
caring 34, 49, 93, 124–136, 137, 158, 164,
    177, 179–180, 191
case load 45–46, 54–58, 61–62, 66, 70, 81,
    86–87, 132, 169–174, 204, 211
cases (multiple experiences) 168, 205–206
case study 9, 18, 27–28, 34–123, 142, 171,
    213
charge nurse/ward sister 2
child care (bought) 45, 57–59, 95,
    105–106, 135, 163
childrens' nursing 9, 49–63, 69, 95–96,
    173–174

children's nurse 9, 49–63, 95–96
clinical experience 41, 43
clinical learning environment 48, 158, 190, 213–214
clinical placements 185, 194, 200, 222
clinical practice 4, 7–8, 34–40, 43–46, 52–59, 62, 65–74, 113–117, 137–138, 144–145, 152–155, 158–159, 167, 171, 181–182, 185–186, 198, 206, 214, 217, 219, 222
clinical skills/nursing skills 64, 171, 198
clinical teaching 3–4, 56
clinical team 36–37, 53–54, 77, 138, 149, 158, 184, 185–188, 196, 205, 220
coaching 56–57, 67, 70, 82, 85, 115–116, 166–171, 197–199, 202, 211, 224, 225, 227
cognitive apprenticeship 197, 199–203
collaboration 39, 43–45, 56, 67–71, 81–84, 95–97, 101–102, 114–117, 166, 181, 194–197, 200–202, 204, 211, 214, 224, 225
commitment 37, 41, 48, 61, 77, 80, 84, 86, 93, 132, 144–145
CFP (Common Foundation Programme) 142, 146
communication 37–39, 46, 65, 77, 93, 97–98, 172, 179
community of practice 16, 48, 51–54, 62, 112, 138, 140, 142, 151–152, 186–190, 200, 208, 215
community care 51, 56–58, 94–95, 109, 144, 162–163, 170, 172, 205
compassion 174
competency 83, 93, 145–146, 153, 156, 158, 166–169, 172, 205, 209, 216, 221
competencies 93, 102, 215
composite focal skills 167–169
confederation 39, 43–45, 56, 67–71, 81–84, 95–97, 101–102, 114–117, 166, 181, 194–197, 200–202, 204, 211, 214, 224, 225, 227
confidence 40–41, 45, 48, 49, 52, 59, 62, 66, 71, 81, 87, 93, 96–97, 111, 113, 115, 119, 143, 145, 149, 151–152, 158, 161–162, 166–167, 179, 181–183, 192, 197, 209
confidential 41, 46

conflict 41, 156, 180
confusion 71–74, 144, 146–149, 186–188, 207
consent 166, 204
course 69, 74, 92, 146, 151, 171–172
contribution 149
craft knowledge 43, 45, 56, 67–70, 81–84, 86, 95–101, 112–114, 167–173, 180, 194, 196–199, 205, 222, 225
critical incidents 70, 162, 172, 208–210
culture shock 51–52, 76–78, 93
curriculum 3, 7–9, 14–18, 67, 92, 99, 108, 146, 171–173, 181, 183, 193–194, 203, 209, 215, 217, 219–222, 226

danger 68, 71, 98–99, 116, 162, 175
data 9, 22–25
data analysis 26–29, 64
death and dying 35–37, 59, 61, 117, 126, 174
debriefing 40, 56–59, 65, 67–68, 71, 84, 112, 116, 171–172, 174, 194, 198, 205–206
debt (financial) 105, 134
debt (emotional) 127, 192
decision making 194
degree course 40, 50, 72–74, 78, 92, 107–108, 142, 146
democratic relationship 191–192
dependency (student) 99, 204
depersonalised 194
despair 77, 84, 86–87
dignity 67, 83, 99
dilemmas 35, 41–42, 46, 110, 116, 118, 131, 144–145, 164, 174–177, 207
diploma in nursing 76, 92, 107, 143, 222
disconfirmation 142–145, 156
disillusion 192
displacement 181
dissonance 156, 208
distress 175
documents 9, 24
dressings (aseptic procedure) 82, 94, 115, 197
dyslexia 87, 147, 211, 217

education 3–9
embarrassment 35, 41, 67–68, 97–98, 115–117, 161–162, 165, 176, 181

emotional labour 35–37, 41–42, 49, 59–61, 65, 83–84, 97–98, 115, 117, 119, 124–136, 159, 162, 172–176, 183, 190, 197, 207–208, 220
emotional membrane 65–67, 75, 84, 134, 173–176
empathy 100, 176, 191
encouragement 70
enrolled nurse 91
entry requirements 14, 92
equilibrium 153–155
essential skills 96, 114, 158, 176, 220
ethics 46, 95, 97–98, 117–118, 174, 176–178, 205, 207
ethnography 18
European Union Directives 14, 94, 142, 221
evaluation 194, 198
evolving cognition 169

failure 45, 77, 86, 104–105
families (students') 51–52, 65, 93, 95, 104, 110, 131, 174, 221–222
fear/fears 35–37, 45, 49, 52, 55, 64–66, 68, 71, 84, 93–94, 100, 102, 110–111, 115, 117, 128–130, 159, 165–166, 175, 190, 192
feelings 35–39, 45, 49, 59–62, 65–66, 84, 86, 117, 129–130, 152, 156, 161, 173–176, 181, 183, 198
field visits (research) 24–26
finances (students) 42, 51, 92, 104–105, 134, 145
flying solo 54, 56–57, 68, 70, 82, 113–117, 156, 165, 170, 185, 197, 203–206, 214
focal skills 168, 222
formal knowledge 171–172, 194, 199, 201, 224
framing questions 202
friends 36–37, 69–70, 73, 88, 175, 198, 207
frustration (students) 179

general/adult nursing 4–49
Grace 91–107
grief 35–37, 156
guilt 177, 186–187, 207

healing 135
healing presence 180
Helen 34–49
holistic care 46, 53, 124–136, 163, 189, 204, 218, 222
holistic skills 31, 124–129, 132–136, 163, 169
humour 85–86, 131, 160

identity 40, 48–49, 62–63, 122–123, 151–153, 181, 188–189, 207, 219, 227
illuminative art 9, 23–24, 34–35, 48–50, 61–63, 71–74, 81, 103, 138, 146, 148
images 93, 124–137, 141–142, 148–149, 155–156, 160, 162, 164, 202, 214, 218
    Grace 92–94
    Helen 34–35
    Jack 88–91
    Marie 40–50
    Nicola 64–67
    Ruth 120–121
impression management 35–37, 48, 53, 62, 118–122, 149–153, 187–188, 208
individualised care 34, 42, 93, 116, 124–129, 132–136, 163
induction 42, 186, 210
injections 45, 82, 96, 101, 162–167
insider 52, 54, 70, 80, 183, 196
insight 58, 68, 71, 180
integration
    personal 76–77
    theory-practice 70, 158, 172, 199
internal speech 201
intra-mental (intrapersonal) 199–201
inter-mental (interpersonal) 199–200
intermission (from course) 142
interpersonal skills 37–39, 64–66, 77, 81, 83, 93–95, 97–99, 119, 124–130, 149, 152, 160–171
interprofessional relationships 7, 57, 70, 81, 126, 180–183, 193, 203, 221
interviews (research method) 9, 23
intimate care 37, 83, 133, 162, 180
I–Thou relationship 42, 56, 66–67, 75, 83, 98–100, 162

Jack 75–91
juggling 45–46

knowledge in use 201–203, 206
knowledge in waiting 201–203

language 199
lay presence 180
learning 4, 43–44, 53–54, 61–62, 66,
    82–84, 88, 94–97, 149, 151–166, 170,
    172–173, 194–196, 201–211,
    213–224, 227
learning agenda 203
learning contracts 24, 38, 67, 85, 87, 102,
    122, 144, 148, 158, 173, 209–210,
    216
learning disabilities 98–99
learning needs 194
learning outcomes 192–193, 201
lecturer practitioner 14, 58, 87–88, 100,
    102, 172, 186, 227
legal aspects/knowledge 174, 180
legitimate participation 40, 43–46, 52–56,
    62, 81–87, 96–97, 112–117, 166–167,
    195–196, 203–204, 210, 223–224
liberation 141
library 58, 158, 209–210
life long learning 222
loving (approach/attitude/nature) 131,
    180

male nurse 75–91
management 5, 45, 46, 86, 116, 125, 159,
    170, 204–205
marginalised 118
Marie 49–63
maternity care 35, 58, 100–101
maze 80, 141, 144, 156
mediating language 203
mental healthcare practice 9, 51–53, 55,
    63–75, 77–78, 127–129, 135, 160,
    165, 172–174, 177, 193, 197
mental health–students' 165
mentor 40, 42, 44–45, 48, 52, 54–57, 59,
    61, 63, 67–71, 84–88, 95–96,
    102–103, 111–112, 126, 145–146,
    148, 153, 156, 163, 167, 173,
    175–176, 182, 185–190, 205,
    209–211, 214, 216, 218
mentorship 9, 16, 40, 44–45, 62, 70, 112,
    145–146, 149, 156, 165, 168, 171,
    185–186, 203, 210, 222–226

menu of experience 193
midwifery 35, 58, 100
mistakes 52, 96
moral knowledge 117
motivation 55–57, 90, 124
multicultural 163

narrative 9, 40–42, 46, 58–59, 69–70, 110,
    142, 184, 185, 206–209, 214, 227
Natalie 129–130, 174, 160, 165
newcomer 69, 99, 109–113, 112, 138, 140,
    181–182, 185, 188, 199
Nicola 63–75
novice 110, 168, 203
nursing degree 42, 146, 213, 219
nursing education 1–9, 213–217, 227
nursing care 34–35, 39–40, 42–44, 54–57,
    91, 95–100, 108, 113–117, 126,
    131–133, 177
nursing knowledge 192
nursing philosophy 93
nursing practice 72, 83–84, 100, 112–117,
    156, 173, 176, 195, 218
nursing skills 38, 43–45, 63, 84–87, 93–97,
    113–117, 193, 195
nursing student 41–42, 61, 66, 73, 90, 138,
    146, 148, 152, 156, 186, 208
nursing tasks 38, 44, 55, 168
nursing theory 43, 83, 135, 179, 213
nursing work 156

observation (research method) 24–26
observing others–students 38, 41, 46, 54,
    55, 68–69, 96–101, 114, 130, 160,
    166
old timer 176, 186
openness 192
oppression 141
outcomes
    UKCC 209, 215
    Course 209
outsider 41, 43–44, 48, 52–54, 69, 76–77,
    109–113, 116–118, 138, 145, 181,
    186–190

paediatrics 45, 59
pain (students') 143, 174
paintings 9, 23–24, 34–35, 49–50, 71–74,
    103, 120–121

partnership with carers/patients 56–58, 127
partnership with mentor 39, 43–45, 56,
    67–71, 81–84, 95–97, 101–102, 114,
    166, 181, 194–197, 200–202, 204,
    211, 214, 224
patient care 35, 38–39, 42, 44–45, 48–49,
    52, 55–57, 66–69, 76, 79, 83–85,
    91–94, 100–101, 108, 113, 116–119,
    122, 124–136, 151, 158, 161,
    165–166, 167–168, 170–171, 193,
    198, 204
patients 94, 122, 124–136, 158, 178
parents
    of student 56–57
    of patient 108
partnership 8–9, 98, 180, 196
past experiences 34–35, 49–50, 52, 55, 57,
    64, 75–78, 91–94, 99, 107–109, 114,
    156, 160, 164, 173, 177
peers 37, 39–40, 42, 46, 50–51, 58–59,
    67–70, 73, 88, 110–112, 127, 174,
    184, 186, 188–189, 206–210, 214,
    216–217, 227
performance 215
peripheral participation (LPP) 43, 56,
    67–71, 97–98, 101, 111–119
personal
    development 37, 67–73, 75, 128
    experience 49–50, 76, 80, 107–108,
        126–129, 133–134, 137, 148, 172
    knowledge 34–35, 49–50, 52, 55, 57, 64,
        75–78, 91–94, 99, 108–109, 114, 156,
        160, 164, 173, 177
    values/beliefs 34–35, 46, 50, 65–66,
        76–79, 82–83, 86, 92–94, 108–109,
        117, 122, 140, 156, 160, 176
philosophy (students') 46, 66, 76, 108–109,
    176, 178
perspective transformation 42–44, 51–53,
    58, 81, 90, 99–101, 109
Petra 172–173
phenomenology 18, 176
placement 16–18, 39, 44, 52–53, 57–58,
    64–70, 79–81, 138, 142, 144,
    151–152, 158, 160, 167, 183, 186,
    209, 217, 220
planning learning experiences 193–195,
    198, 203, 205, 209, 214
poverty 92, 104–107

power-relationship
    nurse–patient 42, 95, 172, 189
    staff–student 77–78
policy 213
practical knowledge 172
practical skills 44–45, 58, 95–97,
    113–119
practise 3, 7, 45, 57, 67, 116, 165, 168,
    174, 208
present-at-hand 169, 179
primary nursing 43, 93, 182
prior-conceptions 34–35, 49–50, 65,
    75–78, 91–94, 200
privacy 94
problem based learning 86, 171, 185, 210,
    214, 216, 222
problem framing 86, 200–201
problem solving 86, 205
professional behaviour 35
professional care 35
professional development 13, 46–49,
    62–63, 70, 74–75, 88–91, 94,
    106–107, 113–117, 122–123, 132,
    185, 210, 214, 226
professional friendship 65–68, 75, 84, 117,
    119, 134, 173–176, 198
professional knowledge 66, 158, 173, 180,
    183–184, 213, 217
professional membrane 65–68, 75, 84, 117,
    119, 134, 173–176, 198
professional practice 54, 61, 67–68, 131,
    159–160, 174, 200, 226
professional relationships 205
professional statutory body 3–6, 9, 167,
    209, 216, 221–222, 225, 226, 228
professional tutor 102
programme 43, 185, 194, 219
project 2000 5–7, 15, 143
psychiatry 64–65
psychomotor skills 44, 169
pupil nurse 91–92
puppy dog 112, 118, 122, 188

quality assurance 7, 30–31, 76, 102, 205,
    215–216, 226

rapport 160
reciprocity 52–53, 111–113, 122, 149,
    180–181, 186–188

record keeping 194
recruitment 6–7, 213, 217–218
referencing work 10–12, 31–33
reflective practice 14, 40, 43, 58–59, 65,
    68–70, 74, 84, 100, 102, 116, 119,
    134, 162–163, 169, 171, 173, 175,
    177, 185, 189, 198, 200, 205, 214,
    216, 222, 225–226
rehabilitation of patients 165
rejection 161
relating to patients/carers 42, 79, 83,
    93–94, 97–99, 101, 119, 127,
    159–164, 168, 214
relationships 65, 131–132, 134–135, 160,
    172
research 2, 9, 13, 18–31, 64, 213, 226–228
research consent
    students 19–20
    patients 19–22
research ethics 20–22
research participants 19–22
responsibility 143, 145, 163, 166
risk (personal) 68
role 35, 40, 42–43, 46, 48, 50, 64–68, 71,
    74, 92, 94, 99, 109–111, 124–127,
    129–133, 136–137, 141, 153, 156,
    181, 187–189, 210, 221
routine 94, 133, 165
Ruth 107–123

safety 42, 205
safety of students' 71, 98, 166, 205
safe-practice 68–69, 97–98, 116, 119, 191,
    205
scaffolding 202–206, 210, 224
science 65, 180, 198, 202, 220
secure base 54–56, 63, 68–71, 81, 88,
    95–97, 112–113, 118, 149, 151,
    191–192, 197
security 44, 162
self awareness 37, 65, 74, 134, 161, 175,
    178, 192–193
self concept 208
self consciousness 36, 39, 68, 74–75,
    160–161, 192
self development 70, 180
self esteem 112, 122
self image 36, 40–41, 48, 53, 66, 73, 82,
    111, 151, 159–160, 208

self knowledge 66
self presentation 53, 119
seminars 39, 42, 92, 172
sense making 71
sensitivity 36–37, 39, 83, 152, 174, 179
sex/sexuality 67, 98–99, 163, 176
shame 190
sign-post 187
single-parent 95, 104–106
situation at hand 168, 171
skills 66, 167, 169, 215
skills laboratory 143, 159, 198
skill mix 218
socio-cultural 199
social learning 196, 200
social support 36–37, 39, 41, 44, 48,
    52–53, 55, 58, 67, 69–70, 75–78, 81,
    88, 104, 106, 110–113, 118, 153,
    186–190, 207–208, 210, 217
socialisation 130, 137–157, 186
spiritual care 124, 126
sponsorship 39–40, 42–43, 45, 52–56,
    69–70, 75–77, 80–81, 84, 96–97,
    100–101, 112–113, 116, 118, 122,
    166–167, 175, 188–193, 204, 210,
    214–215, 223, 224
statutory body 3–6, 9, 167, 209, 216,
    221–222, 225–226, 228
story-telling 40–42, 46, 55, 58–59, 66–67,
    69–70, 84–85, 116, 118, 185,
    206–209, 211, 214, 227
stress 36, 67, 96, 142–144, 163
struggle (to succeed) 165
study 51, 56, 77–79, 87, 101–102, 114,
    145, 148, 158, 205, 209–211
subsidiary skills 168
supernumerary 3, 6, 58, 78–81, 96–97,
    125, 134, 151, 170–172, 178, 184,
    203–206, 210–211, 214, 218, 222,
    226
supervision 4, 16, 34, 43, 54, 67–71, 142,
    156, 166, 175–176, 193, 203, 214, 223

tacit knowledge 43, 168, 222
talk aloud 43, 168, 194, 196, 198, 203,
    210, 225
talking heads 192–203
tasks 35, 42, 160, 165, 169, 215
teachers 34, 102, 107, 213, 227

team member 43, 48, 52–54, 61, 70–71,
    76–77, 80–82, 90, 95–101, 100–101,
    111–113, 118, 126–127, 129, 132,
    141, 151–152, 156, 159, 163,
    181–183, 188, 192, 205, 210
techniques 39, 42–45, 82–84, 95–97, 167,
    221
technical care 170
technical knowledge 159, 164–169, 202
technical skills 43–45, 55–56, 61, 82,
    95–97, 101, 114–117, 119, 134,
    143, 158, 179, 183, 197, 215, 222
telephone 53–54
theory 46, 56, 167, 173, 202–203
theory-practice integration 36, 43, 56–61,
    70, 76–77, 83, 85, 88, 96–97,
    101–102, 122, 131–132, 158,
    198–201, 209–210, 213, 215,
    218–219, 224
therapeutic action 68, 75–76, 83–86, 97,
    99–101, 134, 159, 162, 172, 178, 180,
    183, 191, 215, 218–219
thinking aloud 203
trailing 41, 43–44, 48, 52–53, 76–77,
    111–113, 116–118, 138, 145,
    181
transparency 192
travelling to placements 41

trust 45, 53, 56, 94, 151, 191, 196
two-stage learning 201–203

UKCC/NM Council 6, 8, 9, 14, 142, 167,
    209, 221, 222, 225–226, 228
university student 41–42, 48–51, 61, 71,
    86, 92, 109–110, 114, 129–130, 138,
    146, 148, 156, 211

vacation 167, 223
vocation 42, 218
vulnerability 178

watching others (students) 38, 44, 46,
    54–57, 62, 67, 69, 71, 85, 95–97, 130,
    160, 166
workforce 169
work objects
    patients 34–35, 44, 46
    students 80
workload-mentor 68, 70–71, 187, 189,
    193, 218, 223
workload-student 36, 45–46, 48, 51,
    56–58, 61–62, 69–71, 85, 95, 118,
    125, 135, 159, 179, 182, 204, 218, 223

zone of proximal development 201–204,
    206, 209